Infectious Disease Challenges in Solid Organ Transplant Recipients

Editors

JOSEPH G. TIMPONE Jr
PRINCY N. KUMAR

INFECTIOUS DISEASE CLINICS OF NORTH AMERICA

www.id.theclinics.com

Consulting Editor
HELEN W. BOUCHER

June 2013 • Volume 27 • Number 2

ELSEVIER

1600 John F. Kennedy Boulevard • Suite 1800 • Philadelphia, Pennsylvania, 19103-2899.
http://www.theclinics.com

INFECTIOUS DISEASE CLINICS OF NORTH AMERICA Volume 27, Number 2
June 2013 ISSN 0891–5520, ISBN-13: 978-1-4557-7107-3

Editor: Stephanie Donley
Developmental Editor: Teia Stone

Infectious Disease Clinics of North America (ISSN 0891–5520) is published in March, June, September, and December by Elsevier Inc., 360 Park Avenue South, New York, NY 10010-1710. Periodicals postage paid at New York, NY and additional mailing offices. Subscription prices are $282.00 per year for US individuals, $482.00 per year for US institutions, $139.00 per year for US students, $334.00 per year for Canadian individuals, $596.00 per year for Canadian institutions, $398.00 per year for international individuals, $596.00 per year for international institutions, and $192.00 per year for Canadian and international students. To receive student rate, orders must be accompanied by name of affiliated institution, date of term, and the *signature* of program/residency coordinator on institution letterhead. Orders will be billed at individual rate until proof of status is received. Foreign air speed delivery is included in all *Clinics* subscription prices. All prices are subject to change without notice. **POSTMASTER**: Send address changes to *Infectious Disease Clinics of North America,* Elsevier Health Sciences Division, Subcription Customer Service, 3251 Riverport Lane, Maryland Heights, MO 63043. **Customer Service: 1-800-654-2452 (US). From outside of the US and Canada, call 1-314-447-8871. Fax: 1-314-447-8029. E-mail: JournalsCustomerService-usa@elsevier.com (print support) or JournalsOnlineSupport-usa@elsevier.com (online support).**

Infectious Disease Clinics of North America is also published in Spanish by Editorial Inter-MÅdica, Junin 917, 1er A 1113, Buenos Aires, Argentina.

Reprints. For copies of 100 or more, of articles in this publication, please contact the Commercial Reprints Department, Elsevier Inc., 360 Park Avenue South, New York, New York 10010-1710. Tel. (212) 633-3812, Fax: (212) 462-1935, E-mail: reprints@elsevier.com.

Infectious Disease Clinics of North America is covered in *MEDLINE/PubMed (Index Medicus), Current Contents/ Clinical Medicine, Science Citation Alert, SCISEARCH,* and *Research Alert.*

Printed and bound by CPI Group (UK) Ltd, Croydon, CR0 4YY
Transferred to digital print 2013

Contributors

CONSULTING EDITOR

HELEN W. BOUCHER, MD, FIDSA, FACP
Director, Infectious Diseases Fellowship Program; Associate Professor of Medicine, Division of Geographic Medicine and Infectious Diseases, Tufts Medical Center, Boston, Massachusetts

EDITORS

JOSEPH G. TIMPONE Jr, MD
Associate Professor of Medicine, Division of Infectious Diseases, Georgetown University Hospital, Washington, DC

PRINCY N. KUMAR, MD
Chief, Division of Infectious Diseases, Professor of Medicine and Microbiology, Georgetown University Hospital, Washington, DC

AUTHORS

GAYLE P. BALBA, MD
Assistant Professor of Medicine, Division of Infectious Diseases, Georgetown University Hospital, Washington, DC

GEORGE BEATTY, MD, MPH
Associate Clinical Professor of Medicine, UCSF Positive Health Program, San Francisco General Hospital, San Francisco, California

PETER CHIN-HONG, MD
Associate Professor of Clinical Medicine, Department of Medicine, University of California, San Francisco, California

PEARLIE P. CHONG, MD
Transplant Infectious Diseases Fellow, Division of Infectious Diseases, Department of Medicine, William J. von Liebig Transplant Center, College of Medicine, Mayo Clinic, Rochester, Minnesota

LAURA O'BRYAN COSTER, MD
Assistant Professor of Infectious Diseases, Department of Infectious Diseases, Georgetown University Hospital, Washington, DC

THOMAS M. FISHBEIN, MD
Professor, Departments of Surgery and Pediatrics, Executive Director, Georgetown Transplant Institute, MedStar Georgetown University Hospital, Washington, DC

RAFFAELE GIRLANDA, MD
Assistant Professor of Surgery, Division of Infectious Diseases, Department of Medicine, MedStar Georgetown Transplant Institute, Washington, DC

SARAH P. HAMMOND, MD
Instructor of Medicine, Division of Infectious Diseases, Brigham and Women's Hospital, Harvard Medical School, Boston, Massachusetts

BASIT JAVAID, MD
Medical Director, Division of Transplant Surgery, Georgetown University Hospital, Washington, DC

GEETA S. KARNIK, MD
Senior Infectious Disease Fellow, Department of Infectious Diseases, Georgetown University Hospital, Washington, DC

PRINCY N. KUMAR, MD
Chief, Division of Infectious Diseases, Professor of Medicine and Microbiology, Georgetown University Hospital, Washington, DC

JENNIFER PRIMEGGIA, MD
Assistant Professor of Medicine, Division of Infectious Diseases, Department of Medicine, Washington, DC

RAYMUND R. RAZONABLE, MD
Professor of Medicine, Division of Infectious Diseases, Department of Medicine, The William J. von Liebig Transplant Center, College of Medicine, Mayo Clinic, Rochester, Minnesota

JESSICA ROSEN, MD
Assistant Professor of Medicine and Travel Clinic Director, Division of Infectious Diseases and Travel Medicine, Medstar Georgetown University Hospital, Washington, DC

LAUREN RUDOLPH, BA
Division of Infectious Diseases, Department of Medicine, Georgetown University School of Medicine, Washington, DC

PALI D. SHAH, MD
Assistant Professor of Medicine, Division of Pulmonary and Critical Care Medicine, Johns Hopkins University School of Medicine, Baltimore, Maryland

KIRTI SHETTY, MD
Associate Professor, Department of Surgery, Georgetown University Hospital; Director, Transplant Hepatology, Georgetown Transplant Institute, Georgetown University Hospital, Washington, DC

SHMUEL SHOHAM, MD
Assistant Professor of Medicine, Transplant and Oncology Infectious Diseases Program, Johns Hopkins University School of Medicine, Baltimore, Maryland

PETER STOCK, MD, PhD
Professor of Surgery, Department of Surgery, University of California, San Francisco, California

JOSEPH G. TIMPONE Jr, MD
Associate Professor of Medicine, Division of Infectious Diseases, Department of Medicine, Georgetown University Hospital, Washington, DC

Contents

> Donor-derived infections continue to occur in spite of standard organ donor screening. These infections can be challenging to diagnose and manage for a treating physician. This article reviews the process of organ donor evaluation, limitations of current screening strategies, approach to recipient evaluation in suspected donor-derived infections, and diagnostic and management strategies of selected donor-derived infections.

> Renal transplant recipients continue to have progressive kidney dysfunction and renal graft loss has been attributed to emerging opportunistic infections, specifically BK virus (BKV). BKV is postulated to be selected by the new potent immunosuppressive medications and to be an important factor in graft failure. The prevalence of BKV nephropathy (BKVN) is estimated to be 1% to 10% and renal allograft loss from BKVN has been estimated to occur in up to 50% of affected recipients. With the increasing recognition of BKV infection using PCR assays coupled with the immediate reduction in immunosuppression for BKVN, the incidence of graft failure secondary to BKVN may be decreasing.

> End-stage liver disease and hepatocellular carcinoma from chronic hepatitis C are the most common indications for orthotopic liver transplantation and the incidence of both are projected to increase over the next decade. Recurrent hepatitis C virus infection of the allograft is associated with an accelerated progression to cirrhosis, graft loss, and death. This article presents an overview of the natural history of hepatitis C virus recurrence in liver transplant recipients and guidance on optimal management strategies.

> The most important emerging and rare fungal pathogens in solid organ transplant recipients are the Zygomycetes, *Scedosporium, Fusarium,* and the dark molds. Factors affecting the emergence of these fungi include the combination of intensive immunosuppressive regimens with increasingly widespread use of long-term azole antifungal therapy; employment of aggressive diagnostic approaches (eg, sampling of bronchoalveolar lavage fluid); and changes in patients' interactions with the environment. This article reviews the epidemiology, microbiology, and clinical impact

early postoperative period, serious bacterial infections are more often reported in facial CTA recipients than in hand CTA recipients. Rejection and concomitant viral reactivation of herpes family viruses cause significant morbidity after the immediate postoperative period. Invasive fungal infection is an uncommon complication. Infection prophylaxis practices typically include early antibacterial prophylaxis during the perioperative period and cytomegalovirus, pneumocystis, and toxoplasma prophylaxis for several months after transplantation.

Parasitic diseases are rare infections after a solid organ transplant (SOT). Toxoplasmosis, *Trypanosoma cruzi*, and visceral leishmanias are the 3 main opportunistic protozoal infections that have the potential to be lethal if not diagnosed early and treated appropriately after SOT. Strongyloides *stercoralis* is the one helminthic disease that is life-threatening after transplant. This review addresses modes of transmission, methods of diagnosis, and treatment of the most serious parasitic infections in SOT. The role of targeted pretransplant screening of the donor and recipient for parasitic diseases is also discussed.

More than a quarter of solid-organ transplant recipients are traveling to foreign regions where there are greater health risks than their home country. There may be higher risk of complications from typical travel-related illnesses and risk of opportunistic infections not faced by healthy travelers. Some vaccinations may be contraindicated after solid-organ transplant, and those that are safe may have decreased efficacy. Drug interactions between antirejection regimens and medications for malaria prophylaxis and traveler's diarrhea must be considered. This article discusses how providers can best advise and help protect these high-risk travelers.

Human immunodeficiency virus (HIV) infection is no longer an absolute contraindication for transplantation for patients with advanced kidney and liver failure. This article reviews the outcome data in the solid organ transplantation of HIV-infected patients that led to a change in thinking by the transplant community. Several emerging issues are also reviewed, such as eligibility criteria, selection of optimal immunosuppression agents and antiretroviral therapy in this population, and management of coinfection with hepatitis B and hepatitis C after transplant.

HIV-positive patients are now undergoing solid organ transplantation at increasing rates, with successful outcomes. Transplantation in this unique

patient population presents new challenges in the postoperative management of both antiretroviral regimens and immunosuppressive regimens.
This review highlights the drug-drug interactions between commonly
used immunosuppressive and antiretroviral agents. As more antiretroviral
regimens are cautiously initiated in the posttransplant period, further research is needed to identify drug-drug interactions to minimize toxicities
and improve long-term survival and graft function.

INFECTIOUS DISEASE CLINICS
OF NORTH AMERICA

FORTHCOMING ISSUES

September 2013
Food Borne Illness
David Acheson, MD,
Jennifer McEntire, PhD, and
Cheleste M. Thorpe, MD, *Editors*

December 2013
Sexually Transmitted Diseases
Jeanne Marrazzo, MD, *Editor*

March 2014
Urinary Tract Infections
Kalpana Gupta, MD, *Editor*

RECENT ISSUES

March 2013
**Community-Acquired Pneumonia:
Controversies and Questions**
Thomas M. File Jr, MD, *Editor*

December 2012
Hepatitis C Virus Infection
Barbara McGovern, MD, *Editor*

September 2012
Travel Medicine
Alimuddin Zumla, MD, PhD,
Ronald Behrens, MD, and
Ziad Memish, MD, *Editors*

June 2012
Tropical Diseases
Alimuddin Zumla, MD, and
Jennifer Keiser, MSc, PhD, *Editors*

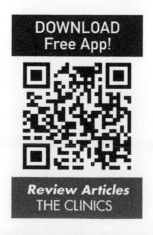

Preface

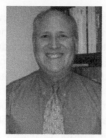 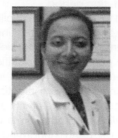

Joseph G. Timpone Jr, MD   Princy N. Kumar, MD
Editors

As a result of advances in immunosuppressive therapies, there has been significant improvement in allograft survival and outcomes in solid organ transplant recipients. However, these advances have come at a price and have lead to new infectious disease challenges in the ever evolving field of solid organ transplantation. The transplant community has benefited greatly from the practice guidelines published in 2009[1]; however, unique challenges in transplant infectious diseases continue to emerge. In this volume of *Infectious Diseases Clinics of North America*, we have attempted to identify clinical problems that have been associated with diagnostic and/or management challenges in the solid organ transplant recipient. These articles provide a comprehensive review of a particular topic, as well as some practical recommendations for clinicians caring for this patient population.

We selected several pathogens that are particularly problematic for allograft function and survival, as in the case of BK polyoma virus infection in renal transplant recipients, and recurrent hepatitis C infection in orthotopic liver transplant recipients. Although there are limited data on how to optimally manage these patients, the authors provide some perspective based on an in-depth review of the literature. Infection due to cytomegalovirus continues to be an extremely important immunomodulatory viral infection that affects both allograft and patient survival in solid organ transplant recipients. The author provides a state-of-the-art review as well as a practical approach to the diagnosis, prevention, and management of this most common viral infection. Although Candida and Aspergillus species remain the most clinically relevant fungal infections in solid organ transplant recipients, due to intensive immunosuppressive regimens coupled with the widespread use of azole therapy, alternative fungal pathogens are becoming increasingly recognized in this patient population. Therefore we have also included an article that unravels some of the "more confusing" fungal pathogens such as Zygomycetes, Scedosporium, Fusarium, and the dematiaceous molds. Multidrug-resistant organisms have unfortunately become a common occurrence in hospitalized patients, and this has certainly trickled into the solid organ transplant patient population. The lung transplant patient population is at particular risk both pretransplantation and posttransplantation, and the authors provide practical advice on patient selection criteria and management. Although donor-derived infections are uncommon,

Infect Dis Clin N Am 27 (2013) xi–xiii
http://dx.doi.org/10.1016/j.idc.2013.03.001
0891-5520/13/$ – see front matter © 2013 Published by Elsevier Inc.

their recognition is crucial and often underdiagnosed. Our authors highlight the diagnosis and management of these rare infections that can result in significant morbidity and mortality in the early posttransplantation period.

The type of allografts that are offered to patients with debilitating and disabling conditions such as short bowel syndrome and limb loss continues to evolve. Within the last 15 years, there has been significant progress in the field of small intestinal and multivisceral transplantation. As these patients have significant pretransplant infectious disease complications and require a higher level of immunosuppression than other transplant recipients, bacterial, fungal, and viral infections are exceedingly common occurrences. The authors attempt to provide a timeline for the types of infection in this population. Composite tissue allotransplantation is in its infancy, as only 50 hand and 20 face transplantations have been performed. The author provides a comprehensive review of the experiences reported thus far within the literature and categorizes the types of infections in this highly specialized field of transplant medicine.

Given the rise of globalization and increased influx of immigrant populations within the transplant pool, we thought it was important to address parasitic infections in the solid organ transplant population. In addition, the success with allograft survival and a tendency for patients to "return to normal" has resulted in an increased number of transplant patients traveling abroad. Our authors have provided an excellent discussion on some of the more clinically relevant parasitic infections, such as *Trypanosoma cruzi*, as well as practical advice for the transplant patient who wishes to travel abroad.

Finally, combination antiretroviral therapy has essentially changed the face of HIV disease in places where there are no obstacles to access these medications. As a result, comorbid conditions, such as cirrhosis due to hepatitis C, and chronic kidney disease due to either HIV itself or other disease comorbidities such as diabetes and hypertension, have become important complications. The early successes with kidney and liver transplantation in HIV-infected patients therefore warranted a state-of-the-art review by experts in this field. Given the complex pharmacology of antiretroviral medications and their potential interactions with many of the immunosuppressive agents, we have provided an article that focuses on this topic.

We are indebted to our expert coauthors, who put an inordinate amount of time into providing a detailed review of the literature to address these very important clinical issues in the field of solid organ transplantation. Finally, a special note of thanks to Dr Helen Boucher, who graciously invited us as guest editors for this very exciting volume of *Infectious Diseases Clinics of North America*.

Joseph G. Timpone Jr, MD
Division of Infectious Diseases
Georgetown University Hospital
3800 Reservoir Road, NW, 5PHC
Washington, DC 20007, USA

Princy N. Kumar, MD
Division of Infectious Diseases
Georgetown University Hospital
3900 Reservoir Road, NW, 5PHC
Washington, DC 20057, USA

E-mail addresses:
timponej@gunet.georgetown.edu (J.G. Timpone)
kumarp@gunet.georgetown.edu (P.N. Kumar)

REFERENCE

1. AST Infectious Diseases Guidelines. 2nd Edition. American Journal of Transplantation 2009;9:S1–281.

Diagnostic and Management Strategies for Donor-derived Infections

Pearlie P. Chong, MD*, Raymund R. Razonable, MD

KEYWORDS

- Donor-derived infections (DDIs) • Organ donor screening
- Potential donor-derived transmission events
- Organ procurement organizations (OPOs)
- Disease Transmission Advisory Committee
- United Network for Organ Sharing (UNOS)
- Organ Procurement and Transplantation Network (OPTN)

KEY POINTS

- Standard organ donor screening has not completely eliminated the risk of donor-derived infections (DDIs).
- The incidence of DDIs is thought to be rare, occurring in less than 1% of organ transplant recipients. It can, however, result in significant morbidity and mortality.
- Treating physicians need to maintain a high index of suspicion for DDIs in organ transplant recipients, especially if they occur during the early post-transplant period.
- Rapid recognition and prompt reporting of DDIs is crucial in enabling early institution of appropriate treatment and minimizing complications.
- Physicians who are involved in the management of organ transplant recipients should be familiar with the process of organ donor screening, as well as the process of reporting DDIs.

INTRODUCTION

Organ transplantation is a potentially life-saving procedure that has become standard of care for the management of numerous diseases. Each year, there are approximately 25,000 organ transplants performed across 250 transplant centers in the United States.[1] As graft survival rates have improved, due in part to better immunosuppression strategies, the number of transplant procedures performed continues to grow. To this end, evaluation of organ-donor suitability is an essential step in ensuring the safety of transplantation.

Funding Sources: None.
Conflict of Interest: None.
Division of Infectious Diseases, Department of Medicine, William J. von Liebig Transplant Center, College of Medicine, Mayo Clinic, 200 First Street Southwest, Rochester, MN 55905, USA
* Corresponding author.
E-mail address: Chong.Pearlie@mayo.edu

Infect Dis Clin N Am 27 (2013) 253–270
http://dx.doi.org/10.1016/j.idc.2013.02.001
0891-5520/13/$ – see front matter Published by Elsevier Inc.

id.theclinics.com

Standard organ donor screening, however, has not completely eliminated the risk of DDIs. Although a rare occurrence, such infections continue to occur, suggesting that there is room for improvement in the current approach to donor screening.[2] Standard screening procedures should be supplemented with specialized testing for donors with identifiable risks. For example, the spectrum of DDIs may be broad, to include parasitic infections such as Chagas disease and malaria, for recipients of organs from donors with diverse geographic exposures.

This article provides an overview of DDIs in solid organ transplant (SOT) recipients, focusing on approaches to diagnosis, prevention, and management strategies of these infections. Traditional DDIs, such as cytomegalovirus (CMV) and Epstein-Barr virus (EBV), are not discussed in this article.

INCIDENCE AND EPIDEMIOLOGY

The true incidence of DDIs is unknown. Current data suggest that potential donor-derived transmission events, including infections and malignancies, likely occur in less than 1% of transplant recipients.[3,4] This is likely an underestimation, however, of the true incidence due to under-recognition and under-reporting. This estimated rate also does not include expected DDIs, such as CMV and EBV. In spite of the rarity of DDIs, significant morbidity and mortality are associated with these events.[3,4] It is, therefore, crucial to consider the donor as the source of any post-transplant infections, especially if they occur during the first month after transplantation.[5]

CLASSIFICATION OF DONOR-DERIVED INFECTIONS AND THE REPORTING PROCESS

The Organ Procurement and Transplantation Network (OPTN), a private, nonprofit organization operated under contract with the US Department of Health and Human Services by the UNOS, establishes national standards to organ procurement and requires that all potential donor-derived transmission events be reported within 24 hours of knowledge or concern.[6] Treating physicians should have a logical approach to the work-up of potential DDIs and be aware that they have an obligation to report suspected and/or proven infections to the OPTN for further investigation. These events are reviewed by the Disease Transmission Advisory Committee (DTAC). DTAC is a web-based network established in 2005 to standardize the reporting and tracking process of donor-derived events, with the aim of decreasing transmission-associated morbidity and mortality. **Table 1** lists the potential DDI transmissions reported to the OPTN as of 2009.

In general, DDIs are classified as expected or unexpected.[7] Expected DDIs occur when routine pretransplant testing reveals donor infection and recipient susceptibility, but, because the benefits of transplantation outweigh the expected risks, this is considered acceptable medical practice. The most common example of expected DDIs is CMV infection transmitted from a CMV-seropositive donor to a CMV-seronegative recipient. Other examples of expected DDIs include EBV and toxoplasmosis.

On the contrary, unexpected DDIs are infections that are unrecognized until after transplantation has occurred. Although rare, these infections have often resulted in significant morbidity and/or mortality. Recent reports of transmission events include lymphocytic choriomeningitis virus (LCMV), rabies virus, West Nile virus (WNV), human immunodeficiency virus (HIV), hepatitis C virus (HCV), *Strongyloides stercoralis*, *Mycobacterium tuberculosis*, *Balamuthia mandrillaris*, and *Trypanosoma cruzi*.[7-16] A suspected event should further be classified as proven, probable, possible, or

Table 1
Potential donor-derived infectious diseases transmissions reported to the OPTN, 2005–2009

Disease	Number of Donor Reports	Number of Recipients with Confirmed Transmission	Number of DDD-Attributable Recipient Deaths
Virus	86	31	8
Bacteria	38	26	7
Fungus	30	26	8
Mycobacteria	26	10	2
Parasite	21	13	4
Total infections	201	106	29

Abbreviation: DDD, donor-derived infectious diseases.

Data from Ison MG, Nalesnik MA. An update on donor-derived disease transmission in organ transplantation. Am J Transplant 2011;11:1123–30.

excluded, according to the classification system developed by the Disease Transmission Advisory Committee in 2007.[3]

EVALUATION AND SCREENING OF POTENTIAL ORGAN DONORS

All organ donors (living and deceased) should be screened for medical conditions that may affect organ function, and for the presence of transmissible diseases and/or malignancies that may result in adverse outcomes in organ recipients. In the United States, the organ procurement organizations (OPOs) responding to an organ donor call from a hospital (called "Host OPO") is responsible for the process of identifying and evaluating potential organ donors as well as the process of organ procurement.[17]

Donor screening practices tend to vary among the various OPOs, but these programs are mandated by OPTN policy to subscribe to minimum requirements (**Box 1**). The host OPO should obtain a medical and behavioral history, focusing on the presence of risk factors for blood-borne pathogens, in particular HIV, hepatitis B

Box 1
Minimum procurement standards for an organ procurement organization (OPO)

1. Review of potential donor's medical and behavioral history

2. Pathogens for which potential donors must be routinely screened:

   - HIV
   - HBV
   - HCV
   - CMV
   - EBV
   - *Treponema pallidum* (syphilis)

3. Donors hospitalized ≥72 hours should have blood and urine cultures obtained.

Modified from 2004 Annual Report of the U.S. Organ Procurement and Transplantation Network and the Scientific Registry of Transplant Recipients: Transplant Data 1994–2003. Department of Health and Human Services. Available at: http://optn.transplant.hrsa.gov/PoliciesandBylaws2/policies/pdfs/policy_2.pdf. Accessed October 11, 2012.

virus (HBV), and HCV (**Box 2**), in addition to the performance of specific screening serologic tests, as outlined in **Box 3**. Donors who meet exclusion criteria set forth by the US Public Health Service 1994 guidelines (**Box 4**) should generally be excluded from donation of organs and tissues. In special situations wherein such organs are considered for donation, informed consent should always be obtained from the potential recipient, and these should be documented in the medical records.

The threshold for acceptance of an organ for transplantation is not well established and continues to evolve as DDIs continue to be reported. In general, transplant teams and patients need to weigh the potential risk of disease transmission against the benefits of organ transplantation. For example, in febrile donors in whom the cause of fever is undefined, especially if encephalitis is present, physicians need to assess carefully if the risk of potential transmission of diseases, such as rabies, WNV, or LCMV, is acceptable. Generally, because of the lack of effective treatment and the potential fatal outcome of certain encephalitides, such as rabies and LCMV, the organs of such donors should be avoided.[18]

Laboratory Screening for Donor-derived Infections

In addition to review of medical history, laboratory screening for selected DDIs should be performed routinely (see **Box 3**). Serology and viral nucleic acid testing (NAT) are the 2 mainstays of laboratory testing of organ donors (discussed later).

Serologic testing

Serologic testing is an indirect method of disease detection because it relies on the ability of IgM and IgG production in response to antigen challenge. This forms the basis of humoral immune response because antigen-presenting cells stimulate immunoglobulin production by activated plasma cells. There is often a lapse between time of infection to production of disease-specific IgM and IgG, so-called "window period". Physicians should keep this in mind when interpreting serologic tests in the context of organ donor screening and diagnosis of DDIs.

Organ donors often require volume resuscitation, which leads to hemodilution and potentially false-negative serology results. All blood samples obtained from donors

---

Box 2
Suggested data to be collected regarding eligibility of organ donors

- Medical history
- Previous infections
- Occupational exposures
- Sexual behavior
- Incarceration
- Tattooing, ear piercing, or body piercing
- Use of illicit drugs
- Transfusions of blood or blood products
- Travel history
- Vaccinations
- Contact with bats, stray dogs, or rodents (including pets)

Data from Grossi PA, Fishman JA. Donor-derived infections in solid organ transplant recipients. Am J Transplant 2009;9(Suppl 4):S19–26.

> **Box 3**
> **Standard screening tests for organ donors**
>
> - HIV antibody
> - HBV serologies (including HBV surface antigen, core antibody, and surface antibody)
> - Hepatitis delta antigen and/or antibody in hepatitis B surface antigen–positive donors
> - HCV antibody
> - Treponemal and nontreponemal testing (TP-HA, TP-PA, FTA-ABS and/or RPR)
> - Toxoplasma antibody
> - CMV antibody
> - EBV antibody panel (EBV viral capsid antigen ± early antigen and nuclear antigen antibody levels)
> - Herpes simplex virus antibody
> - Varicella-zoster virus antibody
> - Blood and urine cultures
>
> Data from Grossi PA, Fishman JA. Donor-derived infections in solid organ transplant recipients. Am J Transplant 2009;9(Suppl 4):S19–26.

are currently required by the OPTN to be assessed for this phenomenon, using an FDA (Food and Drug Administration)–approved hemodilution calculation.[19] Thus, in situations where DDIs are strongly suspected with a suggestive clinical presentation but negative donor serologies, hemodilution should be considered a possible contributing factor. Alternatively, cross-reacting antibodies, newborns carrying maternal antibodies, and improperly performed tests may lead to false-positive serologic test results.

Viral nucleic acid testing

NAT involves the amplification of viral gene products and does not depend on host antibody response. Its major advantage is, therefore, its ability to detect the presence of an infection before antibody production, hence assisting in diagnosis during the window period.

In the United States, NAT has been routinely used to screen for HIV and HCV in blood donors since 1999.[20] It is however, not standard practice during organ donor screening.[21] Its role is currently limited to certain high-risk organ donors with specific behavioral risk factors (see **Box 2**), and OPOs are currently not mandated by the current OPTN policy to perform NAT testing. Recent highly publicized transplant-associated HIV and HCV transmission events have prompted further evaluation of incorporating NAT as part of routine organ donor screening. Using NAT may lead to earlier detection of HIV, HBV, and HCV.

Disadvantages of NAT include significant cost (because testing is performed for single-organ donors compared with batched testing in the blood or tissue donor populations); longer turnaround time, which may result in prolonged cold ischemia time and/or organ loss; increase in false-positive test results, which can lead to erroneous discarding of organs that could otherwise be potentially life saving; and lack of standardization. Some of the major limitations of NAT include the "eclipse period", which is the time between infection to detection of viremia, leading to false-negative test results, and its inability to detect virus level below the lowest limit of detection of the assay. The perceived high sensitivity of NAT may lead to a false sense of security,

---

Box 4
Donor exclusion criteria

Behavior/history exclusionary criteria

1. Men who have had sex with another man in the preceding 5 years

2. Persons who report nonmedical intravenous, intramuscular, or subcutaneous injection of drugs in the preceding 5 years

3. Persons with hemophilia or related clotting disorders who have received human-derived clotting factor concentrates

4. Men and women who have engaged in sex in exchange for money or drugs in the preceding 5 years

5. Persons who have had sex in the preceding 12 months with any of the above person described in items 1–4 above or with a person known or suspected to have HIV infection

6. Persons who have been exposed in the preceding 12 months to known or suspected HIV-infected blood through percutaneous inoculation or through contact with an open wound, nonintact skin, or mucous membrane

7. Inmates of correctional systems

8. Children born to mothers with HIV infection or mothers who meet the behavioral or laboratory exclusionary criteria for adult donors, unless HIV infection can be definitely excluded

Laboratory and other medical exclusionary criteria

1. Persons who cannot be tested for HIV infection because of refusal, inadequate blood samples (eg, hemodilution could result in false-negative tests), or any other reason

2. Persons with a repeatedly reactive screening assay for HIV-1 or HIV-2 antibody, regardless of the results of supplemental assays

3. Persons whose history, physical examination, medical records, or autopsy reports reveal other evidence of HIV infection or high-risk behavior, such as a diagnosis of AIDS, unexplained weight loss, night sweats, blue or purple spots on the skin or mucous membranes typical of Kaposi's sarcoma, unexplained lymphadenopathy lasting >1 month, unexplained temperature >100.5°F (38.6°C) for >10 days, unexplained persistent cough and shortness of breath, opportunistic infections, unexplained persistent diarrhea, male-to-male sexual contact, sexually transmitted diseases, or needle tracks or other signs of parenteral drug abuse

Modified from Guidelines for preventing transmission of human immunodeficiency virus through transplantation of human tissue and organs. Centers for Disease Control and Prevention. MMWR Recomm Rep 1994;43(RR-8):1–17. Available at: http://www.cdc.gov/mmwr/preview/mmwrhtml/00031670.htm. Accessed October 11, 2012.

---

that a negative result translates into nontransmission. Recent transmission events of certain infections, such as LCMV and WNV, have been reported, in spite of negative NAT results, presumably due to the lack of significant viremia as these were performed in normal hosts.[22,23]

Living Donors

There are certain issues that pertain specifically to living donors. Living donors may acquire blood-borne viral infections, including HIV, HBV, and HCV, during the period between initial evaluation and transplant surgery. Thus, it is recommended that living donors be retested for these infections within 7 to 14 days of organ donation. This, however, is currently not uniformly practiced. A recent survey of New York State transplant centers revealed that 3 months or more could have elapsed between a negative HIV enzyme immunoassay (EIA) result and time of transplant surgery.[24] Transplant centers should also routinely provide counseling to HIV-negative prospective living donors at the time of screening, specifically regarding approaches to decrease their risk for acquiring HIV, such as behavioral modification.

The Centers for Disease Control and Prevention (CDC) defines a high-risk donor as someone who carries an increased risk of harboring an infectious disease. The use of organs from high-risk donors is controversial and currently accounts for an average of 6.6% of all transplants, although this tends to vary among OPOs (0%–30%).[18] Specific recommendations for living high-risk donors include the consideration of delaying transplantation (until the time they are tested as negative) and using NAT rather than serologic testing where feasible to screen for blood-borne pathogens.

APPROACH TO RECIPIENT EVALUATION IN SUSPECTED DONOR-DERIVED INFECTIONS

Diagnosis of DDIs can be challenging for many reasons. Classic signs of infection are often absent, and patients may present with atypical syndromes. Due to their immunosuppressed states, diseases often disseminate early and progress rapidly. Often, the only clue may be the presence of disease in multiple recipients of organs from a common donor, and because organs procured from a donor are usually distributed across several institutions, this often leads to delay in disease recognition and treatment.

Treating physicians, therefore, need to maintain a high index of suspicion and think about the possibility of DDIs when faced with a patient who presents with atypical symptom complexes during the early post-transplant period. The local OPO should be contacted immediately, as soon as this is suspected. The OPO should then report the concern to the OPTN, as outlined previously. This eventually alerts the other centers to monitor their transplant recipients for the suspected disease.

SELECTED PATHOGEN-SPECIFIC DIAGNOSTIC AND MANAGEMENT STRATEGIES
Donor-derived Bacterial Infections

Bloodstream infection in organ donors
Organ donors often have risk factors that predispose them to developing bacterial infections. These risk factors include prolonged stay in ICUs; use of medical devices, (such as intravascular catheters, urinary catheters, and endotracheal intubation); and the presence of comorbidities. The OPTN requires that routine blood cultures be obtained from all organ donors hospitalized for at least 72 hours. Positive donor blood culture(s) is therefore not uncommon, although it is usually not recognized until after organ transplantation has occurred.

Historical cases have alerted clinicians to the potentially catastrophic consequences of bacterial transmission from donor to recipient, such as graft infections, arterial anastomotic disruption, poor initial graft function, and sepsis.[25] Recent data have not demonstrated these outcomes, however, and a review of 3 recent retrospective analyses showed zero transmission rates in such recipients.[25–27] It is likely that the modern practice of routine administration of broad-spectrum antimicrobials for perioperative prophylaxis has decreased the rate of bacterial transmission from organ donors, accounting for the lower reported incidence and clinical sequelae of transmission. Likewise, the prompt reporting of positive test results to transplant centers may have led to earlier institution of pathogen-directed treatment that might have averted adverse outcomes.

Management of SOT recipients with donor-derived bloodstream infections involves selection of pathogen-specific antimicrobial agents based on susceptibility results. The optimal duration of antimicrobial treatment is currently unknown, but in general, 7 to 10 days of pathogen-specific antimicrobial therapy is recommended for uncomplicated bloodstream infections.[25] Depending on the isolated pathogen, 14 days of therapy may be considered. In contrast to organ donors with uncomplicated bloodstream infections, current data does not support the use of organs from donors with severe sepsis and multiorgan failure, likely as a result of severe dysfunction in the lungs, heart, liver, and kidneys from these individuals with septic shock.[25]

Coagulase-negative staphylococci (and, if speciated, *Staphylococcus epidermidis*) and *Staphylococcus aureus*, represent some of the more commonly isolated microorganisms from donor blood cultures.[25–27] More recently, however, due to the increasing prevalence of multidrug-resistant organisms in ICUs, asymptomatic colonization and infection of organ donors have also become more common. Whether organs procured from such donors can be safely used remains actively debated. Although cultures are routinely obtained (from blood, urine, respiratory tract, and preservation fluid) at the time of transplantation, results are often not known until transplantation has occurred. This has resulted in poor outcomes, such as allograft loss and multiorgan failure with sepsis as well as death.[28,29] Therefore, some centers may opt not to use organs from donors infected with multidrug-resistant organisms. It seems that prior knowledge of donor infection and/or colonization with multidrug-resistant organisms and antibiotic susceptibility patterns may result in more favorable outcomes,[30] which is most likely due to early institution of appropriate antimicrobial prophylaxis and treatment.

Tuberculosis

Tuberculosis (TB) has an estimated incidence of 1.2% to 6.4% among SOT recipients in developed countries.[31] TB may be acquired via 1 of 3 ways: donor-derived, de novo acquisition from the community, or reactivation of recipient-derived latent infection. Although reactivation of latent TB is the most common cause of infection after transplantation, an estimated 4% of all TB infections in transplant recipients are thought to be donor derived.[8,32–34] When exposed to *Mycobacterium tuberculosis*, SOT recipients have a significantly higher risk of developing infection compared with the general population. In addition, the risk of dissemination and death due to TB is also higher.[35] Given the significant morbidity and mortality associated with post-transplant TB, organ donor and recipient screening should, therefore, be taken seriously.

A consensus report on the diagnosis and management of donor-derived TB was recently published (its recommendations are summarized later).[36] All living donors should undergo clinical evaluation for previously undiagnosed TB or latent TB infection (LTBI) in addition to either a tuberculin skin test (TST) or interferon-gamma release assay (IGRA) as part of routine donor screening process. Screening of deceased donors is, unfortunately, limited to identification of risk factors for TB by history and review of available medical records. In general, IGRAs and TSTs have comparable sensitivity in LTBI detection, except in those who have previously received Bacillus Calmette-Guérin vaccination, where IGRAs are preferred due to better specificity.[37] It was recently proposed that IGRAs may have a potential role in screening deceased donors for TB, but there are important limitations. A negative TST or IGRA should never be used to exclude active TB because 10% to 25% of those with active TB have negative TSTs (using a cutoff induration of 5 mm or greater), and the false-negative rate of TSTs in those with disseminated TB is approximately 50%.[38]

Diagnostic work-up of suspected cases should, therefore, routinely include acid-fast bacilli (AFB) staining and culture as well as nucleic acid amplification testing.

The risk of disease transmission in using organs from donors with a history of or active TB (including patients with LTBI) should be stratified into low to moderate or high-risk groups. Factors that should be taken into consideration during risk assessment include time of diagnosis and whether treatment completion was achieved and documented. In general, organs from donors with confirmed or possible active TB at the time of transplantation should not be used. Chemoprophylaxis with isoniazid should be considered and/or initiated in transplant recipients who received organs from donors with insufficiently treated LTBI. There are currently no data on the optimal timing for organ procurement from a living donor who is actively undergoing treatment of LTBI.

Treatment of active TB in SOT recipients is similar to that of the general population. A 4-drug regimen of isoniazid, a rifamycin, pyrazinamide, and ethambutol is used during the first 2 months pending susceptibility test results, followed by isoniazid and rifampin or rifabutin alone for an additional 4 months.[9] Longer duration of treatment should be considered the following situations: patients with central nervous system or bone and joint involvement; those with severe disseminated disease, as well as cavitary pulmonary disease with positive sputum culture at 2 months of treatment.[9]

Drug-drug interactions are a major challenge in the treatment of active TB in SOT recipients. Rifampin is an extremely potent inducer of cytochrome P3A4, leading to substantial decrease in serum levels of cyclosporine, tacrolimus, and sirolimus. Rejection episodes and subsequent allograft loss have been widely reported in conjunction with rifampin use. Because of the potent sterilizing activity of this drug class, a rifamycin-containing regimen remains strongly preferred. In this regard, rifabutin is a more attractive option, because it is a less potent inducer of cytochrome P3A4. Serum levels of the calcineurin inhibitors should be monitored closely, regardless of whether rifampin or rifabutin is used.

Donor-Derived Viral Infections

Rabies

Rabies is rare in the United States. Its incidence in the general population range from 2 to 6 cases per year.[10,11] Rabies virus transmission is predominantly neurotropic and occurs through bites and/or contact with neural tissue or saliva of infected animals. Transmission in the transplant population has occurred via corneal transplants and through organ and vessel segment transplantation.[39]

The onset of clinical signs and symptoms in SOT recipients occurred within the first 30 days of transplantation in reported cases, in contrast to the general population wherein only 25% of those infected tend to present within the first 30 days of exposure.[39] Although the incubation period seems shorter in SOT recipients, the tempo of disease progression seems similar in both patient populations. All 4 patients developed rapidly progressive encephalitis and died within 13 days of transplantation, similar to that in immunocompetent hosts.[39]

Diagnosis of rabies is challenging, especially in the absence of a documented exposure or suggestive history. Rabies virus serology (IgM and IgG antibodies) can be used for antemortem diagnosis confirmation. It seems that even in the setting of immunosuppression, seroconversion occurs: 3 of all 4 transplant recipients developed both IgM and IgG antibodies, and the other patient had only the IgG antibody to rabies virus.

There is currently no effective antiviral therapy for the treatment of rabies in humans.[40] The US Advisory Committee on Immunization Practices (ACIP) recommendations for rabies postexposure prophylaxis do not contain specific guidelines for transplant recipients or immunosuppressed patients in general.[12,40,41]

Lymphocytic choriomeningitis virus (LCMV)

LCMV is a zoonosis caused by rodent-borne arenavirus. Transmission can occur either by direct contact with or aerosolization of secretions or excretions of infected rodents. As demonstrated by the 2003 and 2005 clusters reported in the literature, LCMV can be transmitted by transplantation.[22]

Infection in immunocompetent hosts is generally benign and rarely fatal. The spectrum of clinical manifestations in these patients ranges from asymptomatic infection to a mild, self-limited viral syndrome to aseptic meningitis. Data on the clinical manifestations and natural history of LCMV in immunocompromised patients are scarce. Immunosuppression is thought to lead to more severe clinical manifestations, because immune control of this viral infection requires cell-mediated immunity.[22,42]

There is currently no FDA-approved test to diagnose LCMV infection. Available assays are likely not sensitive enough to be used for routine organ donor screening purposes, as evidenced by the negative test results of these tests on clinical specimens obtained from the donors in both reported clusters. Immunohistochemical staining may be helpful in the early diagnosis of LCMV infection and frequently demonstrates necrotic and occasional hemorrhagic foci in tissues.[22] Viral inclusions and inflammation are however, frequently absent in the immunocompromised hosts.

Ribavirin has in vitro activity against LCMV but in vivo activity remains unproven.[43–45] Of the 8 SOT recipients in the 2 reported clusters of donor-derived LCMV infection, only 1 received ribavirin therapy and this patient is the only one who survived. Because this patient's immunosuppression was also considerably reduced, the specific contribution of ribavirin to clinical improvement remains unclear at this time.

West Nile virus

WNV infection is commonly acquired through mosquito bites. It can also be transmitted through blood transfusions and transplantation. Two clusters of organ transplant–associated WNV infection have been reported in the literature to date: in 2002, the organ donor had acquired WNV via blood transfusion,[23] whereas in the second report, in 2005, the organ donor was likely infected through mosquito bites, associated with outdoor exposure.[13] Routine screening of organ donors for WNV is currently neither required nor routinely performed in the United States, although the US blood supply has been routinely screened for WNV using NAT since 2003.[46]

The clinical manifestations of WNV infection in organ transplant recipients may vary from that of immunocompetent hosts in the following ways:

1. Higher likelihood of neuroinvasive disease (40 times the risk of the general population)
2. Cerebrospinal fluid (CSF) pleocytosis may be subtle or even absent
3. Prolonged incubation period with asymptomatic viremia

WNV serology and quantitative PCR can be helpful in the diagnosis of WNV infection. Serologic response to infections may be blunted due to underlying immunosuppression; therefore, a negative WNV serology (either serum or CSF) does not rule out the diagnosis. WNV PCR is probably more sensitive than serologic testing and, although not 100% sensitive, can be helpful in detection of asymptomatic viremia, especially if performed on specimens collected close to the time of organ recovery. Organ donors with positive WNV IgM and IgG antibodies but without detectable nucleic acid PCR, however, can still transmit WNV.

Treatment of WNV infection is supportive. Interferon, ribavirin, and intravenous immunoglobulin have not been proven to be effective.[47–49]

HIV

In the United States, screening organ donors for HIV infection has been a requirement since 1985.[50] Transmission of HIV through SOT is in general rare but does occur, suggesting that current screening protocols for HIV infection may be inadequate. The first documented case of HIV transmission in the United States from a living donor was reported in 2009, despite screening with serologic testing.[14] HIV screen by EIA performed in this donor 79 days before actual transplantation was negative. Retrospective HIV NAT testing on the donor's stored serum obtained 11 days pretransplant found a 98% phylogenetic match of the recipient's HIV strain.

This prompted a CDC-led survey of 18 kidney and liver New York State transplant centers to assess current HIV infection screening protocols for prospective living donors.[24] This study found a wide variation in evaluation practices among transplant centers, underscoring a need to standardize this screening process. Results from this survey and the reported case of HIV transmission led to revision of US Public Health Service guidelines (unpublished), which recommends retesting of living donors for blood-borne pathogens, in particular HIV, within 7 to 14 days of donation.

Donor-derived Fungal Infections

The incidence of donor-derived fungal infections is not known but estimated to be rare. Although not common, these infections can be associated with significant complications, such as fungal arteritis with or without mycotic aneurysms, anastomotic infections, fungus ball, and graft site abscesses.[51,52] Unrecognized fungal infections in organ donors at the time of transplantation and contamination of preservation fluid are common modalities of infection transmission. The Infectious Diseases Community of Practice of the American Society of Transplantation recently published guidelines addressing issues related to donor-derived fungal infections.[51]

Candidiasis

Kidney transplant recipients Donor-derived candidiasis is estimated to occur at a frequency of 1:1000 in kidney transplantation.[52] These infections can occur as a result of contamination of preservation fluid, rupture of abdominal viscus in the donor, or, in some cases, donor candidemia. There is evidence that contamination of preservation fluid is likely the main cause of donor-derived candidiasis, because isolates implicated have been genotypically linked to those recovered from the preservation fluid.[52] The predictive value of positive preservation fluid cultures for development of infection remains, however, undefined. Therefore, although few existing data are instructive for obtaining routine preservation fluid cultures at the time of organ transplantation, this practice is currently not mandated.

In the event that *Candida* species is visualized or grown in preservation fluid, or in cases where intestinal perforation was documented in an organ donor, the kidney recipient should undergo further microbiologic and radiographic testing, including obtaining cultures from blood, urine, and all other clinically relevant sites as well as renal allograft imaging with baseline and repeat Doppler ultrasound at 1 week. More detailed studies, such as CT or magnetic resonance angiography, should be considered in cases where the initial Doppler ultrasound is negative, because infection can be associated with various allograft vascular and anastomotic complications.[51]

While awaiting culture and imaging results, empiric antifungal therapy should be initiated, with the drug of choice being fluconazole. Although active against most

Candida species, polyenes are not regarded as first-line therapy due to nephrotoxicity. An echinocandin should be considered if there is high likelihood of non-albicans *Candida* and if lower urinary tract infection has been excluded (because it undergoes extensive metabolism and minimal urinary concentration).

Duration of antifungal therapy is determined by the presence or absence of infection. Antifungal therapy may be discontinued after 2 weeks if there is no clinical or microbiologic evidence of infection. Alternatively, patients with established infection may be treated for 4 to 6 weeks, with at least 6 weeks of treatment in patients with vascular involvement. Repeat imaging should be performed at the end of therapy.[51]

Nonkidney organ transplant recipients Routine antifungal prophylaxis is commonly used in lung transplant recipients.[53] Empiric antifungal therapy should be considered if donor respiratory samples yield *Candida* species, until bronchoscopic evaluation of anastomosis is performed. In patients with risk factors for anastomotic infection, a longer course of antifungal therapy should be considered.[54] Donor-derived candidiasis is unusual, however, after cardiac transplantation.[55]

In liver and pancreatic transplant recipients with visualization or growth of *candida* in preservation fluid, the management of these patients should follow that of kidney transplant recipients. Specifically pertaining to pancreatic transplantation, the act of opening or aspirating duodenal contents during the backbench procedure is associated with the development of *candida* arteritis post-transplantation.[56] This practice should, therefore, be discouraged.

Cryptococcosis

The majority of post-transplant cryptococcal infections are thought to represent reactivation of latent infection. Although relatively rare, transplant-associated cryptococcosis is well documented and should be considered in the following clinical scenarios:

1. Cryptococcosis documented at any site in the first 30 days after transplant
2. Demonstration of cryptococcus at the graft or surgical site
3. Diagnosis of cryptococcal disease in more than 1 recipient from a single donor

Donors with cryptococcal disease or involvement at any site can transmit infection.[57,58] Evaluation and management of SOT recipient diagnosed with cryptococcal disease is as outlined in the Infectious Diseases Society of America 2010 guidelines.[59] Diagnostic evaluation should include CSF analysis, serum and CSF cryptococcal antigen testing, and cultures of blood, urine, CSF, and all clinically infected sites. Patients with mild to moderate disease, in whom central nervous system disease has been excluded, may be treated with fluconazole alone. All other patients, including those with central nervous system or disseminated disease as well as those with moderate to severe pulmonary disease, should receive induction with combination therapy consisting of lipid formulation of amphotericin B and flucytosine for 14 days, followed by consolidation and maintenance with fluconazole. In general, treatment duration is 6 to 12 months. Immunosuppression should be reduced gradually to minimize the risk of immune reconstitution inflammatory syndrome, and physicians should be aware of drug-drug interactions between fluconazole and calcineurin inhibitors.[59]

Although cases of donor-derived *Cryptococcus gattii* have not been documented, the potential for its transmission exists, because *C. gattii* is known to infect individuals with and without identifiable immune defects. The diagnosis and treatment recommendations for *C. gattii* are the same as for *C. neoformans*.[59]

Aspergillus and other molds

Although *Aspergillus* species is the second most common cause of invasive fungal infections in SOT recipients, donor-derived invasive aspergillosis is overall rare.[60–62] Acquisition of unusual molds from contaminated water, such as *Apophysomyces elegans* (an agent of mucormycosis) and *Scedosporium apiospermum*, may occur in donors with specific epidemiologic risk factors, such as near-drowning victims.[63,64] These infections are associated with high rates of graft loss and a multitude of other complications similar to that associated with donor-derived candidiasis, as discussed previously. Diagnosis of invasive mold infections in SOT recipients continue to rely mainly on fungal cultures, as the use of antigen testing, such as galactomannan in this patient population is currently not well studied.

Coccidioidomycosis

Coccidioidomycosis occurs in 4% to 9% of transplant recipients in endemic areas.[65,66] It most commonly occurs during the first year post-transplantation. Although these cases often represent either reactivation of latent infection or *de novo* acquisition of disease, donor-derived coccidioidomycosis has also been described, with the majority of cases occurring in lung, and a few in kidney transplant recipients.[67–72]

All potential organ donors who currently reside or have resided or traveled to endemic areas should be screened for previous exposure to *Coccidioides* species by serologic testing. Universal screening, however, is not recommended for centers outside the endemic areas. Various serologic testing methods exist, and these include EIA, complement fixation, and immunodiffusion. The performance of these assays in transplant recipients have not been studied extensively, and false-negative results have been reported.[72]

Recipients of organs from a donor who is found to be seropositive or to have active infection should undergo clinical evaluation, baseline serologic testing, and prompt initiation of antifungal prophylaxis. Either fluconazole (400 mg daily) or itraconazole (200 mg twice daily) may be used, because both have been used and proved effective.[73,74] The optimal duration of antifungal prophylaxis has not been defined. Lifelong prophylaxis may be considered in lung transplant recipients because granulomas may harbor viable organisms. In non–lung organ transplant recipients, however, discontinuation of prophylaxis after 3 to 6 months may be considered with close monitoring for clinical or serologic evidence of coccidioidomycosis.

Patients with active disease should be treated according to the Infectious Diseases Society of America guidelines.[66] In general, fluconazole or itraconazole is the drug of choice, unless severe pneumonia or disseminated disease is present, in which case amphotericin B should be used initially. Treatment duration should be a minimum of 6 to 12 months, followed by lifelong antifungal prophylaxis once active coccidioidomycosis has been controlled to prevent relapse.[67]

Donor-derived Amoebic and Parasitic Infections

Donor-derived parasitic infections caused by *T cruzi*, *S stercoralis,* and *B mandrillaris* have recently emerged in transplant recipients in the United States.

Chagas disease

Donor-derived Chagas disease is an emerging infection in transplant recipients due to a steady increase of immigrants from Latin America and expansion of organ donor pool.[15,16] Data regarding seroprevalence of *T cruzi* among organ donors are limited but estimated to be approximately 0.25% to 1%.[75,76] Although universal organ donor screening is currently performed in areas with a high prevalence of at-risk individuals (such as Los Angeles and Miami), current guidelines recommend a more targeted screening approach, using one of the FDA–approved or FDA–cleared EIAs or immunofluorescent assays in those who were either born or have resided in Mexico, Central America, or South America.[75]

Whether or not organs from seropositive donors should be used is controversial. Hearts from *T cruzi*–infected donors should be avoided, given the known tropism of this parasite.[77] Alternatively, the use of kidneys and/or livers from seropositive donors can be considered based on some data showing that not all transplants resulted in transmission of Chagas disease.[78,79] Informed consent, however, should be obtained, with close monitoring of transplant recipients, should a decision be made to use these organs. Recipient monitoring should rely primarily on direct detection of *T cruzi* either by PCR, Giemsa-stained peripheral blood smears, or microscopy of fresh buffy coat preparations. Frequency of laboratory monitoring should consist of weekly specimens for 2 months, every 2 weeks for the third month, and monthly thereafter from months 4 to 6 post-transplantation.[75]

Recipients with evidence of *T cruzi* infection should be treated with either benznidazole or nifurtimox, both of which are available for use under Investigational New Drug protocols from the CDC. Benznidazole is the preferred first-line drug in transplant recipients because it is better tolerated and has fewer potential drug interactions when compared to nifurtimox.[75]

SUMMARY

Organ donor screening remains an essential practice in risk reduction of disease transmission associated with organ transplantation. Some of the changes that may be in store in the future of screening for DDIs include multiplex NAT testing, which involves performance of multiple simultaneous assays on small blood samples, will hopefully improve efficiency and turnaround time as well as enforce post-transplant screening for HIV, HBV, and HCV in SOT recipients from high-risk donors as measures to improve patient outcomes. This risk, however, can never be entirely eliminated. Because not all disease transmission through transplantation can be prevented, rapid recognition is critical to facilitate appropriate treatment, minimize complications, and maintain public confidence in the safety of the process of organ transplantation.

REFERENCES

1. Grossi PA, Fishman JA. Donor-derived infections in solid organ transplant recipients. Am J Transplant 2009;9(Suppl 4):S19–26.
2. Humar A, Fishman JA. Donor-derived infection: old problem, new solutions? Am J Transplant 2008;8:1087–8.
3. Ison MG, Hager J, Blumberg E, et al. Donor-derived disease transmission events in the United States: data reviewed by the OPTN/UNOS Disease Transmission Advisory Committee. Am J Transplant 2009;9(8):1929–35.
4. Ison MG, Nalesnik MA. An update on donor-derived disease transmission in organ transplantation. Am J Transplant 2011;11(6):1123–30.
5. Fishman JA. Infection in solid-organ transplant recipients. N Engl J Med 2007; 357(25):2601–14.
6. Minimum procurement standards for an organ procurement organization (OPO). Available at: http://optn.transplant.hrsa.gov/PoliciesandBylaws2/policies/pdfs/policy_2.pdf. Accessed August 24, 2012.

7. Morris MI, Fischer SA, Ison MG. Infections transmitted by transplantation. Infect Dis Clin North Am 2010;24:497–514.

8. Centers for Disease Control and Prevention (CDC). Transplantation-transmitted tuberculosis- Oklahoma and Texas, 2007. MMWR Morb Mortal Wkly Rep 2008; 57(13):333–6.

9. Subramaniam A, Dorman S. Mycobacterium tuberculosis in solid organ transplant recipients. Am J Transplant 2009;9(S4):S57–62.

10. Centers for Disease Control and Prevention (CDC). Human death associated with bat rabies- California, 2003. MMWR Morb Mortal Wkly Rep 2004;53(2):33–5.

11. Centers for Disease Control and Prevention (CDC). First human death associated with raccoon rabies – Virginia, 2003. MMWR Morb Mortal Wkly Rep 2003;52(45): 1102–3.

12. Rupprecht CE, Briggs D, Brown CM, et al, Centers for Disease Control and Prevention (CDC). Use of a reduced (4-dose) vaccine schedule for postexposure prophylaxis to prevent human rabies: recommendations of the advisory committee on immunization practices. MMWR Recomm Rep 2010;59(RR-2):1–9.

13. Centers for Disease Control and Prevention (CDC). West Nile virus infections in organ transplant recipients—New York and Pennsylvania, August-September, 2005. MMWR Morb Mortal Wkly Rep 2005;54(40):1021–3.

14. Centers for Disease Control and Prevention. HIV transmitted from a living organ donor- New York City, 2009. MMWR Morb Mortal Wkly Rep 2011;60(10):297–301.

15. Centers for Disease Control and Prevention (CDC). Chagas disease after organ transplantation- United States, 2001. MMWR Morb Mortal Wkly Rep 2002; 51(10):210–2.

16. Chagas disease after organ transplantation, Los Angeles, California, 2006. MMWR Morb Mortal Wkly Rep 2006;55(29):798–800.

17. OPTN/SRTR 2004 annual report. Richmond (VA): Organ Procurement and Transplantation Network, United Network for Organ Sharing; 2004. Available at: http://www.optn.org/data/annualReport.asp. Accessed August 24, 2012.

18. Kucirka LM, Singer AL, Segev DL. High infectious risk donors: what are the risks and when are they too high? Curr Opin Organ Transplant 2011;16(2):256–61.

19. Delmonico FL. Cadaver donor screening for infectious agents in solid organ transplantation. Clin Infect Dis 2000;31(3):781–6.

20. Stramer SL, Caglioti S, Strong DM. NAT of the United States and Canadian blood supply. Transfusion 2000;40(10):1165–8.

21. Humar A, Morris M, Blumberg E, et al. Nucleic acid testing (NAT) of organ donors: is the 'best' test the right test? A consensus conference report. Am J Transplant 2010;10:889–99.

22. Fischer SA, Graham MB, Kuehnert MJ, et al. Transmission of lymphocytic choriomeningitis virus by organ transplantation. N Engl J Med 2006;354:2235–49.

23. Iwamoto M, Jernigan DB, Guasch A, et al. Transmission of West Nile virus from an organ donor to four transplant recipients. N Engl J Med 2003;348:2196–203.

24. Kwan CK, Al-Samarrai T, Smith LC, et al. HIV screening practices for living organ donors, New York State, 2010: need for standard policies. Clin Infect Dis 2012; 55(7):990–5.

25. Lumbreras C, Sanz F, Gonzalez A, et al. Clinical significance of donor-unrecognized bacteremia in the outcome of solid-organ transplant recipients. Clin Infect Dis 2001;33:722–6.

26. Gonzalez-Segura C, Pascual M, Garcia Huete L, et al. Donors with positive blood culture: could they transmit infections to the recipients? Transplant Proc 2005;37: 3664–6.

27. Freeman R, Ioannis G, Falagas M, et al. Outcome of transplantation of organs procured from bacteremic donors. Transplantation 1999;68(8):1107–11.
28. Goldberg E, Bishara J, Lev S, et al. Organ transplantation from a donor colonized with a multidrug-resistant organism: a case report. Transpl Infect Dis 2012;14: 296–9.
29. Centers for Disease Control and Prevention (CDC). Transmission of multidrug-resistant escherichia coli through kidney transplantation—California and Texas 2009. MMWR Morb Mortal Wkly Rep 2010;59(50):1642–6.
30. Ariza-Heredia EJ, Patel R, Blumberg EA, et al. Outcomes of transplantation using organs from a donor infected with Klebsiella pneumoniae carbapenemase (KPC)-producing K. pneumoniae. Transpl Infect Dis 2012;14:229–36.
31. Munoz P, Rodriguez C, Bouza E. Mycobacterium tuberculosis infection in recipients of solid organ transplants. Clin Infect Dis 2005;40:581–7.
32. Peters TG, Reiter CG, Boswell RL. Transmission of tuberculosis by kidney transplantation. Transplantation 1984;38:514–6.
33. Ridgeway AL, Warner GS, Philips P, et al. Transmission of Mycobacterium tuberculosis to recipients of single lung transplants from the same donor. Am J Respir Crit Care Med 1996;153:1166–8.
34. Kiuchi T, Inomata Y, Uemoto S, et al. A hepatic graft tuberculosis transmitted from a living-related donor. Transplantation 1997;63:905–7.
35. Singh N, Paterson DL. Mycobacterium tuberculosis infection in solid organ transplant recipients: impact and implications for management. Clin Infect Dis 1998; 27:1266–77.
36. Morris MI, Daly JS, Blumberg E, et al. Diagnosis and management of tuberculosis in transplant donors: a donor-derived infections consensus conference report. Am J Transplant 2012;12:2288–300.
37. Pai M, Zwerling A, Menzies D. Systematic review: T-cell based assays for the diagnosis of latent tuberculosis infection: an update. Ann Intern Med 2008;149: 177–84.
38. Sester M, Sotgiu G, Lange C, et al. Interferon-gamma release assays for the diagnosis of active tuberculosis: a systematic review and meta-analysis. Eur Respir J 2011;37:100–11.
39. Srinivasan A, Burton EC, Kuehnert MJ, et al. Transmission of rabies virus from an organ donor to four transplant recipients. N Engl J Med 2005;352:1103–11.
40. Gibbons RV, Rupprecht CE. Postexposure rabies prophylaxis in immunosuppressed patients. JAMA 2001;285(12):1574.
41. Hay E, Derazon H, Bukish N, et al. Postexposure rabies prophylaxis in a patient with lymphoma. JAMA 2001;285(2):166–7.
42. Amman BR, Pavlin BI, Albarino CG, et al. Pet rodents and fatal lymphocytic choriomeningitis in transplant patients. Emerg Infect Dis 2007;13(5):719–25.
43. Moreno H, Gallego I, Sevilla N, et al. Ribavirin can be mutagenic for arenaviruses. J Virol 2011;85(14):7246–55.
44. Enria DA, Maiztegi JI. Antiviral treatment of Argentine hemorrhagic fever. Antiviral Res 1994;23:23–31.
45. Moreno H, Grande-Perez A, Domingo E, et al. Arenaviruses and lethal mutagenesis: prospects for new ribavirin-based interventions. Viruses 2012;4(11): 2786–805.
46. Busch MP, Caglioti S, Robertson E, et al. Screening the blood supply for West Nile virus RNA by nucleic acid amplification testing. N Engl J Med 2005;353:460–7.
47. Gea-Banacloche J, Johnson RT, Bagic A, et al. West Nile virus: pathogenesis and therapeutic options. Ann Intern Med 2004;140:545–53.

48. Planitzer GB, Modrof J, Kreil TR, et al. West Nile virus neutralization by US plasma-derived immunoglobulin products. J Infect Dis 2007;196(3):435.

49. Agrawal AG, Petersen LR. Human immunoglobulin as treatment for WNV infection. J Infect Dis 2003;188(1):1.

50. Rogers MF, Simonds RJ, Lawton KE, et al. Guidelines for preventing transmission of human immunodeficiency virus through transplantation of human tissue and organs. Centers for Disease Control and Prevention. MMWR Recomm Rep 1994; 43(RR-9):1–17.

51. Singh N, Huprikar S, Burdette SD, et al. Donor-derived fungal infections in organ transplant recipients: guidelines of the American Society of Transplantation, Infectious Diseases Community of Practice. Am J Transplant 2012;12:2414–28.

52. Albano L, Bretagne S, Mamzer-Bruneel MF, et al. Evidence that graft-site candidiasis after kidney transplantation is acquired during organ recovery: a multicenter study in France. Clin Infect Dis 2009;48:194–202.

53. Dummer JS, Lazariashvilli N, Barnes J, et al. A survey of antifungal management in lung transplantation. J Heart Lung Transplant 2004;12:1376–81.

54. Hadjiliadis DH, Howell DN, Davis RD, et al. Anastomotic infections in lung transplant recipients. Ann Transplant 2000;3:13–9.

55. Mossad SB, Avery RK, Goormastic M, et al. Significance of positive cultures from donor left atrium and post-preservation fluid in heart transplantation. Transplantation 1997;64:1209–10.

56. Ciancio G, Brke GW, Viciana AL, et al. Destructive allograft fungal arteritis following simultaneous pancreas-kidney transplantation. Transplantation 1996; 61:1172–5.

57. Baddley JW, Schain DC, Gupte AA, et al. Transmission of cryptococcus neoformans by organ transplantation. Clin Infect Dis 2011;52:e94–8.

58. Sun HY, Alexander BD, Lortholary O, et al. Unrecognized pretransplant and donor-derived cryptococcal disease in organ transplant recipients. Clin Infect Dis 2010;51:1062–9.

59. Perfect JR, Dismukes WE, Dromer F, et al. Clinical practice guidelines for the management of cryptococcal disease: 2010 update by the infectious diseases society of America. Clin Infect Dis 2010;50:291–322.

60. Keating MR, Guerrero MA, Daly RC, et al. Transmission of invasive aspergillosis from a subclinically infected donor to three different organ transplant recipients. Chest 1996;109:1119–24.

61. Mueller NJ, Weisser M, Fehr T, et al. Donor-derived aspergillosis from use of a solid organ recipient as a multiorgan donor. Transpl Infect Dis 2010;12:54–9.

62. Shoham S, Hinestrosa F, Moore J, et al. Invasive filamentous fungal infections associated with renal transplant tourism. Transpl Infect Dis 2010;12:371–4.

63. Stas KJ, Louwagie PG, Van Damme BJ, et al. Isolated zygomycosis in a bought living unrelated renal transplant. Transpl Int 1996;9:600–2.

64. Rammaert B, Lanternier F, Zahar JR, et al. Healthcare-associated mucormycosis. Clin Infect Dis 2012;54(Suppl 1):S44.

65. Blair JE, Logan JL. Coccidioidomycosis in solid organ transplantation. Clin Infect Dis 2001;33:1536–44.

66. Galgiani JN, Ampel NM, Blair JE, et al. IDSA guidelines: coccidioidomycosis. Clin Infect Dis 2005;41:1217–23.

67. Miller M, Hendren R, Gilligan P. Posttransplantation disseminated coccidioidomycosiss acquired from donor lungs. J Clin Microbiol 2004;42:2347–9.

68. Tripathy U, yung GL, Kriett JM, et al. Donor transfer of pulmonary coccidioidomycosis in lung transplantation. Ann Thorac Surg 2002;73:306–8.

69. Brugiere O, Forget E, Biondi G, et al. Coccidioidomycosis in a lung transplant recipient acquired from the donor graft in France. Transplantation 2009;88: 1319–20.

70. Vikram HR, Dosanjh A, Blair JE. Coccidioidomycosis and lung transplantation. Transplantation 2011;92:717–21.

71. Carvalho C, Ferreira I, Gaiao S, et al. Cerebral coccidioidomycosis after renal transplantation in a non-endemic area. Transpl Infect Dis 2010;12:151–4.

72. Proia L, Miller R, AST Infectious Diseases Community of Practice. Endemic fungal infections in solid organ transplant recipients. Am J Transplant 2009;9(Suppl 4): S199–207.

73. Blair JE, Douglas DD, Mulligan DC. Early results of targeted prophylaxis for coccidioidomycosis in patients undergoing orthotopic liver transplantation within an endemic area. Transpl Infect Dis 2003;5:3–8.

74. Blair J, Braddy C. Azoles prevent reactivation of prior and clinically quiescent coccidioidomycosis in patients undergoing solid organ transplantation. Presented at the 45th annual Interscience Conference on Antimicrobial Agents and Chemotherapy. Washington, DC, December 16–19, 2005.

75. Chin-Hong PV, Schwartz BS, Bem C, et al. Screening and treatment of chagas disease in organ transplant recipients in the United States: recommendations from the Chagas in Transplant Working Group. Am J Transplant 2011;11:672–80.

76. Nowicki MJ, Chinchilla C, Corado L, et al. Prevalence of antibodies to Trypanosoma cruzi among solid organ donors in Southern California: a population at risk. Transplantation 2008;81:477–9.

77. Kun H, Moore A, Mascola L, et al. Transmission of Trypanosoma cruzi by heart transplantation. Clin Infect Dis 2009;48:1534–40.

78. Riarte A, Luna C, Sabatiello R, et al. Chagas' disease in patients with kidney transplants: 7 years of experience 1989-1996. Clin Infect Dis 1999;29:561–7.

79. De Artega J, Massari PU, Galli B, et al. Renal Transplantation and Chagas' disease. Transplant Proc 1992;24:1900–1.

BK Polyomavirus Infection in the Renal Transplant Recipient

Gayle P. Balba, MD[a],*, Basit Javaid, MD[b], Joseph G. Timpone Jr, MD[a]

KEYWORDS

- BK virus • Nephropathy • Renal transplant • Kidney dysfunction

KEY POINTS

- The incidence of BK virus nephropathy (BKVN) is 1% to 10% of renal transplant recipients and usually occurs within the first few months post-transplant.
- BKVN is associated with an up to 50% rate of allograft failure.
- Renal transplant recipients need to be monitored periodically with BKV urine and serum polymerase chain reaction (PCR).
- Reduction in immunosuppression is the mainstay of therapy for BKVN.
- Adjuvant antiviral therapy is controversial for treatment of BKVN.
- Retransplant is safe in patients with allograft failure due to BKVN.

INTRODUCTION

Although kidney transplant outcomes have greatly improved and new immunosuppressive agents have reduced the rate of graft rejection, a proportion of renal transplant recipients continue to have progressive kidney dysfunction. Renal graft loss has been attributed to emerging opportunistic infections, specifically due to the BK virus (BKV). BKV is postulated to be selected by these new potent immunosuppressive medications and to be an important factor in graft failure over time. The prevalence of BKV nephropathy (BKVN) is estimated to be 1% to 10%, with most cases occurring in the first year post–kidney transplant. Renal allograft loss from BKVN has been estimated to occur in up to 50% of affected recipients.[1] With the increasing recognition of BKV infection using PCR assays coupled with the immediate reduction in immunosuppression for BKVN, the incidence of graft failure secondary to BKVN may be decreasing.

The authors have no conflict of interest to disclosure.
[a] Division of Infectious Diseases, Georgetown University Hospital, 3800 Reservoir Road Northwest, Washington, DC 20007, USA; [b] Division of Transplant Surgery, Georgetown University Hospital, 3800 Reservoir Road Northwest, Washington, DC 20007, USA
* Corresponding author.
E-mail address: Gayle.P.Balba@gunet.georgetown.edu

Infect Dis Clin N Am 27 (2013) 271–283
http://dx.doi.org/10.1016/j.idc.2013.02.002
0891-5520/13/$ – see front matter © 2013 Elsevier Inc. All rights reserved.

VIROLOGY AND PATHOGENESIS

The BKV, a human polyomavirus of the Papovaviridae virus family, was first discovered in 1971.[2] There are 2 types of human polyomaviruses, JC and BK, both named after the initials of patients in whom they were first detected. BKV was isolated from the urine of a recipient of a kidney allograft who developed ureteral stenosis. It has been increasingly recognized as an important opportunistic virus in renal transplantation and has been associated with graft loss from polyomavirus or BKV nephropathy (BKVN).[3]

The polyomaviruses are small (30–45 nm), icosahedral, nonenveloped, double-stranded, circular DNA viruses that replicate in the host nucleus and contain 4 serologic groups and genotypes.[3] The 4 serologic groups and genotypes are categorized as I, II, III, and IV and may have different virulence properties. Group I encodes the prototype strain Dunlop, MM, and GS; group II encodes the SB strain; group III encodes the AS strain; and group IV encodes the MG strains.[3] Three genomic areas have been characterized. The first is the noncoding control region responsible for replication and gene expression, the second early genes encoding regulatory proteins, and the third late genes with the capsid proteins and agnoprotein.[3]

BKV replicates during states of immune suppression and injury. BKV reactivation with viremia and nephropathy is seen predominantly in the renal transplant population. In mouse models, mechanical and chemical injury contributed to acute and reactivation of latent BKV infection.[4] With reactivation, the viral infection spreads cell to cell, causing lysis of infected cells affecting renal tubular cells and interstitial cells.[4]

The exact pathogenesis of BKVN as well as risk factors has yet to be elucidated; however, BKV infection involves components of recipient, graft, and viral factors.[5] Disruption in host immunologic control and viral replication is thought to result in BKVN.

INCIDENCE

BKV is highly seroprevalent in humans, with reported rates of 60% to 80%, with primary infection in childhood by oral and respiratory exposures.[3] Latent infection is established in the renal epithelium (transitional epithelium, renal tubular epithelium, parietal epithelium of Bowman capsule), bladder, and lymphoid cells.[6] Immunocompetent individuals have been demonstrated to intermittently have active replication as well as asymptomatic viral shedding, with an incidence of up to 20%. Immunocompromised patients have increased viral shedding with an incidence between 10% and 60% and studies have demonstrated that the intensity of immunosuppression accounts for BK replication but that the actual immunosuppressive agent did not correlate with replication. The prevalence of BK viruria, BK viremia, and BKVN in renal transplant recipients is estimated to be 30%, 14%, and 8%, respectively.[1] BK-induced nephropathy occurs in from 1% to 10% of renal transplants, with a mean incidence of 4.91%, usually in the first year post-transplant, and may result in graft failure in 15% to 50% of affected patients.[6]

Several prospective studies in which BKV reactivation and replication were monitored in renal transplant recipients have demonstrated both positive BKV viruria and BKV viremia early after transplant even within the first hours post-transplant, with the highest incidence occurring at approximately 1 to 3 months post-transplant.[7] It is thought that BK replication may be a marker of excess immunosuppression.

Thakur and colleagues[8] published a prospective study monitoring BKV reactivation in 33 renal transplant patients, with a 3-year follow-up observation period, and demonstrated that the highest incidence of BK viruria and BK viremia occurred at 1 month post–renal transplant. Mitterhofer and colleagues,[9] however, studied 36 renal transplant recipients prospectively, with the highest levels of viruria and viremia occurring 3 months post-transplant. Most studies have shown that reactivation occurs in the early post-transplant period. BKVN has been rarely reported in recipients of other solid organs although asymptomatic BK viruria is not uncommon.[10] In a recent report of 33 liver transplant patients, 52% had BKV viruria over the 2-year study period.[10]

RISK FACTORS FOR BK VIRUS–ASSOCIATED NEPHROPATHY

Several risk factors for BKV infections have been associated with increased risk of BKVN (**Box 1**). The most important is the degree of immunosuppression within renal transplant recipients, although no specific immunosuppressive regimen has been definitively linked to BK viruria. Other factors thought to be related to increased risk of BKV infection acquired through donor transmission include female gender, deceased donations, ischemia-reperfusion injury, high BKV-specific antibody titers within the donor, HLA mismatch, and African American ethnicity.[7] Because BKV-seropositive donors increase the risk of BKV infection in recipients, BKV infection is

---

Box 1
Risk factors for BK virus nephropathy

Donor-related risk factors

Female gender

Deceased donation

Ischemia-reperfusion injury

High BKV-specific antibody titers

HLA mismatch

African American ethnicity

Recipient-related risk factors

Extremes of age

Male gender

Low or absent BKV-specific T-cell activity

White ethnicity

Risk factors in the post-transplant period

Degree of immunosuppression

Ureteral trauma

Ureteral stents

Diabetes mellitus

Delayed graft function

Cytomegalovirus infection

Treatment of acute rejection

Cumulative steroid exposure

Lymphocyte-depleting antibodies

Tacrolimus combination immunosuppression

hypothesized to originate from the donor kidney.[11] Studies have conflicting evidence regarding the role of BKV serostatus. Shah and colleagues[12] reported that seropositive donors and seronegative recipients were at the highest risk for developing BKVN, at a rate of 43%, whereas Bohl and colleagues[11] reported that seropositive donors and recipients were the highest risk group for developing BKVN, at 50%.[12] In both studies, seronegative donors and recipients developed BKV infection at the lowest rate, of 10%. Bohl and colleagues[11] also found that the absence of HLA-C7 in recipients was associated with an increased risk of infection.

Factors in recipients that increase the risk of BKV infection include older, younger age, male gender, low or absent BKV-specific T cell activity, and white ethnicity.[7] Two pediatric studies have demonstrated BK seronegativity or low antibody titer is a risk factor of BK viruria and BKVN.[13,14] Host factors, especially host humoral and cellular immunity, are thought to determine if BKV viremia results in clinical disease. Hariharan[15] published a study showing trends toward rapid clearance of viremia in subjects with BKV IgG greater than 50 enzyme immunoassay units, hinting that humoral immunity may play an important role in BKVN. Despite adequate humoral immunity, patients may develop BKVN, emphasizing the role of cellular immunity that is typically critical for viral immunity. Comoli and colleagues[16] demonstrated that patients with BKV-associated nephropathy (BKVN) had a reduction in BKV-specific interferon-γ–secreting lymphocytes, suggesting defective cellular immunity was associated with BKVN.

Post-transplant risk factors include ureteral trauma, diabetes mellitus, delayed graft function in renal transplant, cytomegalovirus infection, treatment of acute rejection, cumulative steroid exposure, lymphocyte-depleting antibodies, and tacrolimus combination immunosuppression.[7] In addition, HLA-mismatched and ABO-mismatched patients may have a higher incidence of BKVN. Ureteral stents may also predispose patients to BKVN perhaps by causing ureteral injury.[17]

CLINICAL MANIFESTATIONS OF BK VIRUS

BKVN often begins asymptomatically without any clinical or laboratory signs (**Box 2**). The first signs of disease often are high-level BKV viruria and BKV viremia, without any obvious deterioration in the renal allograft function.[18] BKV viruria may precede BK viremia. Sustained BK viremia has a higher sensitivity and specificity compared with BKV viruria for the diagnosis of BKVN.[19] Persistent BK viremia has been suggested by some observers to correlate with BKVN.[15] BK is found, however, in 10% to 40% of renal transplant recipients without any clinical or histologic evidence of BKVN.[20,21] Urine electron microscopy with negative-staining electron microscopy of urine with cast-like 3-D polyomavirus aggregates has a sensitivity of 100% and specificity of 99%. Urine electron microscopy may determine symptomatic from asymptomatic BK viral replication. Viral cultures are usually used in research settings and can take weeks to months to grow. BKVN has been described, however, in the absence of serum creatinine elevation or other markers of disease activity, such as BK viremia and BK viruria.

BK reactivation in renal transplant recipients is thought to be from reactivation of BKV in tubular epithelial cells of the donor kidney.[11] Typically, BK-induced interstitial nephritis presents with elevated serum creatinine in presence of BK viremia or BK viruria. Urinary abnormalities, such as pyuria, hematuria, and cellular casts with renal tubular cells and inflammatory cells, have also been reported, but are nonspecific. Urine cytology may demonstrate BK-infected cells, called decoy cells, containing an enlarged nucleus with basophilic intranuclear inclusions. Because a majority of renal

---

Box 2
Clinical manifestations of BK virus infection

Asymptomatic

Nephropathy with interstitial nephritis

Hemorrhagic cystitis[a]

Ureteral stenosis

Hydronephrosis

Cystitis

Vasculopathy

Meningoencephalopathy

Retinitis

Pneumonitis

Hemophagocytic syndrome

Multifocal leukoencephalopathy

Systemic lupus erythematosus

[a] Typically this occurs in allogeneic hematopoietic stem cell transplant recipients.

---

transplant recipients with BKVN present with an asymptomatic increase in serum creatinine, BKV urine and serum PCR should be performed whenever unexplained allograft dysfunction is identified.

The other important presentation of BKV is polyomavirus-associated hemorrhagic cystitis, resulting from reactivation of BKV in the bladder, which is more commonly observed in allogeneic hematopoietic stem cell transplant patients and rarely occurs in renal transplant patients.[4] BK viruria occurs in 50% to 100% of hematopoietic bone marrow transplant recipients, usually within 2 months of transplant.[22] Hemorrhagic cystitis affects up to 10% of allogeneic stem cell transplant recipients and presents with dysuria and hematuria.[23] BKV is thought to reactivate in the urothelium and typically occurs greater than 10 days post-transplant.[24]

BKV has also been infrequently reported to cause ureteral stenosis, hydronephrosis, cystitis, vasculopathy, meningoencephalopathy, retinitis, pneumonitis, hemophago-cytic syndrome, and polyomavirus-associated multifocal leukoencephalopathy.[24–30] BKV-related ureteral stenosis has been reported in renal transplant recipients as well as allogeneic stem cell transplant recipients. In a small case series, with 2 cases in renal transplant recipients and 1 in a stem cell transplant recipient, 1 of the 2 renal transplant patients and the stem cell transplant patient survived after ureteral stenosis.[26,31] Hydro-nephrosis has been reported in a stem cell transplant patient secondary to epithelial proliferation within the bladder on both ostii, resulting in bilateral hydronephrosis.[26]

BKV has also been possibly associated with systemic lupus erythematosus by inducing antibodies against DNA and histones and speculated to be associated with neoplasms.[32,33] The extrarenal manifestations, such as meningitis, retinitis, and pneumonitis, have been reported in the nonrenal transplant population. In the case report with retinitis, the patient had advanced AIDS and expired from pneumonia but on postmortem was found to have BKV involvement of the retina.[25] BKV infection resulting in pneumonitis has typically been reported in the nonrenal transplant patient population. Two fatal case reports of pneumonitis have been reported in the literature,

1 patient after hematopoietic stem cell transplant and another with chronic lymphocytic leukemia on chemotherapy.[30,34]

DIAGNOSIS AND MONITORING

Most centers rely on PCR assay of the urine and serum for surveillance of BKV infection and renal biopsy for confirmation of BKVN. The surveillance technique or frequency is center specific. There is wide variation in PCR techniques as well because there is no standardization, and the PCR method is not currently Food and Drug Administration approved for BKV infection.[35] BK viruria precedes BK viremia by approximately 4 weeks. Although threshold values have been suggested for BKV DNA in urine and serum, BK viruria and BK viremia do not always correlate with nephropathy. It has been suggested that urine BKV DNA PCR greater than 10^7 copies/mL may indicate BKVN.[4] Sustained BKV viruria has high sensitivity and specificity of 100% and 94%, respectively, for the development of BK viremia.[19] In patients with suspected BKVN, urine PCR, urine cytology, and serum BKV PCR should be performed.

Persistent viremia has been suggested by some observers to correlate with BKVN.[15] BK is found, however, in approximately 10% to 40% of renal transplant recipients and not all have clinical nephropathy.[20,21] The positive predictive value of BKV viremia for nephropathy is 60%.[15] If BKV load is greater than 10^4 copies/mL within the blood, biopsy should be performed in the setting of allograft dysfunction.[7] A presumptive diagnosis of BKVN can be made in the setting of greater than 2 weeks duration of BK replication (plasma PCR load >10,000 copies/mL) associated with a decline in renal function.[7]

Although noninvasive surveillance and diagnostic studies, such as BKV PCR, to monitor the presence or absence of BKV or the viral load in urine and blood and quantitative assays of urine cytology by light microscopy or electron microscopy offer convenient and sensitive alternatives and could minimize the need for kidney biopsy to establish diagnosis, renal biopsy is the gold standard for diagnosis of BKVN.[4] Renal biopsy is also important in the setting of renal dysfunction to rule out acute rejection.

The definitive diagnosis of BKVN is made by histology/pathology with characteristic cytopathic changes and positive immunohistochemistry test or in situ hybridization for BKV nucleic acids.[7] The immunohistochemistry testing uses antibodies directed against BK (VPI or agnoprotein) or against the cross-reacting simian virus 40 large T antigen.[7] A minimum of 2 biopsy cores, including the medulla, should be taken secondary to the focal nature of BKVN disease and sampling error; diagnosis, may be missed in one-third of biopsies. Histopathology reveals intranuclear basophilic viral inclusion without a surrounding halo; anisonucleosis, hyperchromasia, and chromatin clumping of infected cells; interstitial mononuclear or polymorphonuclear cell infiltrates in the areas of tubular damage; tubular injury with tubular cell apoptosis, cell dropout, desquamation, and flattened epithelial lining; and tubulitis with lymphocyte permeation of the tubular basement membrane.[36,37] Electron microscopy may show viral inclusions and tubular damage with tubular cell necrosis, prominent lysosomal inclusions, luminal protein, and cellular casts (**Fig. 1**).[36,37]

TREATMENT

Reduction in immunosuppressive therapy is the mainstay of treatment and adjunctive therapies may have limited or no value. Two strategies are generally used for BKVN. The first strategy involves reduction or modification in maintenance immunosuppression and the second entails adjunctive use of agents with antiviral activity, which

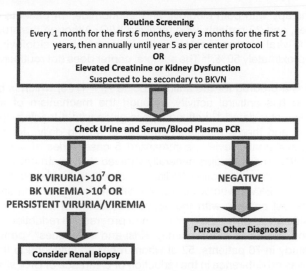

Fig. 1. Flow diagram for monitoring and diagnosis of BKVN.

includes the use of cidofovir, leflunomide, fluoroquinolones, and intravenous immuno-globulin (IVIG).[38,39]

The authors' center's approach is to initially reduce the antiproliferative agents, such as mycophenolate or azathioprine, by 50%, followed by a reduction in the calcineurin inhibitor by 25% to 50%. If a therapeutic response is not achieved, then the antiproliferative agent is discontinued.[7] Another potential strategy involves initially reducing the calcineurin inhibitor by 25% to 50%, followed by reducing the antiproliferative agent by 50%, followed by discontinuation of the antiproliferative agent, if needed. Typically, the discontinuation of the antiproliferative agents (usually mycophenolate or azathioprine) results in resolution of viremia in 95% of patients. Ginevri and colleagues[38] demonstrated that reduction of immunosuppression decreases the risk of BKVN. Preemptive reduction of immmunosuppression alone in the setting of BK viremia often prevents progression to BKVN. Weiss and colleagues[40] demonstrated that withdrawal of immunosuppression compared with reduction alone resulted in improved 1-year graft survival (87.8% vs 56.2%). Successful treatment of BKVN has been suggested to be the clearance of BKV viremia, increase in BKV-specific IgG antibody level, and stabilization of renal function.[20,41]

Goal trough levels for immunosuppressive agents are generally tacrolimus less than 6 ng/mL, cyclosporine less than 150 ng/mL, sirolimus less than 6 ng/mL, and mycophenolate mofetil daily dosing of less than or equal to 1000 mg.[7] In addition, serum creatinine should be monitored once or twice a week, serum BK PCR every 2 weeks, and allograft biopsy in 2 months.[7] Recovery may take from 4 to 8 weeks.

ADJUVANT THERAPY

Drug therapy for BKVN is limited. In patients who continue to have progressive dysfunction, despite reduced immunosuppression, anti-infective agents, such as fluoroquinolone antibiotics, IVIG in those with hypogammaglobulinemia, leflunomide, and cidofovir, may be used. Hilton and Tong[42] reviewed 44 reports describing the use of the 4 agents. There were 184 patients from 27 centers who received cidofovir, 189 patients from 18 centers who received leflunomide, 25 patients who received combination therapy with both cidofovir and leflunomide, 14 patients who received fluoroquinolones, and 29 patients who received IVIG. Although the studies were not comparable, the viral clearance rates were similar between cidofovir, leflunomide, and IVIG, at approximately 50%.[42] The authors' center does not routinely use adjuvant therapy.

Leflunomide is a prodrug for the antimetabolite A77 1726, which is both immunosuppressive and has antiviral activity although the mechanism of action against BKV has not been elucidated.[43] Leflunomide is given with a loading dose of 100 mg orally for 5 days and then a maintenance dose of 40 mg daily. Johnston and colleagues,[38] in a systematic review, summarized 5 case series of leflunomide in the treatment of BKVN. These studies generally showed that treatment with leflunomide stabilized or improved renal function. Williams and colleagues[44] described 17 patients with biopsy-proved BKVN who were treated with reduction of immunosuppression and leflunomide. All patients with the active metabolite of leflunomide (A77 1726) (blood levels >40 μg/mL) cleared the virus or had progressive reductions in the BK viral load in the blood and urine. More recently, Krisi and colleagues[45] performed a large retrospective study in 76 patients, 52 of whom received leflunomide therapy and 24 did not. There was no difference in the reduction or clearance of BKV viremia between the 2 groups. In addition, leflunomide use is limited because hemolysis, transaminitis, thrombotic microangiopathy, and pancytopenia may all occur.[42] More prospective studies need to be performed to determine if leflunomide should be part of the treatment strategy for BKVN.

Cidofovir is a nucleotide analog of cytosine and may have activity against BKV.[46] The utility of cidofovir is unclear because most case studies have concomitantly decreased immunosuppression while giving cidofovir. Cidofovir is usually used in doses from 0.25 mg/kg to 1.0 mg/kg at 1-week to 3-week intervals without probenecid. Johnston and colleagues[42] published a systematic review of all the treatment trials for BK. In their review of the literature, 1 cohort and 11 case series examined the use of cidofovir with immunosuppression for the management of BKV. The studies were mixed regarding clearance of BK viremia and BK viruria. The effect of cidofovir was also variable with some studies showing stabilization of creatinine whereas others found a lack of functional benefit. In addition, cidofovir is a nephrotoxic agent; however, significant nephrotoxicity was not observed at lower doses. Anterior uveitis secondary to cidofovir was surprisingly high and occurred in 12% to 35% of cases.[47] There is a need for randomized trials evaluating cidofovir for BKVN when reduction of immunosuppression does not resolve infection.

The underlying principle behind the use of IVIG therapy in BKVN is that human immunoglobulin preparations may contain anti-BKV antibodies and may potentially transfer protective immunity.[48] Immunoglobulin is given in doses ranging from 0.2 g/kg to 2.0 g/kg and is hypothesized to help with BKVN by supplying anti-BKV antibodies. Serner and colleagues[49] report on a case series of 8 patients with BKVN, with viral clearance of 50% with IVIG use. Other studies, such as that by Wadei and colleagues,[50] did not find that IVIG lead to viral clearance. Case reports have shown stabilization of renal function in the setting of BKVN, clearance of BK viremia, and resolution of BKVN in the pediatric renal transplant population.[50] IVIG was used, however, in the setting of reduced immunosuppression and sometimes other adjuvant agents. The disadvantages of IVIG are expense, aseptic meningitis, thrombotic events, bronchospasm, and nephrotoxicity from sucrose-containing formulas.[51]

Fluoroquinolones inhibit BK growth through the inhibition of DNA topoisomerase activity and simian virus 40 large T antigen helicase. Support for fluoroquinolone use has been from case studies in the hematopoietic stem cell transplant recipients. The fluoroquinolone data are from a single-center observational study in which ciprofloxacin was shown to decrease BK viral load.[52] In this study, 68 patients were randomized to receive ciprofloxacin or a cephalosporin antibiotics after allogeneic hematopoietic stem cell transplant to determine if ciprofloxacin could reduce the rate of BKV viruria and hemorrhagic cystitis. The BKV viruria was lower in the group that received ciprofloacin ($10^5 \times 10^9$), irrespective of corticosteroid use; however, the occurrence of severe hemorrhagic cystitis was not decreased.[52] Large prospective studies evaluating the use of fluoroquinolones in renal transplant recipients are needed before the use of fluoroquinolones can be recommended in this population for the prevention and treatment of BKV infections (**Fig. 2**).

PREVENTION

Current guidelines recommend screening all renal transplant patients with urine BKV PCR or cytology at predetermined intervals.[7,53,54] Renal transplant recipients should be screened for BKV for the first 5 years post-transplant. The authors' center routinely performs BKV screening monthly during the first 6 months post–kidney transplant. Guidelines suggest that screening for BKV using urine and plasma PCR assays should occur at least every 3 months during the first 2 years post–kidney transplant.[7] After that time, screening should be performed annually until year 5 post-transplant.[7] Additionally, BKV PCR testing in the urine and serum should be performed in any renal

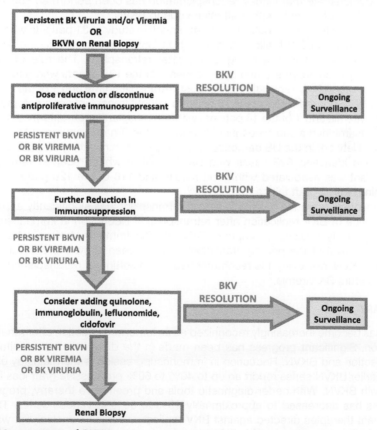

Fig. 2. Management of BKVN.

transplant recipient with a rising serum creatinine that cannot be explained by other causes, such as dehydration, rejection, or calcineurin inhibitor toxicity.

Although there is no prophylaxis other than reduction in immunosuppressive therapy after BK viruria, BK viremia, or BKVN, some recent studies have suggested a role for prophylactic use of fluoroquinolones in renal transplant recipients. Gabardi and colleagues[55] evaluated prophylactic fluoroquinolones for 25 renal transplant patients for the prevention of BK viremia and reported a significantly higher rate of BK viremia (22.5% vs 4%; $P = .03$) in patients who did not receive the 1-month ciprofloxacin or levofloxacin course. A similar study by Koukoulaki and colleagues,[56] however, did not find any benefit of prophylactic administration of ciprofloxacin on BKV replication in a prospective study of 32 renal transplant patients.[57] Wojciechowski and colleagues[58] retrospectively compared the impact of 30 days of ciprofloxacin prophylaxis in 236 kidney transplant recipients over a 12-month period and found a lower rate of BKV infection at 3 months but not at 12 months. At this time, the optimal duration and effectiveness of fluoroquinolones prophylaxis are uncertain.

RETRANSPLANTATION

It is estimated that 300 renal graft failures occur annually secondary to BKVN.[59] Consensus guidelines for retransplant after BKVN, in particular, the need for clearance of viremia and transplant nephrectomy, are lacking. Case series and retrospective reviews demonstrate that kidney retransplantation has been performed successfully in 80% to 90% of patients with graft failure due to BKVN.[7]

Geetha and colleagues[59] published a retrospective study of 31 patients who underwent retransplant for BKVN allograft loss, with 11 (35%) patients developing BK viruria and BK viremia and 2 developing BKVN after retransplant. The role of allograft nephrectomy is controversial and in this series 3 of the 13 patients who had allograft nephrectomy had BKV replication in the post-retransplant time and 1 of the 13 developed BKVN compared with 8 of the 18 patients without transplant nephrectomy developing BK viremia and 1 of the 18 patients without transplant nephrectomy developing BKVN.[59] Dharnidharka and colleagues[60] evaluated the Organ Procurement and Transplantation Network in the US database for kidney transplant with graft loss attributed to BKV and identified 823 cases with BKVN, 126 of which received retransplant. Retransplant was associated with good results and 118 of the 126 grafts were still functioning, with 1 graft failure from BKV.[60]

Documented clearance of viremia before retransplant was significantly associated with absence of BKV replication after retransplant.[59] Reduction in immunosuppression is generally advised to improve BKV-specific immunity before retransplant. Surgical removal of the primary transplant has not been shown to protect against recurrent BKVN; however, it is recommended in the setting of retransplantation with ongoing serum BK viremia.[7]

SUMMARY

BKVN has become increasingly recognized as an important infection after renal transplantation. Significant progress has been made in the diagnosis and monitoring of BKV infection and BKVN. Reduction in immunosuppression is the mainstay of treatment. Earlier BKVN series report an up to 40% to 60% progressive graft loss in renal grafts with BKVN. With better diagnostic tools and preemptive therapy, progressive graft loss has decreased to approximately 15% to 50% in various series. The role of adjuvant therapies directed against BKV replication remains unclear but warrants further study in larger controlled clinical trials.

REFERENCES

1. Hirsch HH, Brennan DC, Drachenberg BC, et al. Polymovavirus associated nephropathy in renal transplantation: interdisciplinary analyses and recommendations. Transplantation 2005;79:1277–86.
2. Gardner SD, Field AM, Coleman DV, et al. New human papovavirus (BK) isolated from urine after renal transplanation. Lancet 1971;1253–7.
3. Hirsch HH, Steiger J. Polyomavirus BK. Lancet Infect Dis 2003;3:611–23.
4. Bohl DB, Brennan DC. BK virus nephropathy and kidney transplant. Clin J Am Soc Nephrol 2007;2:S36–46.
5. Comoli P, Binggell S, Ginevri F, et al. Polyomavirus-associated nephropathy: update on BK virus-specific immunity. Transpl Infect Dis 2006;8:86–94.
6. Patel R. Infections in the recipients of kidney transplants. Infect Dis Clin North Am 2001;15(3):901–52.
7. Hirsch HH, Randhawa R, AST infectious diseases community of practice. BK virus in solid organ transplant recipients. Am J Transplant 2009;9:S136–46.
8. Thakur R, Arora S, Nada R, et al. Prospective monitoring of BK virus reactivation in renal transplant recipients in North India. Transpl Infect Dis 2011;13(6): 575–83.
9. Mitterhofer AP, Pietropaolo V, Barile M, et al. Meaning of early polyomavirus-BK replication post kidney transplant. Transplant Proc 2010;42:1142–5.
10. Kusne S, Vilchez RA, Zanwar P, et al. Polyomavirus JC urinary shedding in kidney and liver transplant recipients associated with reduced creatinine clearance. J Invest Dermatol 2012;206(6):875–80.
11. Bohl DL, Storch GA, Ryschkewitsch C, et al. Donor origin of BK virus in renal transplant and role of HLA C7 in susceptibility to sustained viremia. Am J Transplant 2005;5:2213–21.
12. Shah K. Human polyomavirus BKV and renal disease. Nephrol Dial Transplant 2000;15(6):754–5.
13. Ali AM, Gibson IW, Birk P, et al. Pretransplant serologic testing to identify the risk of polyoma BK viremia in pediatric kidney transplant recipients. Pediatr Transplant 2011;15(8):827–34.
14. Smith JM, Mcdonald RA, Finn LS, et al. Polyomavirus nephropathy in pediatric kidney transplant recipients. Am J Transplant 2004;4:2109–17.
15. Hariharan S. BK virus nephritis after renal transplant. Kidney Int 2006;69:655–62.
16. Comoli P, Azzi A, Maccario R, et al. Polyomavir BK specific immunity after kidney transplantation. Transplantation 2004;78:1229–32.
17. Abraham T, Dropulic LK, Rahman MH, et al. Ureteral stents: a novel risk factor for polyomavirus nephropathy. Transplantation 2007;84:433–6.
18. Hirsch HH, Knoweles W, Dickenmann M, et al. Prospective study of polyomavirus type BK, replication and nephropathy in renal transplant recipients. N Engl J Med 2002;347:488–96.
19. Babel N, Fendt J, Karaivano S, et al. Sustained BK viruria as an early marker for the development of BKV-associated nephropathy: analysis of 4128 urine and serum samples. Transplantation 2009;88:89–95.
20. Brennan DC, Agha I, Bohl E, et al. Incidence of BK with tacrolimus verus cyclosporine and impact of preemptive immunosuppression reduction. Am J Transplant 2005;5:582–94.
21. Hussain S, Orentas R, Walczak J, et al. Prevention of BKV nephritis by monitoring BK viremeia in renal transplant recipients. A prospective study. Graft 2004;7: 28–30.

22. O'Donnell PH, Swanson K, Josephson MA, et al. BK vivus infection is associated with hematuria and renal impairment in recipients of allogeneic hematopoetic stem cell transplants. Biol Blood Marrow Transplant 2009;15(9):1038–48.

23. Dropulic LK, Jones RJ. Polyomavirus BK infection in blood and marrow transplant recipients. Bone Marrow Transplant 2008;41(1):11–8.

24. Jiang M, Abend JR, Johnson SF, et al. The role of polyomavirus in human disease. Virology 2009;384(2):266–73.

25. Bratt G, Hamarin AL, Grandien M, et al. BK virus as the cause of meningoencephalitis retinitis and nephritis in a patient with AIDS. AIDS 1999;13:1071–5.

26. Basara N, Rasche FM, Schwalenberg T, et al. Hydronephrosis resulting from bilateral ureteral stenosis: a late complication of polyoma BK virus cystitis? J Transplant 2010;2010:1–6.

27. Hedquist BG, Bratt G, Hammarin AL, et al. Identification of BK virus in a patient with acquired immune deficiency syndrome and bilateral atypical retinitis. Ophthalmology 1999;106:129–32.

28. Pedrogiannis-Halotis T, Saloulas G, Kirby J, et al. BK-related polymomavirus vasculopathy in a renal transplant recipient. N Engl J Med 2001;345:1250–5.

29. Esposito L, Hirsh H, Basse G, et al. BK virus-related hemophagocytic syndrome in a renal transplant patient. Transplantation 2007;83(3):365.

30. Akazaw Y, Terada Y, Yamane T, et al. Fatal BK virus pneumonia following stem cell transplantation. Transpl Infect Dis 2012;14(6):E142–6.

31. Coleman DV, Mackenzie EF, Gardner SD. Human Polyomavirus (BK) infection and ureteric stenosis in renal allograft recipients. J Clin Pathol 1978;31(4):338–47.

32. Abend JR, Jiang M, Imperiale MJ. BK virus and human cancer: innocent until proven guilty. Semin Cancer Biol 2009;19(4):252–60.

33. Sundsfjord A, Rosenqvist H, Van Ghelue M, et al. BK and JC viruses in patients with systemic lupus erythematous: prevalent and persistent sequence stability of the viral regulatory regions and nondetectable viremia. J Infect Dis 1999;180(1): 1–9.

34. Galan A, Rauch CA, Otis CN. Fatal BK polyoma viral pneumonia associated with immunosuppression. Hum Pathol 2005;36(9):1031–4.

35. Rennert H, Jenkins SG, Azurin C, et al. Evaluation of BK virus viral load assay using the QIAGEN Artus BK virus RG PCR Test. J Clin Virol 2012;54(3):260–4.

36. Drachenberg CB, Hirsh HH, Ramos E, et al. Polyomavirus disease in renal transplantation: review of pathological findings and diagnostic methods. Hum Pathol 2005;36(12):1245–55.

37. Dranchenberg CB, Papdimitriou JC, Hirsch HH, et al. Histologic patterns of polymovavirus nephropathy: correlation with graft outcome and viral load. Am J Transplant 2004;4(12):2082–92.

38. Johnston O, Jaswal D, Gill JS, et al. Treatment of polyomavirus infection in kidney transplant recipients: a systematic review. Transplantation 2010;89(9):1057–70.

39. Ginevir F, Azzi H, Hirsch HH, et al. Prospective monitoring of polymoavirus BK replication and impact of preemptive intervention in pediatric kidney recipients. Am J Transplant 2007;7:2727–35.

40. Weiss AS, Gralla J, Chan L, et al. Aggressive immunosuppression minimization reduces graft loss following diagnosis of BK virus-associated nephropathy: a comparison of two reduction strategies. Clin J Am Soc Nephrol 2008;3:1812–9.

41. Hariharan S, Cohen EP, Vasudev B, et al. BKV specific antibodies and BKV DNA in renal transplant recipients with BKV nephritis. Am J Transplant 2005;5:2719–24.

42. Hilton R, Tong CY. Antiviral therapy for polymovavirus-associated nephropathy after renal transplant. J Antimicrob Chemother 2008;62:855–9.

43. Bernhoff E, Tylden GD, Kjerpeseth LJ, et al. Leflunoide inhibition of BK virus replication in renal tubular epithelial cells. J Virol 2010;84:2150–6.
44. Williams JW, Javaid B, Gillen D, et al. Leflunomide for polyomavirus type BK nephropathy. N Engl J Med 2005;352:1157–8.
45. Krisi JC, Taber DJ, Pilch N, et al. Leflunomide efficacy and pharmacodynamics for the treatment of BK viral infection. Clin J Am Soc Nephrol 2012;7(6):1003–9.
46. Lamoth F, Pascual M, Erard V, et al. Low-dose cidofovir for the treatment of polymovavirus-associated nephropathy: two case reports and review of the literature. Antivir Ther 2008;13:1001–9.
47. Lopez V, Solia E, Gutierrez C, et al. Anterior uveitis associated with treatment with intravenous cidofovir in kidney transplant patients with BK nephropathy. Transplant Proc 2006;38:2412–3.
48. Randhawa RS, Schonder K, Shapiro R, et al. Polyomavirus BK neutralizing activity in human immunoglobulin preparations. Transplantation 2010;89(12):1462–5.
49. Serner A, House AA, Jevnikar AM, et al. Intravenous immunoglobulin as a treatment for BK virus associated nephropathy. On year follow up of renal allograft recipients. Transplantation 2006;81:117.
50. Wadei HM, Rule AD, Lewin M, et al. Kidney transplant function and histological clearance of virus following diagnoses of plymoavirus associated nephropathy (PVAN). Am J Transplant 2006;6:1025.
51. Jordan SC, Toyoda M, Kahwaji J, et al. Clinical aspects of intravenous immunoglobulin use in solid organ transplant recipients. Am J Transplant 2011;11: 196–202.
52. Leung AY, Chan MT, Yuen KY, et al. Ciprofloxacin decreased polyoma BK virus load in patients who underwent allogeneic hematopoietic stem cell transplantation. Clin Infect Dis 2005;40:528–37.
53. Blanckaert K, De Vriese AS. Current recommendations for diagnosis and management of polyoma BK virus nephropathy in renal transplant recipients. Nephrol Dial Transplant 2006;21(12):3364–7.
54. Dall A, Hariharan S. BK virus nephritis after renal transplantation. Clin J Am Soc Nephrol 2008;3(Suppl 2):S68–75.
55. Gabardi S, Waikar S, Martin S, et al. Evaluation of fluoroquinolones for the prevention of BK viremia after renal transplant. Clin J Am Soc Nephrol 2010;5:1298–304.
56. Koukoulaki M, Apostolou T, Hadjiconstantinou V, et al. Impact of prophylactic administration of ciprofloxacin on BK polyoma virus replication. Transpl Infect Dis 2008;10:449–51.
57. Thamboo TP, Jeffery KJ, Friend PJ, et al. Urine cytology screening for polyoma virus infection following renal transplantation: the Oxford experience. J Clin Pathol 2007;60(8):927–30.
58. Wojciechowski D, Chanda R, Chandran S, et al. Ciprofloxacin prophylaxis in kidney transplant recipients reduces BK virus infection at 3 months but not at 1 Year. Transplantation 2012;94(11):1117–23.
59. Geetha D, Sozio SM, Ghanta M, et al. Results of repeat renal transplantation after graft loss from BK virus nephropathy. Transplantation 2011;92(7):781–6.
60. Dharnidharka VR, Cherikh WS, Neff R, et al. Retransplantation after BK virus nephropathy in prior kidney transplant: an OPTN database analysis. Am J Transplant 2010;10(5):1312–5.

Management of Recurrent Hepatitis C in Orthotopic Liver Transplant Recipients

Geeta S. Karnik, MD[a],*, Kirti Shetty, MD[b,c]

KEYWORDS

- Hepatitis C virus • Liver transplant • Recurrence • Immunosuppression
- Direct-acting antivirals

KEY POINTS

- End-stage liver disease and hepatocellular carcinoma (HCC) from chronic hepatitis C are the most common indications for orthotopic liver transplantation (OLT) and the incidence of both are projected to increase over the next decade.
- Recurrent hepatitis C virus (HCV) infection of the allograft is associated with an accelerated progression to cirrhosis, graft loss, and death.
- Multiple host, donor and viral factors are associated with rapid fibrosis progression.
- Treatment for HCV recurrence is challenging and produces sustained viral response (SVR) rates of approximately 30-50%.
- Timing of HCV treatment initiation, agents, and management are areas of ongoing study.

INTRODUCTION

Hepatitis C virus (HCV) is an enveloped, spherical positive-stranded RNA virus that is a member of the Flaviviridae family. Hepatitis C virus infection is a global health problem affecting 180 million people worldwide and has become the leading indication for orthotopic liver transplantation (OLT) in the United States. As of 2011, HCV accounts for 25% of all adult liver transplants performed in the United States and this percentage is expected to increase further.[1] The Centers for Disease Control and Prevention

Funding Sources: None.
Conflict of Interest: None.
[a] Department of Infectious Diseases, Georgetown University Hospital, 3800 Reservoir Road Northwest, 5PHC, Washington, DC 20007, USA; [b] Department of Surgery, Georgetown University Hospital, 3800 Reservoir Road Northwest, Washington, DC 20007, USA; [c] Transplant Hepatology, Georgetown Transplant Institute, Georgetown University Hospital, 3800 Reservoir Road Northwest, 2 Main, Washington, DC 20007, USA
* Corresponding author.
E-mail address: Geeta.S.Karnik@gunet.georgetown.edu

Infect Dis Clin N Am 27 (2013) 285–304
http://dx.doi.org/10.1016/j.idc.2013.02.003
0891-5520/13/$ – see front matter © 2013 Elsevier Inc. All rights reserved.

id.theclinics.com

has reported a marked birth cohort effect on HCV prevalence. Even though persons born during 1945 to 1965 comprise an estimated 27% of the population, they account for approximately three-fourths of all HCV infections in the United States and 73% of HCV-associated mortality.[2] According to a recent analysis of the Organ Procurement and Transplantation (OPTN) database, persons within that same birth cohort account for 81% of all new liver transplant registrants with HCV.[3] The maturation of the HCV-infected population and an anticipated increase in the rates of cirrhosis and hepatocellular carcinoma (HCC) is therefore one of the most significant challenges to confront the transplant community.

Although OLT is an effective treatment to reduce rates of morbidity and mortality in this population, recurrent HCV infection is an inevitable consequence in patients with a detectable viral load. HCV infection of the allograft occurs at the time of transplantation and may be associated with accelerated development of chronic liver disease and cirrhosis, leading to graft failure and loss. Forman and colleagues[4] in their analysis of the OPTN registry found the 5-year survival was only 64% among anti-HCV-positive recipients compared with 75% among anti-HCV-negative patients undergoing OLT and there was a significant increased risk of death and allograft failure (hazard ratio 1.23 and 1.30) among those HCV-positive recipients.

Antiviral therapy has been shown to modify the natural history of recurrent hepatitis C, but survival outcomes in the setting of HCV recurrence remain significantly compromised. Recent advances in the treatment of HCV, particularly the advent of direct-acting antiviral agents (DAA), now offer the promise of HCV eradication. However, the use of these agents in a transplant population awaits further elucidation of safety and efficacy. This review focuses on specific concerns within the OLT patient population and guidance on optimal management strategies.

NATURAL HISTORY OF HEPATITIS C RECURRENCE AFTER LIVER TRANSPLANTATION

The transplanted liver serves as a favorable target for the HCV. Individuals who are viremic at the time of transplantation experience universal recurrence of disease. The degree of histologic injury and natural history after infection remains variable.

Viral Kinetics of Hepatitis C Recurrence

A temporary decline in serum HCV RNA is observed in the anhepatic phase. Viral replication, however, resumes within a few hours and infection of the hepatic allograft occurs within 24 hours of reperfusion. Levels of HCV RNA have been shown to reach 1 to 2 logs higher than pretransplant levels at 3 months safter transplantation.[5] At the end of the first postoperative year, levels of HCV RNA are on average 10- to 20-fold higher than pretransplant levels.[6]

Histologic Findings of Hepatitis C Recurrence

The diagnosis of HCV recurrence is based on the presence of HCV RNA in serum combined with histologic changes, confirmed by liver biopsy. Recurrent HCV is characterized by hepatocellular damage, infiltration of inflammatory cells, and remodeling that leads to a more accelerated course of fibrosis progression than that seen in nontransplant patients. Human hepatocytes are thought to be the primary target cells supporting HCV replication in vivo. Acute hepatitis (biochemical and histologic) generally occurs in the first 3 to 4 months, before the establishment of chronic hepatitis and its sequela. Once reinfection is established, about 50% to 70% recipients eventually develop chronic liver disease.[7,8]

Cholestatic hepatitis C (CHC) is a rare variant of early recurrence and occurs in less than 10% of HCV-infected transplanted recipients. CHC is characterized by very high serum levels of HCV RNA ($\geq 10^6$ IU/mL) and evidence of pronounced cholestasis with levels of alkaline phosphatase and glutamyltransferase greater than 5 times the upper limits of normal. Pathognomonic histology includes ballooning of hepatocytes, varying degrees of bile duct proliferation, and areas of confluent necrosis. Graft failure in the setting of CHC occurs in 50% of patients within a few months of onset.[9,10]

Clinical Course of Hepatitis C Recurrence

Progression to cirrhosis occurs in 20% to 40% of OLT recipients with HCV recurrence within 5 years.[11] Once cirrhosis develops, patient survival decreases to 41% and 10% at 1 to 3 years, respectively. The first episode of decompensation may occur in less than 1 year. After 5 to 10 years allograft failure occurs in 10% of patients.[12] The development of decompensated cirrhosis and graft failure because of recurrent hepatitis C is now the most frequent cause of death and need for retransplantation in HCV-infected recipients.

RISK FACTORS ASSOCIATED WITH SEVERITY OF POSTTRANSPLANT HCV RECURRENCE

Given the variable natural history of recurrent hepatitis C, defining risk factors for severity of progression remains an important area of research. Several studies have sought to identify factors impacting the severity and timing of HCV recurrence (**Table 1**). Several variables have been associated with progressive HCV recurrence

Table 1
Factors associated with the risk of HCV recurrence and disease progression following liver transplantation

Variable	Risk of Recurrent Hepatitis C and Disease Progression	Reference
Donor factors		
Donor age ≥65	Increased	13–17
Prolonged ischemia	Increased	18
Host factors		
Recipient age ≥50	Increased	24
HCV viral load ≥1 million IU/mL	Increased	19–22
Race/gender	Uncertain	23,25–27
HIV coinfection	Increased	30–36
CMV coinfection	Increased	23,28,29
DM/metabolic syndrome	Increased	38,39
IL28B polymorphism (CT or TT genotype)	Increased	72,73,103–105
Immunosuppression		
Steroids (high doses or bolus or fast taper)	Increased	40–45
Cyclosporine vs tacrolimus	Uncertain	46–58
MMF and T-cell depleting agents	Increased severity of disease with OKT3 and Campath; MMF equivocal	59–63
Sirolimus	Decreased (preliminary analysis)	63–66

Abbreviations: CMV, cytomegalovirus; DM, diabetes mellitus; HCV, hepatitis C; HIV, human immunodeficiency virus; MMF, mycophenolate mofetil.

and reduced survival. Outcome is impacted by factors related to the donor, surgery, host, environment, and level of immunosuppression.

Donor-related and Surgical Predictors of Recurrence

Increasing age of the donor has been independently associated with disease progression.[13,14] Accelerated damage is speculated to be due to increased telomere shortening and fibrogenesis associated with mature donor livers. Older donor age has also been shown to impact the success of posttransplantation antiviral therapy.[15–17] However, in an era marked by a shortage of donor organs and increasing donor age, the decision to use older livers is ultimately dependent on the transplant center, severity of recipient liver disease, and wait times. Prolonged cold and warm ischemia times have also been identified as risk factors for early recurrence because of posttransplant preservation injury.[18]

Host-related Predictors of Recurrence

Multiple host-related factors have been suggested as predictors of severe recurrence of HCV in those undergoing OLT for HCV. Pretransplant viral titers have been associated with poor patient and graft survival.[19] Other studies have demonstrated a lack of correlation between posttransplant viral titers and histologic severity of disease.[20,21] Similarly, HCV genotype and quasi-species have been shown to have a variable effect on recurrence.[22] The interplay between viral kinetics and patient genetic factors warrants further investigation to understand factors better that determine disease and patient outcomes.

Recipient factors including age greater than 50 years, male gender, and donor-recipient mismatch (white donors to black recipients) are also reported to be associated with a higher risk of developing severe recurrence of HCV and impaired outcomes.[23–27] Particular areas of interest in the literature surround the impact of coinfection with cytomegalovirus (CMV) and human immunodeficiency virus (HIV) as well as the presence of metabolic syndrome.

Impact of CMV coinfection

CMV infection is common following liver transplantation, occurring in approximately one-quarter of HCV-infected liver transplant recipients.[23] Reported implications of postoperative infection with CMV on HCV recurrence have varied. However, most studies have demonstrated an association of CMV disease with a more severe recurrence of HCV.[28] Bosch and colleagues[29] recently published data from a large retrospective cohort (N = 347), which looked at this question and demonstrated an independent association between the development of CMV infection within the first year of transplantation and increased risk of severe recurrence of hepatitis C. CMV coinfection seems to be an independent risk factor for graft failure.

Impact of HIV coinfection

Persons coinfected with HIV and HCV represent a unique patient population both before and following liver transplantation. The advent of highly active antiretroviral therapy has increased the overall survival of coinfected HIV/HCV individuals. Nevertheless, natural history studies of coinfected individuals have demonstrated that an accelerated rate of hepatic fibrosis progression and liver disease is currently the leading cause of death in this population.[30] Consequently, OLT is becoming an increasingly necessary treatment option. Studies do suggest that although liver transplantation in coinfected HIV/HCV patients is safe, rates of survival are lower than in HCV monoinfected individuals.[31–34] Several studies have indicated that these coinfected individuals experience an earlier and more severe recurrence of HCV.

Duclos-Vallee and colleagues[35] observed a high level of viral replication along with early histologic features of acute hepatitis and rapid progression of liver fibrosis.

Miro and colleagues[36] in a prospective multicenter study conducted in Spain demonstrated in 84 coinfected HCV/HIV liver recipients a significantly lower 5-year post-OLT rate of survival than monoinfected individuals (54% vs 71%, respectively, $P = .008$). Most recently Terrault and colleagues[37] published outcome data from the Solid Organ Transplantation in HIV multicenter US cohort study comparing patient and graft survival in HCV/HIV coinfected patients to outcomes in monoinfected individuals. The 3-year rates of patient and graft survival were 60% (47%–71%) and 53% (40%–64%), respectively, for coinfected HIV/HCV patients and 79% (72%–84%) and 74% (66%–79%) for HCV-infected recipients ($P<.001$). In addition, the 3-year incidence of treated acute rejection was found to be 1.6-fold higher for the coinfected HCV/HIV patients versus the monoinfected HCV/HIV patients. Interestingly, the cumulative rates of HCV recurrence did not differ between the 2 groups. Cholestatic HCV was not found to be more common in the coinfected group.

Impact of diabetes mellitus and metabolic syndrome

Hepatitis C in both the transplant and the nontransplant setting seems to have a reciprocal effect associated with insulin resistance (IR): not only is HCV infection linked with onset or exacerbation of IR, but IR may also contribute to rates of morbidity and mortality associated with an HCV infection. A meta-analysis of 7 retrospective studies including 1889 liver transplant recipients revealed that HCV-positive recipients had a significantly higher rate of new-onset posttransplant diabetes mellitus (DM) than HCV-negative recipients (54% vs 38%; odds ratio 2.5).[38] Similarly, as in the nontransplant HCV setting, IR and DM are risk factors for fibrosis progression in HCV-positive liver transplant recipients. A study in 160 HCV-positive liver transplant recipients found that those with IR were twice as likely to develop fibrosis stage ≥ 3 at 5 years posttransplant as those with normal insulin sensitivity (43% vs 21%; $P = .016$).[39] Early recognition, prevention, and treatment of posttransplant obesity and diabetes may impact long-term posttransplant survival.

Immunosuppression Regimens—Impact on Viremia and Recurrence

The management of liver transplantation in patients with HCV is complicated by the need to balance immunosuppression to prevent rejection, while allowing for adequate immune control of HCV replication. Whether specific immunosuppression regimens differentially affect HCV recurrence remains an area of ongoing study.

Steroids

Several studies have confirmed an association between steroid bolus therapies for acute rejection episodes and the development of severe recurrence of hepatitis C.[40–42] In particular, pulse intravenous steroids for acute cellular rejection is associated with 1 to 2 log increases in level of HCV RNA and accelerated progression of recurrent HCV. Although several studies have been conducted analyzing the effects of absolute steroid-free protocols, there seems to be no clinical advantage or impact on recurrence.[43] However, a slow rather than a rapid taper is preferred in general practice.[44] Vivarelli and colleagues[45] performed a randomized trial of rapid versus slow steroid tapering in conjunction with tacrolimus. The rates of histologic recurrence at 1-year follow-up were significantly higher in the rapid tapering group.

Calcineurin inhibitors

Two calcineurin inhibitors tacrolimus (TAC) and cyclosporine (CSA) are currently approved for immunosuppression after liver transplantation and form the backbone of most regimens. The optimal immunosuppression agent remains a topic of ongoing controversy.[46]

In theory, CSA may be a more attractive agent in the setting of HCV for several reasons. Cyclophilin A, the target of CSA, also serves the hepatitis C virus as an essential host factor for viral replication. CSA has been shown to suppress HCV RNA replication in vitro.[47,48] However, in vivo trials of CSA did not demonstrate suppression of HCV viremia in patients after liver transplantation.[49] CSA has also been shown to impact the efficacy of antiviral therapy for recurrent HCV with those patients maintained on CSA more likely to achieve a sustained virologic response (SVR) than those on TAC.[50] TAC, on the other hand, has been shown to interfere with interferon (IFN) signaling and thus reduce the antiviral activity of IFN in vitro.[51] However, a recent study examining the effect of both TAC and CSA in a replicon model of HCV did not find evidence of either TAC or CSA interfering with IFN-mediated inhibition of HCV replication and virion production in vitro.[52]

Most retrospective studies comparing the use of TAC and CSA showed no difference in disease severity of HCV recurrence.[53–55] Two large prospective studies have examined this issue in the clinical setting. Levy and colleagues,[56] in a 12-month follo–up analysis of data from a multicenter prospective, randomized trial, reported a higher rate of mortality and graft loss in patients who had received TAC compared with CSA, but with similar rates of histologic HCV recurrence in both groups. Berenguer and colleagues[53] also published a prospective study in 2010 comparing protocol liver biopsies and found no difference in severe recurrent HCV or overall survival in those receiving CSA compared with those receiving TAC. Final results are awaited from the REFINE (Randomized Evaluation of Fibrosis due to Hepatitis C after De Novo Liver Transplant) study, a multicenter randomized comparison of CSA and TAC in 450 HCV-positive liver transplant recipients, whereby the primary outcome was rate of fibrosis stage ≥ 2 at 1-year posttransplant. At this point, several prospective and retrospective studies, along with experimental models, do not provide either mechanistic or clinical evidence to support the use of one calcineurin inhibitor versus the other in the management of HCV infected OLT recipients.[57,58]

Mycophenolate mofetil and T-cell depleting therapies

There are limited data on the impact of azathioprine, mycophenolate mofetil (MMF), and T-cell-depleting agents on hepatitis C recurrence. Although small studies have suggested a slightly higher risk of HCV recurrence associated with MMF, the overall impact of MMF seems to be neutral or beneficial.[59–61] On the other hand, OKT3 is a murine monoclonal antibody of the immunoglobulin IgG2a isotype and administration seems to be a significant risk factor for the rapidity and severity of histologic recurrence of HCV.[62] The lymphoablative agent Alemtuzumab has also been shown to exacerbate HCV recurrence. Data on the impact of Thymoglobulin on HCV recurrence are lacking, but this agent should probably be used with great caution in this setting.[63]

Sirolimus

Sirolimus is an immunosuppressant from the class termed mammalian target of rapamycin (mTOR) inhibitors, which inhibit the mTOR signal transduction pathway and prevent IL-2 stimulation of T lymphocytes. In addition to its regulation of the cell cycle, mTOR affects several different cellular processes that impact fibrogenesis by hepatic stellate cells. Two different animal models have demonstrated that sirolimus slows disease progression to advanced liver fibrosis and will prolong survival in a setting of cirrhosis.[64–66]

Based on the theoretical benefits of sirolimus as an anti-fibrotic agent, McKenna and colleagues[67] compared the rate of fibrosis progression in HCV patients maintained on sirolimus versus calcineurin-based immunosuppressant regimens. Multivariate analysis demonstrated sirolimus as an independent predictor of minimal fibrosis at 1 and 2 years. This comparison is the first study among liver transplant recipients with HCV to describe the positive impact of sirolimus in respect to reduced fibrosis and rate of progression. Further evaluation in the setting of a randomized controlled trial is merited.

Our understanding of the impact of immunosuppression on HCV recurrence continues to evolve and many experts speculate timing of immunosuppression might be more important than the specific regimen. Furthermore, in the era of the new direct-acting antiviral agents against HCV, the choice of immunosuppressant will be affected not only by these considerations but also by potential drug interactions.

ASSESSING THE RATE OF PROGRESSION OF RECURRENT HEPATITIS C

Progression of fibrosis following HCV recurrence after liver transplantation strongly determines a patient's prognosis. It is important to identify patients who are at increased risk for disease recurrence and fibrosis early in their course.

Serum Biomarkers

Several serum fibrosis markers have been described for the early prediction of HCV disease recurrence. Carrion and colleagues[68] found that a composite score of 3 markers (hyaluronic acid, amino-terminal pro-peptide of type II procollagenase, and tissue inhibitor of matrix metalloproteinase type 1) was helpful in discriminating between mild and progressive HCV recurrence. Other useful markers have included serum chemokine CXC ligand 10 (CXXL10) and YKL-40, also known as human cartilage glycoprotein.[69,70] The clinical utility of these markers is hindered by the observation that serum biomarkers may be affected by concurrent illness.

Genetic Biomarkers

Genetic markers may be a more robust marker of disease. do O and colleagues recently published their experience with a genetic risk score comprising allele variants in 7 genes. This cirrhosis risk score (CRS) has been shown to predict severe fibrosis in HCV-infected individuals within a nontransplant setting and has been validated in another study. do O and colleagues[71] demonstrated that in their population of 137 post-OLT HCV patients, the odds ratio for severe fibrosis at 1 year was 4.7 for patients with a high CRS versus patients with a low CRS. This effect was independent of other known clinical risk factors.

Gene polymorphisms in the interleukin 28B (IL28B) gene predict the treatment response of recurrent HCV to IFN therapy (see later section entitled *Role of IL28B gene in Recurrent Hepatitis C Virus Infection*). There are conflicting reports about the correlation of these polymorphisms with fibrosis progression. Charlton and colleagues[72] showed that at 1 year of transplantation 32% of patients with the IL28B CC genotype had a fibrosis stage of 2 or higher, compared with 12% with IL28CC genotype ($P = .024$). Eurich and colleagues,[73] on the other hand, demonstrated an association between graft inflammation and outcomes of therapy related to IL28B, but no definite correlation with fibrosis.

Histologic Fibrosis Assessment

Liver biopsy with trichrome staining is considered to be the gold standard for monitoring disease progression. The natural history of histologic progression of fibrosis has been described by several groups that perform protocol biopsies. Linear fibrosis progression rates of 0.8 fibrosis stage units per year have been described by one group,[74] whereas other researchers have described a nonlinear fibrosis progression, with mean fibrosis scores of 1.2 at 1 year and 1.7 at 2 years following OLT.[7]

The first 6 months following OLT are important determinants of long-term outcome. The presence of significant necroinflammatory changes seen on biopsy during the acute hepatitis phase is associated with worse outcomes. Posttransplant surveillance and protocol biopsies are now widely accepted at most transplant centers as an effective means of assessing disease status and progression. At the authors' centers and others, patients transplanted for hepatitis C undergo protocol liver biopsies annually, or more often if dictated by clinical indicators. However, liver biopsy is an invasive procedure and can be affected by sampling errors. The addition of the hepatic venous pressure gradient can improve diagnostic accuracy. Blasco and colleagues[75] demonstrated that the presence of portal hypertension with a hepatic venous pressure gradient greater than 6 mm Hg 1 year after OLT identified 12 (80%) of the 15 patients with severe HCV recurrence, whereas only 9 (60%) had significant fibrosis on biopsy specimen testing.

Therefore, multiple studies have also investigated the utility of noninvasive testing such as ultrasound transient elastography or magnetic resonance elastography.[76–79] Both are promising alternatives to liver biopsy for the detection of hepatic fibrosis and liver stiffness caused by recurrent HCV after OLT. Until further studies validate these methods, the use of noninvasive tools to assess liver fibrosis is used as an adjunct to liver biopsy. It is important to identify progression of post-OLT HCV promptly because initiation of antiviral therapy may be beneficial in preventing graft loss.

APPROACHES TO ANTIVIRAL THERAPY IN RECURRENT HCV INFECTION

Treatment of established HCV recurrence is based on available treatment modalities for treating HCV in the nontransplant setting. In 2011, the standard of care for patients infected with HCV genotype 1 became a combination of an oral HCV NS3/4A serine protease inhibitor, boceprevir (BOC) or telaprevir (TVR), along with pegylated interferon (PEG-IFN) and oral ribavirin (RBV). Evolving treatment strategies for post-OLT HCV include these direct-acting antiviral agents, but much of the published data focuses on the use of PEG-IFN and RBV. The main goal of antiviral treatment is the permanent eradication of HCV and achievement of an SVR, but therapy can also provide stabilization of disease progression and prevention of graft loss. Published reports on antiviral therapy are difficult to compare directly given varying definitions of recurrence, choice of antiviral agents, and study endpoints. In general, the following approaches to antiviral therapy have been described (**Fig. 1**).

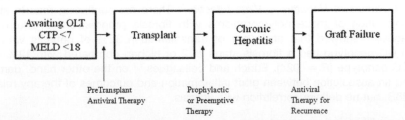

Fig. 1. Potential time points for therapeutic intervention to prevent or eradicate hepatitis C virus infection or slow disease progression. CTP, Child-Turcotte-Pugh score; OLT, orthotopic liver transplantation; MELD, model end stage liver disease.

Pretransplant Antiviral Therapy

Achievement of SVR before OLT in patients with HCV can prevent posttransplant recurrence of HCV in selected patients.[80] However, treatment in patients with advanced liver disease with PEG-IFN and RBV yields relatively low rates of SVR (11%–13%).[81] Furthermore, treatment is often poorly tolerated and associated with serious adverse effects. The International Liver Transplant Society consensus panel concluded that treatment should be limited to cirrhotic patients with Child-Turcotte-Pugh score of less than 7 or model end-stage liver disease score less than 18 and is contraindicated when Child-Turcotte-Pugh score is greater than 11 or model end-stage liver disease score is greater than 25.[7]

Preemptive Antiviral Therapy

Preemptive therapy refers to the initiation of therapy in the early posttransplant period when HCV viral loads are lower than pretransplant levels, and histologic disease is absent or minimal. Even though there is a theoretical advantage to such an approach, there is limited clinical feasibility and utility. Preemptive studies have shown an SVR ranging from 13% to 35%.[82] In May of 2011 Bzowej and colleagues[83] published data from the PHOENIX trial—the largest randomized controlled trial investigating the efficacy of "prophylactic antiviral" therapy following OLT. This trial was designed to examine the efficacy and safety of an escalating-dose regimen of PEG-IFN alfa-2a and RBV in patients treated before significant histologic recurrence, within 26 weeks of OLT, in comparison to an observational cohort. SVR was achieved by 12 of 54 treated patients (22.2%) and by 3 of 14 observation patients who later switched to treatment (21.4%). This study was disappointing to advocates of prophylactic therapy because, on an intent-to-treat basis, significant HCV recurrence at 120 weeks was similar in the prophylaxis (61.8%) and observation arms (65.0%, $P = .725$).

Limitations to initiating antiviral therapy immediately posttransplant include significant anemia, fluctuating renal function, and physical or neurologic limitations. High rates of discontinuation are noted due to drug interactions, pancytopenia, and intercurrent illness. Overall, it is not clear as to whether preemptive therapy for recurrent HCV offers improved outcomes and this approach awaits further study.

Treatment for Established Recurrent HCV Disease

In accordance with the 2003 International Liver Transplantation Society the standard approach for established recurrent hepatitis C in post-OLT patients has been to start combined PEG-IFN and RBV for grade III-IV inflammation or stage II fibrosis.[7] Multiple studies in the past decade have investigated the efficacy and safety of PEG-IFN and RBV to treat recurrent HCV. Results of antiviral therapy for established recurrence have been disappointing with rates of SVR that are significantly lower than in nontransplant populations. Potential explanations for this include higher HCV viral load following liver transplantation, higher frequency of genotype 1 patients, and inability to tolerate full-dose therapy. Baseline variables associated with SVR in OLT recipients are similar to that in the nontransplant patient population. Mild fibrosis, young age, low baseline level of viremia, HCV genotypes 2 and 3, and donor/recipient IL28B CC polymorphisms are associated with higher rates of SVR (**Box 1**).

Many studies evaluating IFN-based therapies are uncontrolled, use variable doses and duration of therapy, and are of a sample size too limited to perform multivariate analyses to identify predictors of response. In 2008 Berenguer[84] published a systematic review that included 19 studies and more than 600 patients with established recurrent hepatitis C after OLT treated with PEG-IFN and RBV. Their analysis revealed

> **Box 1**
> **Pretreatment variable associated with higher rates of sustained viral clearance in treatment of established recurrent HCV disease following orthotopic liver transplantation**
>
> - Genotype 2 or 3
> - Baseline HCV viral load <1 million IU/mL
> - Fibrosis stage ≤2
> - Donor age ≤60
> - IL28B CC polymorphism
> - No evidence of insulin resistance/DM
> - Adherence to therapy
> - Longer duration of therapy
> - Rapid virologic response
> - Early virologic response

a pooled SVR of 30% (range 8%–50%). The rate of discontinuation was 27% and 73% of the patients required dose reductions in therapy secondary to anemia.

Recent controlled and randomized trials using PEG-IFN/RBV in the treatment of HCV recurrence treatment are summarized in **Table 2**.[85–94] The dose of IFN used in these studies ranged from 1.5 to 5 MU 3 times weekly. Doses of RBV ranged from 400 to 1200 mg daily. Tolerance was variable among the studies. As expected, the development of severe side effects was the principal limiting factor. Anemia, leucopenia, and thrombocytopenia were the most common reasons cited for treatment discontinuation and dose reduction. Many of the researchers speculated that dose reductions and discontinuations likely contributed to the lower response rates observed.

The optimal duration of treatment of recurrent HCV disease is unknown. Duration of therapy in the studies highlighted in **Table 2** ranged from 48 to 52 weeks. Longer treatment durations are thought to enhance probability of achieving SVR, yet it is not always clinically feasible in the setting of limitations such as those previously described.[95] Growth factors to manage cytopenias and maintain optimal doses of antiviral therapy have been shown to be important in maximizing response to therapy.

Another area of concern regarding therapy for HCV recurrence is whether IFN therapy serves as a major risk factor for rejection. Berenguer and colleagues' systematic review revealed minimal acute or chronic rejection episodes less than 5%. Although doubts remain regarding the true risk of rejection during therapy for hepatitis C recurrence, low rates of rejection have been consistently reported (see **Table 2**).

Although rates of virologic response after therapy for recurrent HCV in OLT remain low, achievement of SVR in these patients remains a goal and is associated with improved graft[89,96] and overall patient survival.[97] Even in the absence of complete SVR, the histologic benefits of undergoing antiviral therapy have been shown. Ikegami and colleagues[98] demonstrated that, despite full virologic response, activity grade and fibrosis stage had significantly improved in patients who received IFN plus RBV. It is well recognized that antiviral therapy is important in improving outcomes following OLT for HCV recurrence.

Table 2
Summary of recent data regarding treatment of established recurrent HCV with combination Pegylated interferon and ribavirin therapy 2003–2012 (controlled trials only)

Author, Year	Study Design	Treatment Arm (N)	PEG-IFN Dose	RBV Dose (mg/d)	Duration (wk)	SVR in Tx Arm (%)	RBV Dose Reduction (%)	EPO use (%)	Rejection (N)	Discontinue (%)
Samuel et al,[85] 2003	RCT	28	2b: 1.5–3 µg/kg/wk	800–1200	48	6 (21)	7 (25)	NA	0	12 (43)
Castells et al,[86] 2005	CT	24	2b: 1.5 µg/kg/wk	400–800	48	8 (35)	14 (58)	14 (58)	1	0
Angelico et al,[87] 2007	RCT	21	2a: 90–180 mcg/kg/wk	200–800 (dose-escalating)	52	7 (33)	8 (33)	NA	1	7 (33)
Carrion et al,[88] 2007	RCT	54	2b: 1.5 µg/kg/wk	400–1200	48	18 (33)	36 (66)	46 (85)	4	21 (39)
Picciotto et al,[89] 2007	CT	61	2b: 1.0 µg/kg/wk	600–800	24–48	17 (28)	48 (79)	NA	1	9 (15)
Lodato et al,[90] 2008	CT	53	2b: 1.0 µg/kg/wk	800–1000	52	58 (44)	NA	24 (35)	0	12 (23)
Hashemi et al,[91] 2011	CT	30	2A: 90–180 mcg/kg/wk	800–1500 (dose-escalating)	48	18 (60)	16 (53)	23 (77)	2	11 (37)
Perrakis et al,[92] 2011	CT	16	2b: 0.8–1.6 µg/kg/wk	800–1200	60	4 (25)	2 (12)	4 (25)	0	4 (25)
Belli et al,[93] 2012	RCT	73	2b: 0.5–1.5 µg/kg/wk	400–1200	52	15 (41)	6 (17)	26 (36)	3	13 (36)
Gordon et al,[94] 2012	CT	125	2b: 1.5 µg/kg/wk	400–1200 (dose-escalating)	48	36 (29)	69 (55)	25 (20)	4	38 (30)

Abbreviations: EPO, erythropoietin; HCV, hepatitis C virus; PEF-IFN, pegylated interferon; RBV, ribavirin; SVR, sustained viral response; Tx, treatment.

ROLE OF IL28B GENE IN RECURRENT HCV INFECTION

The IL28B gene encodes for IFN-λ3. In chronic hepatitis C, single-nucleotide polymorphisms of chromosome 19, in the region of the IL28B gene, are strongly associated with the probability of achieving SVR with IFN therapy.[99] In particular, genotype 1–infected HCV infected patients carrying the favorable CC genotype at rs12979860 have an approximately twofold increase in SVR to PEG-IFN and RBV, compared with those with the less favorable CT or TT genotypes.[100]

Understanding the role of IL28B gene in OLT recipients is an evolving area of study. Recipient and donor liver IL28B genotype have been shown to be strongly and independently associated with IFN-based treatment response in patients after OLT and to determine outcomes.[72,101,102] It is speculated that optimal graft/recipient matching depending on IL28 alleles may be a strategy to improve antiviral therapy sensitivity and rates of SVR. However, at this point prospective studies evaluating IL28B genotype and SVR in the context of DAA-containing regimens are currently awaited.

NEW TREATMENT OPTIONS IN THE ERA OF DIRECT-ACTING ANTIVIRALS AND PROTEASE INHIBITORS

The science behind hepatitis C drug development is continuing to move forward rapidly. Recent advancement in HCV treatment is focused on developing therapeutic agents that target multiple stages of the HCV lifecycle to inhibit viral replication directly. In 2011 with the Federal Drug Administration approval of 2 new landmark agents, the oral HCV NS3/4A serine protease inhibitors BOC and TVR, the standard of care for patients with HCV genotype 1 infection has become a combination of one of these DAAs along with PEG-IFN and RBV. The development of DAAs has increased the rate of SVR from approximately 40% to 70% among nontransplanted patients with HCV genotype 1.[103,104]

Challenges to combined treatment strategies for HCV following liver transplantation include not only the large pill burden and overlapping toxicities but also the complexity of drug interactions. Protease inhibitors are substrates of the CYP3A4 system, as are the calcineurin inhibitors. Both BOC and TVR interact with the cytochrome P450, family 3, subfamily A (CYP3A) as both inhibitors and substrates. TVR increases TAC blood levels by approximately 70-fold.[105]

Clinical trials are underway to determine safety and efficacy of DAA in conjunction with PEG-IFN and RBV for hepatitis C in patients awaiting and having undergone liver transplantation. Currently, the Georgetown Transplant Institute, in conjunction with another transplant center, is treating a cohort of patients with HCV cirrhosis listed for transplantation with triple therapy comprising PEG-IFN, RBV, and a DAA following a strict treatment protocol. The authors' preliminary results in 32 patients have shown promise, with 90% and 70% of individuals completing 4 and 12 weeks of therapy, respectively. At week 12, 71% of patients had an undetectable viral load. However, early discontinuation was necessary in 25% of patients, and 10% of patients had serious adverse events, including hepatic decompensation and need for expedited liver transplantation.[106] The authors therefore urge caution with such an approach, and further study is warranted in carefully controlled settings.

Preliminary data on triple therapy with BOC or TVR in combination with PEG-IFN and RBV have also shown improved on-treatment virologic responses in patients with genotype 1 severe hepatitis C recurrence after liver transplantation. At the 2012 European Association for the Study of the Liver, Coilly and colleagues[107] presented preliminary data from their multicenter experience studying the efficacy and safety of protease inhibitors for severe HCV recurrence after liver transplantation.

At the 8-week mark, triple therapy with either BOC or TVR produced rates of virologic response of 56% and 70%, respectively.

Werner and colleagues[108] recently published their experience with treatment of recurrent HCV using triple therapy (PEG-IFN/RBV/TVR). In a 12-week intention-to-treat analysis, 8 of the 9 patients were found to be HCV RNA negative. This interim efficacy data are promising and will require further validation in larger populations.

As anticipated, studies using DAAs in conjunction with PEG-IFN and RBV in the setting of liver transplantation found anemia to be the most frequent adverse event. Coilley and colleagues[107] noted that erythropoietin treatment was required in 93% of patients. Also, concerns regarding viral breakthrough, emergence of viral resistance, and the effects of multiple drug interactions remain to be resolved.

Currently, more than 100 new HCV inhibitors are under preclinical and clinical investigation. These agents have demonstrated promising antiviral efficacy in transplant patients. It is hoped that the most promising of these will eventually become part of the authors' therapeutic armamentarium against this virus and may then be deployed within the challenging arena of the posttransplant patient with HCV recurrence.

RETRANSPLANTATION FOR RECURRENT HCV

In the United States, retransplantations account for 10% of all OLTs, with recurrent HCV infection comprising approximately 30% of retransplant volumes.[1] In general, retransplantation accrues greater cost and 20% reduction in survival, but it is not clear whether HCV-positive patients suffer significantly worse outcomes. McCashland and colleagues[109] in their multicenter US study compared the following 3 groups: (1) HCV-infected retransplant recipients, (2) non-HCV-infected retransplant recipients, and (3) HCV-infected transplant recipients with recurrence, managed without retransplant. Survivals were similar in both retransplant groups (1 year 69% in the HCV vs 73% in the non-HCV group and at 3 year 49% vs 55%, respectively). The group that did not undergo retransplantation had a significantly lower 3-year survival (47%). Even though this study suggests that retransplantation for HCV may be a reasonable option, it is important to keep in mind that the patients selected for this option were carefully screened to optimize outcomes. Predictors of poor outcome after retransplantation include recipient age over 50 years, creatinine greater than 2.0 mg/dL, serum bilirubin greater than 10 mg/dL, and comorbidities.[110,111]

In summary, retransplantation remains a controversial issue and limited data are available to assess the impact of HCV recurrence in a subsequent allograft. Most transplant programs, including ours, use a selective case-by-case approach in limiting this option to patients with favorable clinical characteristics.

SUMMARY

Hepatitis C recurrence continues to be a major challenge in liver transplantation. Reinfection of the allograft by HCV is almost universal with at least 25% patients progressing to liver cirrhosis within 5 to 10 years. Once cirrhosis is established, transplanted patients demonstrate an accelerated natural history with complications, including increased incidence of graft loss and mortality. Allograft failure secondary to HCV recurrence accounts for two-thirds of graft failures. OLT recipients with HCV have a reduced 5-year graft and rates of patient survival in comparison with HCV-negative recipients.

With a growing demand for OLT and an increasing shortage of organs, there is a need to improve strategies for managing HCV recurrence after OLT. Although there is no consensus on the ideal diagnostic or therapeutic strategy for this challenging group of patients, the principles of management include optimal donor selection, early identification of HCV recurrence, diligent and aggressive use of antiviral therapy, and close attention to immunosuppression management. Viral eradication is now increasingly a feasible option with the advent of DAAs and may offer these patients a chance at improved graft and overall survival. It is hoped that future research studies will optimize strategies further for the prevention and treatment of HCV in a transplant population.

REFERENCES

1. Organ Procurement and Transplantation Network (OPTN) and Scientific Registry of Transplant Recipients (SRTR). OPTN/SRTR 2010 Annual data report. Department of Health and Human Services, Health Resources and Services Administration, Healthcare Systems Bureau, Division of Transplantation; 2011. Available at: http://optn.transplant.hrsa.gov/data/annualreport.asp. Accessed October 6, 2012.
2. Smith B, Morgan R, Beckett G, et al. Recommendations for the identification of chronic hepatitis C virus infection among persons born during 1945-1965. MMWR Recomm Rep 2012;61:1–32.
3. Biggins S, Bambha K, Terrault N, et al. Projected future increase in aging HCV-infected liver transplant candidates: a potential effect of HCC. Liver Transpl 2012;10:1471–8.
4. Forman L, Lewis J, Berlin J, et al. The association between hepatitis C infection and survival after orthotopic liver transplantation. Gastroenterology 2002;122: 889–96.
5. Weisner R, Sorrell M, Villamil F, et al. Report of the first International Liver Transplantation Society expert panel consensus conference on liver transplantation and hepatitis C. Liver Transpl 2003;9:1–9.
6. Sreekumar S, Gonzalez-koch A, Maor-Kendler Y, et al. Early identification of recipients with progressive histological recurrence of hepatitis C after liver transplantation. Hepatology 2000;32:1125–30.
7. Neumann U, Berg T, Bahra M, et al. Fibrosis progression after liver transplantation in patients with recurrent hepatitis C. J Hepatol 2004;41:830–6.
8. Gane E. The natural history and outcome of liver transplantation in hepatitis C virus-infected recipients. Liver Transpl 2003;9:S28–34.
9. Doughty A, Spencer J, Cossart Y, et al. Cholestatic hepatitis after liver transplantation is associated with persistently high serum hepatitis C virus RNA levels. Liver Transpl Surg 1998;4:15–21.
10. Narang T, Ahrens W, Russo M. Post-liver transplant cholestatic hepatitis C: a systematic review of clinical and pathological findings and application of consensus criteria. Liver Transpl 2010;16:1228–35.
11. Demtris A. Evolution of hepatitis C virus in liver allografts. Liver Transpl 2009; 15:35.
12. Berenguer M, Prieto M, Rayon J, et al. Natural history of clinically compensated HCV related graft-cirrhosis following liver transplantation. Hepatology 2000;32: 852–8.
13. Berenguer M, Prieto M, San Juan F, et al. Contribution of donor age to the recent decrease in patient survival among HCV infected liver transplant recipients. Hepatology 2002;36:202–10.
14. Rayhill S, Wu Y, Katz D, et al. Older donor livers show early severe histological activity, fibrosis, and graft failure after liver transplantation for hepatitis C. Transplantation 2007;84:331–9.

15. Berenguer M. What determines the natural history of recurrent hepatitis C after liver transplantation. J Hepatol 2005;42:448–56.
16. Perez-Daga J, Ramirez-Plaza C, Suarez M, et al. Impact of donor age on the results of liver transplantation in hepatitis C virus positive recipients. Transplant Proc 2008;40:2959–61.
17. Condron S, Heneghan M, Patel K, et al. Effect of donor age on survival of liver transplant recipients with hepatitis C virus infection. Transplantation 2005;80: 145–8.
18. Watt K, Lyden E, Gulizia J, et al. Recurrent hepatitis C posttransplant: early preservation injury may predict poor outcome. Liver Transpl 2006;12:134–9.
19. Cescon M, Grazi G, Cucchetti A, et al. Predictors of sustained virological response after antiviral treatment for hepatitis C recurrence following liver transplantation. Liver Transpl 2009;15:782–9.
20. Roche B, Samuel D. Risk factors for hepatitis C recurrence after liver transplantation. J Viral Hepat 2007;14:89–96.
21. Charlton M, Seaberg E, Wiesner R, et al. Predictors of patient and graft survival following liver transplantation for hepatitis C. Hepatology 1998;28:823–30.
22. Feray C, Gigou M, Samuel D, et al. Influence of the genotypes of hepatitis C virus on the severity of recurrent liver disease after liver transplantation. Gastroenterology 1995;108:1088–96.
23. Burak K, Kremers W, Batts K, et al. Impact of cytomegalovirus infection, year of transplantation, and donor age on outcomes after liver transplantation for hepatitis C. Liver Transpl 2002;8:362–9.
24. Selzner M, Kashfi A, Selzner N, et al. Recipient age affects long term outcome and hepatitis C recurrence in old donor livers following transplantation. Liver Transpl 2009;15:1288–95.
25. Belli L, Burroughs A, Burra P, et al. Liver transplantation for HCV cirrhosis: improved survival in recent years and increased severity of recurrent disease in female recipients: results of a long term retrospective study. Liver Transpl 2007;13:733–40.
26. Layden J, Cotler S, Grim S, et al. Impact of donor and recipient race on survival after hepatitis C-related liver transplantation. Transplantation 2012;93:444–9.
27. Moeller M, Zalawadia A, Alrayes A, et al. The impact of donor race on recurrent hepatitis C after liver transplantation. Transplant Proc 2010;42:4175–7.
28. Rosen H, Chou S, Corless C, et al. Cytomegalovirus viremia: risk factor for allograft cirrhosis after liver transplantation for hepatitis C. Transplantation 1997;64: 721–6.
29. Bosch W, Heckman M, Pungpapong S, et al. Association of cytomegalovirus infection and disease with recurrent hepatitis C after liver transplantation. Transplantation 2012;93:723–8.
30. Weber R, Sabin C, Friis-Moller N, et al. Liver-related deaths in persons infected with the HIV: the D: A:D study. Arch Intern Med 2006;166:1632–41.
31. de Vera M, Dvorchik I, Tom K, et al. Survival of liver transplant patients co-infected with HIV and HCV is adversely impacted by recurrent hepatitis C. Am J Transplant 2006;6:2983–93.
32. Duclos-Vallee J, Feray C, Sebagh M, et al. Survival and recurrence of hepatitis C after liver transplantation in patients co-infected with human immunodeficiency virus and hepatitis C virus. Hepatology 2008;47:407–17.
33. Mindikoglu A, Regev A, Magder L. Impact of human immunodeficiency virus on survival after liver transplantation: analysis of united network for organ sharing database. Transplantation 2008;85:359–68.

34. Baccarani U, Adani GL, Bragantini F, et al. Long-term outcomes of orthotopic liver transplantation in human immunodeficiency virus-infected patients and comparison with human immunodeficiency virus-negative cases. Transplant Proc 2011;43:1119–22.

35. Duclos-Vallee JC, Vittecoq D, Teicher E, et al. Hepatitis C virus viral recurrence and liver mitochondrial damage after liver transplantation in HIV-HCV co-infected patients. J Hepatol 2005;42(3):341–9.

36. Miro J, Montejo M, Castells L, et al. Outcome of HCV/HIV-co-Infected liver transplant recipients: a prospective and multicenter cohort study. Am J Transplant 2012;12:1866–76.

37. Terrault N, Roland M, Schiano T, et al. Outcomes of liver transplant recipients with hepatitis C and human immunodeficiency virus co-infection. Liver Transpl 2012;18:716–26.

38. Chen T, Jia H, Li J, et al. New onset diabetes mellitus after liver transplantation and hepatitis C virus infection: meta-analysis of clinical studies. Transpl Int 2009; 22:408–15.

39. Veldt B, Poterucha J, Watt K, et al. Insulin resistance, serum adipokines and risk of fibrosis progression in patients transplanted for hepatitis C. Am J Transplant 2009;9:1406–13.

40. Weiler N, Thrun I, Hoppe-Lotichius M, et al. Early steroid-free immunosuppression with FK506 after liver transplantation: long-term results of a prospectively randomized double-blinded trial. Transplantation 2010;90:1562–6.

41. Marubashi S, Umeshita K, Asahara T, et al. Steroid-free living donor liver transplantation for HCV - a multicenter prospective cohort study in Japan. Clin Transplant 2012;26:857–67.

42. Sgourakis G, Radtke A, Fouzas I, et al. Corticosteroid-free immunosuppression in liver transplantation: a meta-analysis and meta-regression of outcomes. Transpl Int 2009;22:892–905.

43. Klintmalm G, Davis G, Teperman L, et al. A randomized, multicenter study comparing steroid-free immunosuppression and standard immunosuppression for liver transplant recipients with chronic hepatitis C. Liver Transpl 2011;17:1394–403.

44. Berenguer M, Aguilera V, Prieto M, et al. Significant improvement in the outcome of HCV-infected transplant recipients by avoiding rapid steroid tapering and potent induction immunosuppression. J Hepatol 2006;44:717–22.

45. Vivarelli M, Burra P, La Barba G, et al. Influence of steroids on HCV recurrence after liver transplantation: a prospective study. J Hepatol 2007;47:793–8.

46. Berenguer M. Hot topic in hepatitis C virus research: the type of immunosuppression does not matter. Liver Transpl 2011;17:24–8.

47. Firpi RJ, Zhu H, Morelli G, et al. Cyclosporine suppresses hepatitis C virus in vitro and increases the chance of a sustained virological response after liver transplantation. Liver Transpl 2006;12:51–7.

48. Watashi K, Hijikata M, Hosaka M, et al. Cyclosporin A suppresses replication of hepatitis C virus genome in cultured hepatocytes. Hepatology 2003;38:1282–8.

49. Haddad E, McAlister V, Renouf E, et al. Cyclosporin versus tacrolimus for liver transplanted patients. Cochrane Database Syst Rev 2006;4:51–61.

50. Selzner N, Renner EL, Selzner M, et al. Antiviral treatment of recurrent hepatitis C after liver transplantation: predictors of response and long-term outcome. Transplantation 2009;88:1214–21.

51. Hirano K, Ichikawa T, Nakao K, et al. Differential effects of calcineurin inhibitors, tacrolimus and cyclosporine a, on interferon-induced antiviral protein in human hepatocyte cells. Liver Transpl 2008;14:292–8.

52. Pan Q, Metselaar H, de Ruiter P, et al. Calcineurin inhibitor tacrolimus does not interfere with the suppression of hepatitis C virus infection by interferon-alpha. Liver Transpl 2010;16:520–6.
53. Berenguer M, Aguilera V, San Juan F, et al. Effect of calcineurin inhibitors in the outcome of liver transplantation in hepatitis C virus-positive recipients. Transplantation 2010;90:1204–9.
54. Berenguer M, Royuela A, Zamora J. Immunosuppression with calcineurin inhibitors with respect to the outcome of HCV recurrence after liver transplantation: results of a meta-analysis. Liver Transpl 2007;13:21–9.
55. Irish W, Arcona S, Bowers D, et al. Cyclosporine versus tacrolimus treated liver transplant recipients with chronic hepatitis C: outcomes analysis of the UNOS/OPTN database. Am J Transplant 2011;11:1676–85.
56. Levy G, Grazi G, Sanjuan F, et al. 12 month follow up analysis of a multicenter randomized, prospective trial in de novo liver transplant recipients (LIS2T) comparing cyclosporine microemulsion (C2 monitoring) and tacrolimus. Liver Transpl 2006;12:1464–72.
57. McAlister V, Haddad E, Renouf E, et al. Cyclosporin versus tacrolimus as primary immunosuppressant after liver transplantation: a meta-analysis. Am J Transplant 2006;6:1578–85.
58. Kim R, Mizuno S, Sorensen J, et al. Impact of calcineurin inhibitors on hepatitis C recurrence after liver transplantation. Dig Dis Sci 2012;57:568–72.
59. Wiesner R, Rabkin J, Klintmalm G, et al. A randomized double-blind comparative study of mycophenolate mofetil and azathioprine in combination with cyclosporine and corticosteroids in primary liver transplant recipients. Liver Transpl 2001;7:442–50.
60. Wiesner R, Shorr J, Steffen B, et al. Mycophenolate mofetil combination therapy improves long-term outcomes after liver transplantation in patients with and without hepatitis C. Liver Transpl 2005;11:750–9.
61. Manzia T, Angelico R, Toti L, et al. Long-term, maintenance MMF monotherapy improves the fibrosis progression in liver transplant recipients with recurrent hepatitis C. Transpl Int 2011;24:461–8.
62. Rosen H, Shackleton C, Higa L, et al. Use of OKT3 is associated with early and severe recurrence of hepatitis C after liver transplantation. Am J Gastroenterol 1997;92:1453–7.
63. Horton P, Tchervenkov J, Barkun J, et al. Antithymocyte globulin induction therapy in hepatitis C-positive liver transplant recipients. J Gastrointest Surg 2005;9:896–902.
64. Akselband Y, Harding M, Nelson P. Rapamycin inhibits spontaneous and fibroblast growth factor beta-stimulated proliferation of endothelial cells and fibroblasts. Transplant Proc 1991;23:2833–6.
65. Biecker E, De Gottardi A, Neef M, et al. Long-term treatment of bile duct-ligated rats with rapamycin (sirolimus) significantly attenuates liver fibrosis: analysis of the underlying mechanisms. J Pharmacol Exp Ther 2005;313:952–61.
66. Neef M, Ledermann M, Saegesser H, et al. Low-dose oral rapamycin treatment reduces fibrogenesis, improves liver function, and prolongs survival in rats with established liver cirrhosis. J Hepatol 2006;45:786–96.
67. McKenna G, Trotter J, Klintmalm E, et al. Limiting hepatitis C virus progression in liver transplant recipients using sirolimus-based immunosuppression. Am J Transplant 2011;11:2379–87.
68. Carrion J, Fernandez-Varo G, Bruguera M, et al. Serum fibrosis markers identify patients with mild and progressive hepatitis C recurrence after liver transplantation. Gastroenterology 2010;138:147–58.

69. Berres M, Trautwein C, Schmeding M, et al. Serum chemokine CXC ligand 10 (CXCL10) predicts fibrosis progression after liver transplantation for hepatitis C infection. Hepatology 2011;53:596–603.
70. Pungpapong S, Nunes D, Krishna M, et al. Serum fibrosis markers can predict rapid fibrosis progression after liver transplantation for hepatitis C. Liver Transpl 2008;14:1294–302.
71. do O NT, Eurich D, Schmitz P, et al. A 7-gene signature of the recipient predicts the progression of fibrosis after liver transplantation for hepatitis C virus infection. Liver Transpl 2012;18:298–304.
72. Charlton M, Thompson A, Veldt B, et al. Interleukin-28B polymorphisms are associated with histological recurrence and treatment response following liver transplantation in patients with hepatitis C virus infection. Hepatology 2011; 53:317–24.
73. Eurich D, Boas-Knoop S, Ruehl M, et al. Relationship between the interleukin-28b gene polymorphism and the histological severity of hepatitis C virus-induced graft inflammation and the response to antiviral therapy after liver transplantation. Liver Transpl 2011;17:289–98.
74. Firpi R, Abdelmalek M, Soldevila-Pico C, et al. One-year protocol liver biopsy can stratify fibrosis progression in liver transplant recipients with recurrent hepatitis C infection. Liver Transpl 2004;10:1240–7.
75. Blasco A, Forns X, Carrion JA, et al. Hepatic venous pressure gradient identifies patients at risk of severe hepatitis C recurrence after liver transplantation. Hepatology 2006;43:492–9.
76. Adebajo C, Talwalkar J, Poterucha J, et al. Ultrasound-based transient elastography for the detection of hepatic fibrosis in patients with recurrent hepatitis C virus after liver transplantation: a systematic review and meta-analysis. Liver Transpl 2012;18:323–31.
77. Rigamonti C, Donato M, Fraquelli M, et al. Transient elastography predicts fibrosis progression in patients with recurrent hepatitis C after liver transplantation. Gut 2008;57:821–7.
78. Bellido-Munoz F, Giraldez-Gallego A, Roca-Oporto C, et al. Monitoring the natural evolution and response to treatment of post liver transplant recurrent hepatitis C using transient elastography: preliminary results. Transplant Proc 2012;44:2082–6.
79. Lee V, Miller F, Omary R, et al. Magnetic resonance elastography and biomarkers to assess fibrosis from recurrent hepatitis C in liver transplant recipients. Transplantation 2011;92:581–6.
80. Testillano M, Fernandez JR, Suarez MJ, et al. Survival and hepatitis C virus recurrence after liver transplantation in HIV- and hepatitis C virus-coinfected patients: experience in a single center. Transplant Proc 2009;41(3):1041–3.
81. Everson GT, Terrault NA, Lok AS, et al. A randomized controlled trial of pretransplant antiviral therapy to prevent recurrence of hepatitis c after liver transplantation. Hepatology 2012. [Epub ahead of print].
82. Roche B, Samuel D. Liver transplantation in viral hepatitis: prevention of recurrence. Best Pract Res Clin Gastroenterol 2008;22:1153–69.
83. Bzowej N, Nelson DR, Terrault NA, et al. PHOENIX: a randomized controlled trial of peginterferon alfa-2a plus ribavirin as a prophylactic treatment after liver transplantation for hepatitis C virus. Liver Transpl 2011;17:528–38.
84. Berenguer M. Systematic review of the treatment of established recurrent hepatitis C with pegylated interferon in combination with ribavirin. J Hepatol 2008;49:274–87.

85. Samuel D, Bizollon T, Feray C, et al. Interferon-alpha 2b plus ribavirin in patients with chronic hepatitis C after liver transplantation: a randomized study. Gastroenterology 2003;124:642–50.
86. Castells L, Vargas V, Allende H, et al. Combined treatment with pegylated interferon (alpha-2b) and ribavirin in the acute phase of hepatitis C virus recurrence after liver transplantation. J Hepatol 2005;43:53–9.
87. Angelico M, Petrolati A, Lionetti R, et al. A randomized study on peg-interferon alfa-2a with or without ribavirin in liver transplant recipients with recurrent hepatitis C. J Hepatol 2007;46:1009–17.
88. Carrion J, Navasa M, Garcia-Retortillo M, et al. Efficacy of antiviral therapy on hepatitis C recurrence after liver transplantation: a randomized controlled study. Gastroenterology 2007;132:1746–56.
89. Picciotto F, Tritto G, Lanza A, et al. Sustained virological response to antiviral therapy reduces mortality in HCV reinfection after liver transplantation. J Hepatol 2007;46:459–65.
90. Lodato F, Berardi S, Gramenzi A, et al. Clinical trial: Peg-interferon alfa-2b and ribavirin for the treatment of genotype-1 hepatitis C recurrence after liver transplantation. Aliment Pharmacol Ther 2008;28:450–7.
91. Hashemi N, Araya V, Tufail K, et al. An extended treatment protocol with pegylated interferon and ribavirin for hepatitis C recurrence after liver transplantation. World J Hepatol 2011;3:198–204.
92. Perrakis A, Yedibela S, Schuhmann S, et al. The effect and safety of the treatment of recurrent hepatitis C infection after orthotopic liver transplantation with pegylated interferon alpha2b and ribavirin. Transplant Proc 2011;43:3824–8.
93. Belli L, Volpes R, Graziadei I, et al. Antiviral therapy and fibrosis progression in patients with mild-moderate hepatitis C recurrence after liver transplantation. A randomized controlled study. Dig Liver Dis 2012;44:603–9.
94. Gordon F, Kwo P, Ghalib R, et al. Peginterferon-alpha-2b and ribavirin for hepatitis C recurrence postorthotopic liver transplantation. J Clin Gastroenterol 2012;46:700–8.
95. Bertuzzo V, Cescon M, Morelli M, et al. Long-term antiviral treatment for recurrent hepatitis C after liver transplantation. Dig Liver Dis 2012;44:861–7.
96. Bizollon T, Pradat P, Mabrut J, et al. Benefit of sustained virological response to combination therapy on graft survival of liver transplanted patients with recurrent chronic hepatitis C. Am J Transplant 2005;5:1909–13.
97. Kornberg A, Kupper B, Tannapfel A, et al. Sustained clearance of serum hepatitis C virus-RNA independently predicts long-term survival in liver transplant patients with recurrent hepatitis C. Transplantation 2008;86:469–73.
98. Ikegami T, Taketomi A, Soejima Y, et al. The benefits of interferon treatment in patients without sustained viral response after living donor liver transplantation for hepatitis C. Transplant Proc 2009;41:4246–52.
99. Ge D, Fellay J, Thompson AJ, et al. Genetic variation in IL28B predicts hepatitis C treatment-induced viral clearance. Nature 2009;461:399–401.
100. Tanaka Y, Nishida N, Sugiyama M, et al. Genome-wide association of IL28B with response to pegylated interferon-alpha and ribavirin therapy for chronic hepatitis C. Nat Genet 2009;41:1105–9.
101. Duarte-Rojo A, Veldt B, Goldstein D, et al. The course of posttransplant hepatitis C infection: comparative impact of donor and recipient source of the favorable IL28B genotype and other variables. Transplantation 2012;94:197–203.

102. Fukuhara T, Taketomi A, Motomura T, et al. Variants in IL28B in liver recipients and donors correlate with response to peg-interferon and ribavirin therapy for recurrent hepatitis C. Gastroenterology 2010;139:1577–85.
103. Poordad F, McCone J, Bacon BR, et al. Boceprevir for untreated chronic HCV genotype 1 infection. N Engl J Med 2011;364:1195–206.
104. Jacobson I, McHutchison J, Dusheiko G, et al. Telaprevir for previously untreated chronic hepatitis C virus infection. N Engl J Med 2011;364:2405–16.
105. Garg V, van Heeswijk R, Lee JE, et al. Effect of telaprevir on the pharmacokinetics of cyclosporine and tacrolimus. Hepatology 2011;54:20–7.
106. Verna E, Shetty K, Brown R, et al. Use of direct acting antiviral therapy prior to liver transplantation: urban cohort patients with HCV cirrhosis. Hepatology 2012; 56:218–22.
107. Coilly A, Roche B, Botta-Fridlund D, et al. Efficacy Efficacy and safety of protease inhibitors for severe Hepatitis C recurrence after liver transplantation: a first multicentric experience. Antimicrob Agents Chemother 2012;56:5728–34.
108. Werner C, Egetemeyr D, Lauer U, et al. Short report: telaprevir-based triple therapy in liver transplanted HCV patients: a 12 week pilot study providing safety and efficacy. Liver Transpl 2012;18(12):1464–70.
109. McCashland T, Watt K, Lyden E, et al. Retransplantation for hepatitis C: results of a U.S. multicenter retransplant study. Liver Transpl 2007;9:1246–53.
110. Carmiel-Haggai M, Fiel M, Gaddipati H, et al. Recurrent hepatitis C after retransplantation: factors affecting graft and patient outcome. Liver Transpl 2005;11: 1567–73.
111. Carrion J, Navasa M, Forns X. Retransplantation in patients with hepatitis C recurrence after liver transplantation. J Hepatol 2010;53:962–70.

Emerging Fungal Infections in Solid Organ Transplant Recipients

Shmuel Shoham, MD

KEYWORDS

- Solid organ transplant • Zygomycetes • *Scedosporium* • *Fusarium*

KEY POINTS

- The leading emerging fungal pathogens in transplant recipients are the Zygomycetes, *Scedosporium/Pseudallescheria*, *Fusarium*, and the dark molds.
- Amphotericin B products are the treatment of choice for mucormycosis.
- Identifying emerging fungi to the species level and performing susceptibility testing can help guide therapy.
- When there is evidence for an active infection, even low-virulence fungi that are isolated from the respiratory tract or sinuses generally require treatment.
- Treatment frequently necessitates a combined approach that includes antifungal therapy, debridement of infected material, and efforts to improve host defenses.

INTRODUCTION

Development of invasive fungal infections in solid organ transplant (SOT) recipients depends on the interplay between host and fungal factors. Changes in either of these variables can favor emergence of infections in new populations and/or by previously nonpathogenic fungi.

Managing SOT recipients with emerging fungal infections can be a daunting task. Most clinicians have very limited personal experience in treating these infections. Therapy frequently requires a multidisciplinary approach that includes toxic medications and invasive procedures, and these infections have the potential for devastating outcomes, including graft loss or death. The medical literature describing such infections is difficult to interpret, as it consists mostly of anecdotal experiences and small case series. Adding to the complexity is the evolving nomenclature of many of these fungi. The goals of this review are to demystify these infections and to serve as a resource for clinicians contending with emerging fungal infections in SOT recipients.

Disclosures: Research funding from Astellas, Merck, and Pfizer. Member of the Merck Scientific Advisory Board: The Johns Hopkins University, in accordance with its conflict of interest policies, is managing the terms of this arrangement.
Transplant and Oncology Infectious Diseases Program, Johns Hopkins University School of Medicine, 1830 East Monument Street, Room 450-D, Baltimore, MD 21205, USA
E-mail address: sshoham1@jhmi.edu

Infect Dis Clin N Am 27 (2013) 305–316
http://dx.doi.org/10.1016/j.idc.2013.02.004
0891-5520/13/$ – see front matter © 2013 Elsevier Inc. All rights reserved.

id.theclinics.com

OVERVIEW

Emerging fungi are increasingly recognized as potential pathogens in SOT recipients, and account for 7% to 10% of invasive fungal infections in this population.[1–4]

Microbiology

Clinically significant emerging fungi include[1–3,5–11]:

- Zygomycetes (eg, *Rhizopus*, *Mucor*, *Absidia*, and *Mycoladu*s species)
- *Scedosporium* (eg, *Scedosporium apiospermum*, *Scedosporium auranticum*, and *Scedosporium prolificans*)
- *Fusarium* (eg, *Fusarium solani* and *Fusarium oxysporum*)
- Dark molds, also called dematiaceous fungi (eg, *Ochroconis*, *Cladophialophora*, *Rhinocladiella*, *Bipolaris*, and *Fonsecaea* species)
- *Paecilomyces*, *Acremonium*, and *Trichoderma*
- Yeast-like organisms (eg, *Trichosporon*, *Cryptococcus gattii*, and *Rhodotorula* species)

Environment

The emerging fungi are typically found in diverse environmental sources such as soil, water, decaying vegetation, and sewage. Patients come into contact with these fungi either via inhalation of airborne spores or, less commonly, by touching a contaminated source. The environmental microbiology and, hence, patients' exposures, can vary by geographic locale. For example, risk for infection attributable to the Zygomycetes and to *Scedosporium* species are particularly high in the Middle East and Australia, respectively.[12,13]

Certain occupations and living circumstances can put patients at higher risk. Exposures to construction sites, farming operations, sandblasting work, air-conditioning filters, and flooded sites are important in this regard. Risks for contact with potentially pathogenic fungi and ways to reduce patients' exposure should be discussed with transplant recipients. If an infection is suspected, inquiring about a patient's travel, occupation, and activities may provide important epidemiologic clues. Sometimes exposures can occur within the health care setting.[14,15] Outbreaks of mucormycosis have been associated with contaminated adhesive bandages, wooden tongue depressors, ostomy bags, water circuitry damage, and adjacent building construction. Fusariosis may be acquired from contaminated hospital drains and showerheads.

Patterns of fungal exposure may also be affected by environmental disruptions such as natural disasters and by the development of new ecological niches. Infections caused by the Zygomycetes and *Scedosporium* species may be seen after floods, tornados, and tsunamis.[16,17] The risk of transmitting such organisms may be relevant when evaluating potential organ donors who have suffered drowning accidents.[18,19] The role of new ecological niches has been demonstrated in the recent outbreak of *Cryptococcus gattii* in the Pacific Northwest region of North America.[20] Starting in 2004, cases of *C gattii* infections have been identified in this region,[21] and approximately one-fifth of those affected in that outbreak have been SOT recipients. With regard to climate change, some have hypothesized that global warming may increase the prevalence of fungal diseases by increasing the geographic range of currently pathogenic species and by selecting for adaptive thermotolerance in species that are currently unable to survive at human body temperature.[22]

Host Factors

Multiple arms of the immune system are impaired in transplant recipients. The first lines of defense are intact anatomic barriers. If there is exposure to an emerging fungal pathogen when such barriers are disrupted and there is ongoing high-level immunosuppression, a "perfect storm" can develop, resulting in invasive infection. This process can occur in any SOT recipient, but lung transplant recipients are at highest risk.[1,3,23–25] Factors favoring fungal infections in lung transplant recipients include ongoing exposure of the graft to environmental fungi, underlying chronic respiratory disease, and concomitant sinus and airway abnormalities impeding fungal clearance. Patients with impaired cutaneous barriers caused by traumatic injury or an invasive medical procedure are also at risk. Skin infections due to the *Zygomycetes*, *Scedosporium*, *Fusarium*, and the dark molds have been described in such circumstances.[14,26–28]

Primary Site of Infection (by Route of Exposure):
- Inhalation of airborne spores: Most likely sites are the sinuses, airways, and/or lung parenchyma. Disease may then extend to involve adjacent sites or disseminate to distant organs.
- Direct inoculation: The most likely site is the skin and adjacent soft-tissue structures.
- Donor derived (eg, zygomycosis via contamination of the preservation fluid or from the organ itself): Infection can be localized to the transplanted organ and the graft anastomosis or disseminate widely. Such cases are associated with high rates of graft loss and mortality, and may be particularly problematic in commercial transplantation.[19,29,30]

An additional factor in the evolution of infection attributable to emerging fungi may be the impact of antifungals used for prophylaxis and therapy. Decreased susceptibility to 1 or more commonly used antifungals is common in emerging fungi. For example, the Zygomycetes are not susceptible to voriconazole and to the echinocandins. Use of these agents has been associated with increased risk for development of mucormycosis in some, but not all studies.[31–33] *Trichosporon* and *Fusarium* species are frequently resistant to amphotericin B (AmB), and *Scedosporium prolificans* may be resistant to all commonly used antifungal agents. It is likely that development of infections with these fungi is related to antifungal selection pressure.

SPECIFIC FUNGI
Mucormycosis

Infections attributable to the Zygomycetes are the best characterized of the emerging fungal infections in SOT recipients.[1–3] Exposure is generally via inhalation, but may also occur at the skin or gastrointestinal tract. Direct contact with soil or water following natural disasters or near drowning episodes, and exposure to contaminated medical devices (as already described), are additional routes to infection.[14]

Clinically important Zygomycetes include species of *Rhizopus*, *Mucor*, *Rhizomucor*, *Cunninghamella*, *Absidia*, *Apophysomyces*, and *Mycocladus*. The predominant infecting organism can vary by geographic site of exposure.[34] In addition, pathogenic potential may differ by organism. For example, *Mycocladus corymbifer* pulmonary infection has been associated with higher rates of disseminated disease.[35]

Epidemiology[6]:
- Zygomycosis accounts for approximately 2% of fungal infections in SOT recipients.

- Lung and liver transplant recipients are the most affected.
- Infections tend to occur at a median of 6 months after transplant, except in liver transplant recipients, in whom infection can occur in the first month.
- Risk factors in SOT recipients include renal failure, diabetes mellitus, exposure to high doses of corticosteroids, and prior use of voriconazole.
- "Traditional" risk factors for mucormycosis (eg, ketoacidosis, prolonged and profound neutropenia, and deferoximine) are infrequently seen in SOT recipients.

Clinical Presentations[6,35–37]:
- Lungs are the most common sites of infection. Disease presents as consolidation/mass lesions nodules and cavities.
- Infection at the sinuses and nose may remain localized or extend to orbits, brain, and other intracranial structures.
- Primary cutaneous infection occurs at sites of surgical wounds or drains, intravenous catheter sites, and after skin trauma. The typical appearance is of black necrotic lesions surrounded by cellulitis, thrombophlebitis, or extension to deeper structures.
- Disseminated disease can involve virtually any organ including the lungs, pericardium, myocardium, endocardium, brain, liver, esophagus, stomach, small and large intestine, kidney, retroperitoneum, thyroid gland, and skin.

Diagnosis usually requires an invasive procedure such as biopsy, fine-needle aspiration, bronchoscopy, or surgical exploration, but occasionally the organism can be grown from expectorated sputum.[37] On direct staining the Zygomycetes tend to appear as broad, ribbon-like, nonseptate hyphae. Not infrequently, the organisms are identified on either histology or culture, but not both. Increasingly the polymerase chain reaction is being used to detect Zygomycetes.[34]

Outcomes depend on timely initiation of appropriate antifungal therapy, the host immune status, and the site and extent of infection. The cornerstones of management are effective antifungal therapy, improvement in host defenses, and surgical resection of necrotic tissue generated by this angioinvasive fungus.

Medical therapy alone can be attempted in some patients with pulmonary infection. However, surgery is typically required if there is extensive necrosis, infection at lung transplant anastomosis, or a threat to major vascular structures. Debridement of airway or sinus disease may be performed endoscopically.

Antifungal Treatment Options:
- Drugs of choice: Lipid-formulation AmB (5.0–7.5 mg/kg/d)
- Combination of an echinocandin + lipid-formulation amphotericin B may be considered based on data from animal studies and retrospective reports.
- Posaconazole may be considered for maintenance once clinical stability has been achieved and for salvage therapy in patients intolerant to or failing AmB.[38–40]

Dark (Dematiaceous) Molds

The dark molds are a diverse group of pigmented fungi that are associated with a variety of infections.[41] Their nomenclature can be confusing, and many organisms have undergone name changes in recent years. Invasive infection is called phaeohyphomycosis. Colonization of the respiratory tract and sinuses is common and does not necessarily indicate infection. Such colonization may be particularly common in lung transplant candidates and recipients. Infections tend to occur late, often several years after transplantation. The site of infection depends on the mode of exposure and the fungal species (see later discussion). Certain species tend to cause cutaneous infections at sites of inoculation, presenting as papules, nodules, or pustules, whereas others cause pulmonary or disseminated (including central nervous system [CNS]) disease.[7,8,42–48]

Phaeohyphomycosis by Site and Organism:
- Primary skin: *Alternaria, Curvularia, Exophiala*
- Pulmonary: *Ochroconis gallopavum, Cladophialophora bantiana, Exophiala, Alternaria, Curvularia,* and *Fonsecaea*
- CNS: *Cladophialophora bantiana, Ochroconis gallopavum, Rhinocladiella mackenziei, Exophiala dermatitidis, Bipolaris,* and *Fonsecaea*

The diagnosis can be straightforward as in the case of symptomatic disease, with evidence of the fungus in histopathology and culture. However, simply growing these molds in culture (particularly from the nose or sinuses) does not necessarily imply infection. In tissue these fungi may be identified by the golden-brown coloration in the walls of the hyphae.[44] The presence of melanin can be highlighted by Fontana-Masson staining.

Treatment depends on the infecting organism and site of infection. In general, surgical excision or debridement is recommended whenever feasible; this may even be sufficient for isolated cutaneous disease. Conversely, when disease is limited to the respiratory tract, medical management alone may suffice. Voriconazole, posaconazole, or itraconazole are typically the first-line agents, but there may also be a role for AmB and the echinocandins.[48,49] Susceptibility testing can be useful to guide therapy.

Fusarium

Among SOT patients, fusariosis predominantly affects lung transplant recipients. Such infections account for less than 1% of fungal infections in SOT recipients.[1,3] Most of the infections are caused by *Fusarium solani* and *Fusarium oxysporum*, and to a lesser extent *Fusarium proliferatum, Fusarium moniliforme,* and *Fusarium sacchari*.[15] Exposure is primarily via inhalation of airborne conidia or by contact with contaminated material (eg, soil, plants, and organic matter). *Fusarium* may also be found in water-distribution systems, tap water, sinks, and showerheads.[15]

The clinical spectrum includes superficial, localized, and disseminated infections.[50] The specific presentation depends on portal of entry, extent of immunosuppression, and transplant type.[51–56]

Clinical Presentations:
- Primary skin infection form direct inoculation: Present as superficial or localized infection (eg, nodules, ulcers, cellulitis, subcutaneous abscess) and usually very responsive to therapy.
- Respiratory tract and sinus infection: Results from inhalation and typically occurs in lung transplant recipients.
- Secondary dissemination to multiple organs including the gastrointestinal tract, liver, heart valves, kidneys, lung, CNS, and skin.

Diagnosis[53,57,58]:
- Targetoid skin lesions with darkish discoloration are a clue to disseminated fusariosis. Skin biopsy can establish the diagnosis.
- Occasionally the organism grows in blood cultures.

- The role of nonculture-based diagnostic tests (eg, β-glucan and galactomannan) is currently evolving, but these may be useful as adjunctive tests.

Treatment options and outcomes depend on site and extent of infection, and on the species.[59] Identification of the organism to the species level and antifungal susceptibility testing can help guide therapy. Surgical excision or debridement should be performed whenever possible.

Treatment Options[56]:
- *F solani* and *Fusarium verticillioides*: AmB
- Other species: voriconazole
- Limited skin disease: excision alone might suffice
- Combination therapy (AmB + voriconazole) for invasive infection while awaiting identification and susceptibility testing and in severe cases

Scedosporium/Pseudallescheria

Infections attributable to *Scedosporium* and *Pseudallescheria* species can be particularly difficult to treat. The organisms are frequently resistant to multiple antifungal agents, and outcomes of invasive infections can be devastating. The nomenclature is complicated and is still evolving. The teleomorph (sexual form) is referred to as *Pseudallescheria* and the asexual form (anamorph) as *Scedosporium*. The predominant species are *Scedosporium apiospermum* (teleomorph: *Pseudallescheria apiosperma*), *Scedosporium aurantiacum*, *Pseudallescheria boydii* (anamorph: *Scedosporium boydii*), *Scedosporium dehoogii*, and *Scedosporium prolificans*.[60,61]

These organisms are typically found in soil and contaminated water, including in urban environments.[12] Exposure is generally via inhalation of airborne spores, but may also occur after contact with contaminated water. Patients with cystic fibrosis are often colonized with *Scedosporium* even before transplant. Infections are predominantly seen in lung transplant recipients, but occur across the spectrum of organ transplants.[3,62] Primary sites of infection include the respiratory tract, sinuses, and skin. Infection may progress or disseminate to involve additional organs including bone, join, brain, eye, ear, and vocal cords.[62]

Treatment recommendations are listed here; however, antifungal susceptibility testing of all clinical isolates is essential for guiding therapy[63–67]:

Treatment Options:
- *S apiospermum*: voriconazole ± echinocandin
- *S aurantiacum*: voriconazole
- *S prolificans*: resistant to multiple antifungal agents, but there may be a role for voriconazole + echinocandin, AmB + terbinafine, or voriconazole + terbinafine
- Surgical debridement should be considered whenever feasible, particularly in cases of multidrug-resistant fungal infection

Paecilomyces

Paecilomyces species, particularly *Paecilomyces lilacinus*, have emerged as a cause of fungal infections in highly immunocompromised patients. These environmental fungi are generally found in the air and in soil, but have also been associated with an outbreak of infection related to contaminated skin lotion.[68] The predominant clinical presentation in SOT recipients is subacute skin infection.[69] *Paecilomyces* can sometimes cause such infections in association with other fungi or mycobacteria.[70,71] The

Table 1
Emerging fungal pathogens in SOT

Category	Important Species
Zygomycetes	Species of *Rhizopus, Mucor, Absidia*, and *Mycoladus*
Dematiaceous molds	Species of *Ochroconis, Cladophialophora, Rhinocladiella, Bipolaris*, and *Fonsecaea*
Scedosporium/Pseudallescheria	*S apiospermum, S auranticum*, and *S prolificans*
Fusarium	*F solani* and *F oxysporum*
Other filamentous fungi	Species of *Paecilomyces, Acremonium*, and *Trichoderma*
Yeasts	Species of *Trichosporon, Rodotorula*, and *Cryptococcus gattii*

antifungal agent with the best track record for *P lilacinus* infections is voriconazole, but susceptibility testing may help guide therapy.[72,73]

Trichosporon

Trichosporon species, particularly *Trichosporon asahii* and *Trichosporon mucoides*, can cause systemic infection in SOT recipients.[74,75] These yeasts are found in diverse settings including soil, water, and vegetables, and as commensals of the human skin and gastrointestinal tract. Clinical presentations include fungemia and widely disseminated infection. The significance of *Trichosporon* funguria in renal transplant recipients is unclear, and may not require antifungal therapy.[76] When treatment is indicated, as in systemic disease, azoles are the mainstay of treatment.[74,75,77] However, resistance to azoles and AmB is common, and antifungal susceptibility testing is necessary to help guide therapy.[10]

Miscellaneous Rare Fungi

There are multiple rare fungi that have been described as causes of infection in SOT recipients at the case-report level, including *Acremonium, Scopulariopsis*, and

Table 2
Clinical characteristics of emerging fungi

Infection	Characteristic Transplant Recipient	Median Time to Infection	Typical Sites of Infection
Mucormycosis	All, but especially liver, lung, kidney	Liver transplant: 2–3 mo, others ~18–24 mo	Respiratory tract/sinuses/central nervous system
Dematiaceous molds	All	≥18–24 mo	Respiratory, sinuses/central nervous system, skin
Scedosporiosis	Lung	≥18–24 mo	Respiratory tract
Fusariosis	All, but especially liver, lung	Range from 1–3 to ≥9 mo	Respiratory tract sinus, skin
Paecilomyces	All, but especially heart, lung	≥12–18 mo	Respiratory tract, sinus, skin
Trichosporon	All, but especially kidney, liver	Within first few weeks or ≥18–24 mo	Endovascular/bloodstream surgical wounds

Trichoderma species.[78–80] As general rules, surgical excision should be attempted when possible and therapy should be guided by susceptibility testing.

SUMMARY

Development of invasive fungal infections depends on the confluence of host factors and environmental exposure. Changes in either of these parameters can favor emerging fungal infections, and we are now in the midst of such changes. Current trends in transplantation include increasingly diverse patient populations, use of novel and potent immunosuppressive regimens, and expanded use of antifungal agents for prophylaxis and treatment. When coupled with environmental disruptions including natural disasters, new ecological niches, and perhaps climate change, we can expect an ongoing evolution of fungal epidemiology in SOT recipients and an increasingly important role for emerging fungi (**Tables 1** and **2**).

REFERENCES

1. Neofytos D, Fishman JA, Horn D, et al. Epidemiology and outcome of invasive fungal infections in solid organ transplant recipients. Transpl Infect Dis 2010; 12(3):220–9.
2. Pappas PG, Alexander BD, Andes DR, et al. Invasive fungal infections among organ transplant recipients: results of the Transplant-Associated Infection Surveillance Network (TRANSNET). Clin Infect Dis 2010;50(8):1101–11.
3. Park BJ, Pappas PG, Wannemuehler KA, et al. Invasive non-Aspergillus mold infections in transplant recipients, United States, 2001-2006. Emerg Infect Dis 2011;17(10):1855–64.
4. Kubak BM, Huprikar SS. Emerging and rare fungal infections in solid organ transplant recipients. Am J Transplant 2009;9(Suppl 4):S208–26.
5. Stelzmueller I, Lass-Floerl C, Geltner C, et al. Zygomycosis and other rare filamentous fungal infections in solid organ transplant recipients. Transpl Int 2008; 21(6):534–46.
6. Singh N, Aguado JM, Bonatti H, et al. Zygomycosis in solid organ transplant recipients: a prospective, matched case-control study to assess risks for disease and outcome. J Infect Dis 2009;200(6):1002–11.
7. Shoham S, Pic-Aluas L, Taylor J, et al. Transplant-associated *Ochroconis gallopava* infections. Transpl Infect Dis 2008;10(6):442–8.
8. Rosow L, Jiang JX, Deuel T, et al. Cerebral phaeohyphomycosis caused by *Bipolaris spicifera* after heart transplantation. Transpl Infect Dis 2011;13(4):419–23.
9. Grossi P, Farina C, Fiocchi R, et al. Prevalence and outcome of invasive fungal infections in 1,963 thoracic organ transplant recipients: a multicenter retrospective study. Italian Study Group of Fungal Infections in Thoracic Organ Transplant Recipients. Transplantation 2000;70(1):112–6.
10. Netsvyetayeva I, Swoboda-Kopec E, Paczek L, et al. *Trichosporon asahii* as a prospective pathogen in solid organ transplant recipients. Mycoses 2009;52(3): 263–5.
11. Riedel DJ, Johnson JK, Forrest GN. *Rhodotorula glutinis fungemia* in a liver-kidney transplant patient. Transpl Infect Dis 2008;10(3):197–200.
12. Harun A, Gilgado F, Chen SC, et al. Abundance of *Pseudallescheria/Scedosporium* species in the Australian urban environment suggests a possible source for scedosporiosis including the colonization of airways in cystic fibrosis. Med Mycol 2010;48(Suppl 1):S70–6.

13. Einollahi B, Lessan-Pezeshki M, Pourfarziani V, et al. Invasive fungal infections following renal transplantation: a review of 2410 recipients. Ann Transplant 2008;13(4):55–8.

14. Rammaert B, Lanternier F, Zahar JR, et al. Healthcare-associated mucormycosis. Clin Infect Dis 2012;54(Suppl 1):S44–54.

15. Anaissie EJ, Kuchar RT, Rex JH, et al. Fusariosis associated with pathogenic *Fusarium* species colonization of a hospital water system: a new paradigm for the epidemiology of opportunistic mold infections. Clin Infect Dis 2001;33(11): 1871–8.

16. Weddle G, Gandy K, Bratcher D, et al. *Apophysomyces trapeziformis* infection associated with a tornado-related injury. Pediatr Infect Dis J 2012;31(6):640–2.

17. Garzoni C, Emonet S, Legout L, et al. Atypical infections in tsunami survivors. Emerg Infect Dis 2005;11(10):1591–3.

18. Katragkou A, Dotis J, Kotsiou M, et al. *Scedosporium apiospermum* infection after near-drowning. Mycoses 2007;50(5):412–21.

19. Alexander BD, Schell WA, Siston AM, et al. Fatal *Apophysomyces elegans* infection transmitted by deceased donor renal allografts. Am J Transplant 2010;10(9): 2161–7.

20. Mak S, Klinkenberg B, Bartlett K, et al. Ecological niche modeling of *Cryptococcus gattii* in British Columbia, Canada. Environ Health Perspect 2010; 118(5):653–8.

21. Centers for Disease Control and Prevention (CDC). Emergence of *Cryptococcus gattii*—Pacific Northwest, 2004-2010. MMWR Morb Mortal Wkly Rep 2010;59(28): 865–8.

22. Garcia-Solache MA, Casadevall A. Global warming will bring new fungal diseases for mammals. MBio 2010;1(1). pii:e00061–10.

23. Carneiro HA, Coleman JJ, Restrepo A, et al. *Fusarium* infection in lung transplant patients: report of 6 cases and review of the literature. Medicine (Baltimore) 2011; 90(1):69–80.

24. Cooley L, Spelman D, Thursky K, et al. Infection with *Scedosporium apiospermum* and *S. prolificans*, Australia. Emerg Infect Dis 2007;13(8):1170–7.

25. Castiglioni B, Sutton DA, Rinaldi MG, et al. *Pseudallescheria boydii* (Anamorph *Scedosporium apiospermum*). Infection in solid organ transplant recipients in a tertiary medical center and review of the literature. Medicine (Baltimore) 2002; 81(5):333–48.

26. Gallelli B, Viviani M, Nebuloni M, et al. Skin infection due to *Alternaria* species in kidney allograft recipients: report of a new case and review of the literature. J Nephrol 2006;19(5):668–72.

27. Talbot TR, Hatcher J, Davis SF, et al. *Scedosporium apiospermum* pneumonia and sternal wound infection in a heart transplant recipient. Transplantation 2002;74(11):1645–7.

28. Palmore TN, Shea YR, Childs RW, et al. *Fusarium proliferatum* soft tissue infection at the site of a puncture by a plant: recovery, isolation, and direct molecular identification. J Clin Microbiol 2010;48(1):338–42.

29. Shoham S, Hinestrosa F, Moore J Jr, et al. Invasive filamentous fungal infections associated with renal transplant tourism. Transpl Infect Dis 2010;12(4):371–4.

30. Tomazic J, Pirs M, Matos T, et al. Multiple infections after commercial renal transplantation in India. Nephrol Dial Transplant 2007;22(3):972–3.

31. Chamilos G, Marom EM, Lewis RE, et al. Predictors of pulmonary zygomycosis versus invasive pulmonary aspergillosis in patients with cancer. Clin Infect Dis 2005;41(1):60–6.

32. Llata E, Blossom DB, Khoury HJ, et al. A cluster of mucormycosis infections in hematology patients: challenges in investigation and control of invasive mold infections in high-risk patient populations. Diagn Microbiol Infect Dis 2011;71(1): 72–80.

33. Saegeman V, Maertens J, Meersseman W, et al. Increasing incidence of mucormycosis in University Hospital, Belgium. Emerg Infect Dis 2010;16(9): 1456–8.

34. Ruping MJ, Heinz WJ, Kindo AJ, et al. Forty-one recent cases of invasive zygomycosis from a global clinical registry. J Antimicrob Chemother 2010;65(2): 296–302.

35. Sun HY, Aguado JM, Bonatti H, et al. Pulmonary zygomycosis in solid organ transplant recipients in the current era. Am J Transplant 2009;9(9):2166–71.

36. Sun HY, Forrest G, Gupta KL, et al. Rhino-orbital-cerebral zygomycosis in solid organ transplant recipients. Transplantation 2010;90(1):85–92.

37. Almyroudis NG, Sutton DA, Linden P, et al. Zygomycosis in solid organ transplant recipients in a tertiary transplant center and review of the literature. Am J Transplant 2006;6(10):2365–74.

38. Alexander BD, Perfect JR, Daly JS, et al. Posaconazole as salvage therapy in patients with invasive fungal infections after solid organ transplant. Transplantation 2008;86(6):791–6.

39. van Burik JA, Hare RS, Solomon HF, et al. Posaconazole is effective as salvage therapy in zygomycosis: a retrospective summary of 91 cases. Clin Infect Dis 2006;42(7):e61–5.

40. Kontoyiannis DP. Invasive mycoses: strategies for effective management. Am J Med 2012;125(Suppl 1):S25–38.

41. Revankar SG, Sutton DA. Melanized fungi in human disease. Clin Microbiol Rev 2010;23(4):884–928.

42. Raparia K, Powell SZ, Cernoch P, et al. Cerebral mycosis: 7-year retrospective series in a tertiary center. Neuropathology 2010;30(3):218–23.

43. Qureshi ZA, Kwak EJ, Nguyen MH, et al. *Ochroconis gallopava*: a dematiaceous mold causing infections in transplant recipients. Clin Transplant 2012;26(1): E17–23.

44. Harrison DK, Moser S, Palmer CA. Central nervous system infections in transplant recipients by *Cladophialophora bantiana*. South Med J 2008;101(3):292–6.

45. Taj-Aldeen SJ, Almaslamani M, Alkhalf A, et al. Cerebral phaeohyphomycosis due to *Rhinocladiella mackenziei* (formerly *Ramichloridium mackenziei*): a taxonomic update and review of the literature. Med Mycol 2010;48(3):546–56.

46. Lief MH, Caplivski D, Bottone EJ, et al. *Exophiala jeanselmei* infection in solid organ transplant recipients: report of two cases and review of the literature. Transpl Infect Dis 2011;13(1):73–9.

47. Vermeire SE, de Jonge H, Lagrou K, et al. Cutaneous phaeohyphomycosis in renal allograft recipients: report of 2 cases and review of the literature. Diagn Microbiol Infect Dis 2010;68(2):177–80.

48. Boyce RD, Deziel PJ, Otley CC, et al. Phaeohyphomycosis due to *Alternaria* species in transplant recipients. Transpl Infect Dis 2010;12(3):242–50.

49. Nakai T, Uno J, Otomo K, et al. In vitro activity of FK463, a novel lipopeptide antifungal agent, against a variety of clinically important molds. Chemotherapy 2002; 48(2):78–81.

50. Cocuroccia B, Gaido J, Gubinelli E, et al. Localized cutaneous hyalohyphomycosis caused by a *Fusarium* species infection in a renal transplant patient. J Clin Microbiol 2003;41(2):905–7.

51. Sampathkumar P, Paya CV. *Fusarium* infection after solid-organ transplantation. Clin Infect Dis 2001;32(8):1237–40.
52. Halpern M, Balbi E, Carius L, et al. Cellulitis and nodular skin lesions due to *Fusarium* spp in liver transplant: case report. Transplant Proc 2010;42(2):599–600.
53. Kleinschmidt-Demasters BK. Disseminated *Fusarium* infection with brain abscesses in a lung transplant recipient. Clin Neuropathol 2009;28(6):417–21.
54. Lodato F, Tame MR, Montagnani M, et al. Systemic fungemia and hepatic localizations of *Fusarium solani* in a liver transplanted patient: an emerging fungal agent. Liver Transpl 2006;12(11):1711–4.
55. Guinvarc'h A, Guilbert L, Marmorat-Khuong A, et al. Disseminated *Fusarium solani* infection with endocarditis in a lung transplant recipient. Mycoses 1998; 41(1–2):59–61.
56. Nucci M, Anaissie E. *Fusarium infections* in immunocompromised patients. Clin Microbiol Rev 2007;20(4):695–704.
57. Ostrosky-Zeichner L, Alexander BD, Kett DH, et al. Multicenter clinical evaluation of the (1–>3) beta-D-glucan assay as an aid to diagnosis of fungal infections in humans. Clin Infect Dis 2005;41(5):654–9.
58. Cuetara MS, Alhambra A, Moragues MD, et al. Detection of (1–>3)-beta-D-glucan as an adjunct to diagnosis in a mixed population with uncommon proven invasive fungal diseases or with an unusual clinical presentation. Clin Vaccine Immunol 2009;16(3):423–6.
59. Lortholary O, Obenga G, Biswas P, et al. International retrospective analysis of 73 cases of invasive fusariosis treated with voriconazole. Antimicrob Agents Chemother 2010;54(10):4446–50.
60. Gilgado F, Cano J, Gene J, et al. Molecular phylogeny of the *Pseudallescheria boydii* species complex: proposal of two new species. J Clin Microbiol 2005; 43(10):4930–42.
61. Gilgado F, Cano J, Gene J, et al. Molecular and phenotypic data supporting distinct species statuses for *Scedosporium apiospermum* and *Pseudallescheria boydii* and the proposed new species *Scedosporium dehoogii*. J Clin Microbiol 2008;46(2):766–71.
62. Troke P, Aguirrebengoa K, Arteaga C, et al. Treatment of scedosporiosis with voriconazole: clinical experience with 107 patients. Antimicrob Agents Chemother 2008;52(5):1743–50.
63. Figueiredo RT, Fernandez PL, Dutra FF, et al. TLR4 recognizes *Pseudallescheria boydii* conidia and purified rhamnomannans. J Biol Chem 2010;285(52):40714–23.
64. Lackner M, de Hoog GS, Verweij PE, et al. Species-specific antifungal susceptibility patterns of *Scedosporium* and *Pseudallescheria* species. Antimicrob Agents Chemother 2012;56(5):2635–42.
65. Cuenca-Estrella M, Alastruey-Izquierdo A, Alcazar-Fuoli L, et al. In vitro activities of 35 double combinations of antifungal agents against *Scedosporium apiospermum* and *Scedosporium prolificans*. Antimicrob Agents Chemother 2008;52(3): 1136–9.
66. Rodriguez MM, Calvo E, Serena C, et al. Effects of double and triple combinations of antifungal drugs in a murine model of disseminated infection by *Scedosporium prolificans*. Antimicrob Agents Chemother 2009;53(5):2153–5.
67. Meletiadis J, Mouton JW, Meis JF, et al. In vitro drug interaction modeling of combinations of azoles with terbinafine against clinical *Scedosporium prolificans* isolates. Antimicrob Agents Chemother 2003;47(1):106–17.
68. Orth B, Frei R, Itin PH, et al. Outbreak of invasive mycoses caused by *Paecilomyces lilacinus* from a contaminated skin lotion. Ann Intern Med 1996;125(10):799–806.

69. Pastor FJ, Guarro J. Clinical manifestations, treatment and outcome of *Paecilomyces lilacinus* infections. Clin Microbiol Infect 2006;12(10):948–60.

70. Lavergne RA, Cassaing S, Nocera T, et al. Simultaneous cutaneous infection due to *Paecilomyces lilacinus* and *Alternaria* in a heart transplant patient. Transpl Infect Dis 2012;14:E156–60.

71. Kim JE, Sung H, Kim MN, et al. Synchronous infection with *Mycobacterium chelonae* and *Paecilomyces* in a heart transplant patient. Transpl Infect Dis 2011; 13(1):80–3.

72. Ounissi M, Abderrahim E, Trabelsi S, et al. Hyalohyphomycosis caused by *Paecilomyces lilacinus* after kidney transplantation. Transplant Proc 2009;41(7):2917–9.

73. Van Schooneveld T, Freifeld A, Lesiak B, et al. *Paecilomyces lilacinus* infection in a liver transplant patient: case report and review of the literature. Transpl Infect Dis 2008;10(2):117–22.

74. Lacasse A, Cleveland KO. *Trichosporon mucoides* fungemia in a liver transplant recipient: case report and review. Transpl Infect Dis 2009;11(2):155–9.

75. Biasoli MS, Carlson D, Chiganer GJ, et al. Systemic infection caused by *Trichosporon asahii* in a patient with liver transplant. Med Mycol 2008;46(7):719–23.

76. Lussier N, Laverdiere M, Delorme J, et al. *Trichosporon beigelii* funguria in renal transplant recipients. Clin Infect Dis 2000;31(5):1299–301.

77. Nettles RE, Nichols LS, Bell-McGuinn K, et al. Successful treatment of *Trichosporon mucoides* infection with fluconazole in a heart and kidney transplant recipient. Clin Infect Dis 2003;36(4):E63–6.

78. Wuyts WA, Molzahn H, Maertens J, et al. Fatal *Scopulariopsis* infection in a lung transplant recipient: a case report. J Heart Lung Transplant 2005;24(12):2301–4.

79. Beaudreuil S, Buchler M, Al Najjar A, et al. Acute septic arthritis after kidney transplantation due to *Acremonium*. Nephrol Dial Transplant 2003;18(4):850–1.

80. Chouaki T, Lavarde V, Lachaud L, et al. Invasive infections due to *Trichoderma* species: report of 2 cases, findings of in vitro susceptibility testing, and review of the literature. Clin Infect Dis 2002;35(11):1360–7.

Management Strategies for Cytomegalovirus Infection and Disease in Solid Organ Transplant Recipients

Raymund R. Razonable, MD

KEYWORDS

- Cytomegalovirus • Graft failure • Allograft rejection • Valganciclovir • Viral load
- Polymerase chain reaction • Nucleic acid testing

KEY POINTS

- Cytomegalovirus (CMV) is the most common viral pathogen that infects solid organ transplant recipients. Infection may be asymptomatic or it can lead to a febrile illness or tissue-invasive disease, which most commonly affects the gastrointestinal tract.
- Transplant recipients at highest risk of CMV disease are those without preexisting CMV-specific immunity and those who have received severe pharmacologic immunosuppression. Hence, CMV-seronegative patients who received organ allograft from CMV-seropositive donors, and those who received lymphocyte-depleting drugs, are considered at highest risk.
- CMV is associated with poor allograft and patient survival after transplantation. Its prevention is therefore key in the management of every transplant recipient. The 2 methods for prevention are antiviral prophylaxis and preemptive therapy. Both strategies are effective in preventing CMV disease. Antiviral prophylaxis may also prevent the indirect effects of CMV infection but is associated with late-onset CMV disease, especially among CMV D+/R− recipients.
- Nucleic acid testing is the most commonly used method for the diagnosis of CMV infection after transplantation. The recent availability of an International Standard for Quantification, by the World Health Organization, should help standardize reporting among various nucleic acid amplification tests. The other method commonly used for the diagnosis of CMV infection is pp95 antigenemia. Histopathology to document tissue-invasive CMV disease may be necessary in certain situations.
- Valganciclovir is the drug of choice for the prevention of CMV disease. The duration of antiviral prophylaxis varies depending on the risk profile and organ transplant type. Recent trials suggest that longer durations of prophylaxis may be better in CMV disease prevention for high-risk kidney and lung transplant recipients.

Continued

Disclosures: None.
Conflict of Interest: None.
Division of Infectious Diseases, The William J von Liebig Transplant Center, Mayo Clinic, Marian Hall 5, 200 First Street Southwest, Rochester, MN 55905, USA
E-mail address: razonable.raymund@mayo.edu

Infect Dis Clin N Am 27 (2013) 317–342
http://dx.doi.org/10.1016/j.idc.2013.02.005
0891-5520/13/$ – see front matter © 2013 Elsevier Inc. All rights reserved.

Continued

- Valganciclovir and intravenous ganciclovir are the drugs of choice for the treatment of CMV disease. Valganciclovir is used for mild to moderate cases, whereas intravenous ganciclovir should be used for the treatment of severe and life-threatening CMV disease, those with gastrointestinal involvement when absorption is questionable, and those with very high viral load. The duration of treatment should be guided by clinical viral load monitoring. It is generally recommended that treatment be continued until viral load is no longer detected in the blood.
- Drug-resistant CMV is an emerging concern, and is heralded by persistence or increase in viral load or recurrence of clinical symptoms. Resistance should be documented by genotypic assays to determine the mutation involved in UL54 and UL97 genes. Treatment of drug-resistant CMV is difficult, and often involves nephrotoxic drugs. The choice of definitive therapy should be guided by genotypic assay.

INTRODUCTION

Cytomegalovirus (CMV), a double-stranded DNA virus, is one of the most common infections that adversely affect the outcome of solid organ transplantation (SOT). It is the fifth member of the human herpesvirus family (human herpesvirus 5) and 1 of the 3 human β-herpes viruses (together with human herpesvirus 6 [HHV-6] and HHV-7). CMV is widely distributed and infects most people.[1] In the United States, the CMV seroprevalence rate is about 50%,[2] although the rate varies depending on age, gender, ethnicity, and socioeconomic status. Worldwide, the seroprevalence rate ranges from as low as 30% in industrialized and developed countries to as high as 97% in developing nations.[2,3]

Infection with CMV is acquired from exposure to infected saliva and other body secretions.[1] Primary CMV infection in immunocompetent individuals manifests as an asymptomatic or self-limited febrile illness.[1] In some, CMV infection may mimic an infectious mononucleosislike illness characterized by fever and lymphadenopathy. A robust CMV-specific humoral and cell-mediated immunity develops during infection in immunocompetent individuals.[4] Despite this immunity, CMV infection is not eradicated and the virus establishes lifelong latency in various cells of an infected individual.[2,3]

Human cells harboring latent virus serve as reservoirs for viral reactivation and as vehicles for transmission of CMV infection. In healthy individuals, CMV reactivates intermittently throughout life; however, these episodes are controlled by a functioning immune system and do not generally result in clinical illness.[5] In individuals with suppressed immune function, such as transplant recipients, these reactivation events may lead to a potentially severe clinical disease. In addition, latently infected cells serve as carriers that transmit infection to susceptible individuals. This characteristic serves as the major mechanism of primary CMV infection in SOT recipients.[6,7]

This article reviews the epidemiology, clinical manifestations, and diagnosis of CMV disease in SOT recipients. Advances in its prevention and treatment are discussed, together with novel antiviral therapeutics and vaccines.

EPIDEMIOLOGY AND MECHANISMS OF CMV INFECTION AND DISEASE

CMV is the most common viral infection affecting SOT recipients.[6] Without antiviral prophylaxis, CMV infection occurs in up to 75% of SOT recipients.[8] The incidence varies depending on the type of transplanted organ. Recipients of lungs and intestinal transplants have the highest risk, whereas recipients of heart and liver have moderate risk, and recipients of kidney transplants have the lowest risk of CMV infection and disease (**Table 1**).[8–11] CMV serostatus of the donor and recipient, which reflects previous infection and the presence (or absence) of preexisting CMV-specific immunity, greatly influences the risk of CMV disease.[9–11] CMV disease risk is dependent on the overall state of immunosuppression, with incidence rates highest among patients with severely impaired immunity,[12] such as those receiving lymphocyte-depleting agents for treatment of rejection.[8,13]

CMV infection may occur after SOT as (1) primary infection, (2) reactivation infection, or (3) superinfection. Primary CMV infection occurs when a CMV-seronegative SOT recipient receives an allograft from a CMV-seropositive donor (CMV D+/R–). CMV D+/R– mismatched category, which is estimated in 20% of SOT patients, is the highest-risk group for CMV disease.[1] CMV disease that occurs in CMV D+/R– individuals could be clinically severe because of the absence of preexisting CMV-specific immunity. CMV-seronegative SOT recipients may further acquire primary CMV infection from infected individuals in the community (through natural transmission), or from transfusion of blood from CMV-seropositive donors. To reduce the risk from acquiring CMV through blood transfusion, CMV-seronegative SOT recipients should receive leuko-reduced blood products or those obtained from CMV-seronegative blood donors.[14]

Among CMV-seropositive SOT recipients (CMV R+), CMV disease may occur either as (1) reactivation (when endogenous latent virus in the recipient reactivates to cause infection) or (2) superinfection (when latent virus in donor cells reactivates to cause CMV infection).[7,15] Transmission of multiple CMV strains from the donor may occur, and superinfection may be more common than endogenous latent viral reactivation.[7,15] Generally, secondary infections (through reactivation and superinfection) cause CMV disease of lesser severity (compared with primary infection) because patients have preexisting CMV-specific immunity that mitigates viral replication. Studies on viral dynamics show the slower viral replication cycle in CMV R+ recipients compared with the very rapid viral replication in CMV D+/R– SOT recipients.[16–18] In 1 study, the growth rate of CMV in CMV R+ individuals (0.61 units/d) was significantly slower than in CMV D+/R– individuals (1.82 units/d).[16]

Without prevention strategy, CMV infection and disease typically occur during the first 3 months after SOT.[19–23] However, this onset of infection has been delayed by

---

Table 1
Risk factors for CMV infection in SOT recipients

Traditional Risk Factors	Recently Described Risk Factors
CMV D+/R–	Toll-like receptor 2 polymorphism
Lack of CMV-specific CD4+ T cells	Toll-like receptor 4 polymorphism
Lack of CMV-specific CD8+ T cells	Mannose-binding lectin deficiency
Allograft rejection	Chemokine and cytokine defects (interleukin 10,
High viral replication	monocyte chemotactic protein 1, C-C chemokine
Type of organ transplant	receptor type 5)
Mycophenolate mofetil	
Muromonab-CD3	
Antithymocyte globulin	
Alemtuzumab	
HHV-6	
HHV-7	
Renal insufficiency	

antiviral prophylaxis. In patients receiving antiviral prophylaxis, CMV infection and disease occurs during the first 3 months after completing CMV prophylaxis.[19–23] Beyond this period, the risk of CMV disease is generally low, although sporadic cases continue to occur, especially in SOT recipients with a higher degree of immunosuppression.[24] Hence, clinicians should continue to consider CMV as a potential cause of compatible clinical illness that occurs beyond the traditional high-risk period.[24,25] In our clinical experience, these very-late-onset cases generally present with gastrointestinal symptoms, and in some cases, they may not be detected in the blood.[24]

CLINICAL MANIFESTATIONS OF CMV DISEASE

CMV infection in SOT recipients can be symptomatic or asymptomatic. Asymptomatic CMV infection is indicated only by the presence of CMV in the blood, in the absence of any signs and symptoms. CMV infection can be shown by (1) viral nucleic acid testing (NAT), (2) CMV pp65 antigenemia, and (3) viral culture. The clinical impact of asymptomatic CMV infection is debated, and some data suggest that it increases the risk of allograft failure and all-cause mortality.[26]

Symptomatic CMV infection is termed CMV disease, which could be categorized into CMV syndrome or tissue-invasive CMV disease.[27,28] CMV syndrome is the more common clinical manifestation, and is characterized by fever, malaise, flulike illness, leukopenia, or thrombocytopenia (**Table 2**).[10,11,22] In some cases, there is evidence of end-organ disease (termed tissue-invasive CMV disease), which most commonly involves the gastrointestinal tract.[10,11,29] Gastrointestinal CMV disease generally manifests with diarrhea and abdominal pain.[29] There is a predilection to involve the transplanted allograft so that CMV pneumonitis, hepatitis, nephritis, myocarditis, and pancreatitis are observed more commonly among lung, liver, kidney, heart, and pancreas recipients, respectively.[1] This allograft predilection may be caused by (1) the practice of obtaining tissue biopsies if there is evidence of allograft dysfunction, (2) the fact that the allograft harbors the virus that reactivates during periods of immunosuppression, and (3) aberrant immune response within the allograft.[8] CMV pneumonitis is particularly severe among lung recipients, and often with long-lasting effects on lung function.[9] Virtually any organ system can be involved by

Table 2	
Direct and indirect effects of CMV in SOT recipients	
Direct Effects	**Indirect Effects**
CMV syndrome	Acute allograft rejection
Tissue-invasive CMV disease	Chronic allograft rejection
Gastrointestinal disease	Bronchiolitis obliterans
Pneumonitis	Transplant vasculopathy
Hepatitis	Tubulointerstitial fibrosis
Central nervous system disease	Opportunistic and other infections
Retinitis	Fungal superinfection
Nephritis	Nocardiosis
Pancreatitis	Bacterial superinfection
Myocarditis	Epstein-Barr virus and posttransplant
Others (any organ may be involved)	lymphoproliferative disorder
Mortality	Hepatitis C recurrence
	Other viruses (HHV-6, HHV-7)
	New-onset diabetes mellitus
	Thrombosis
	Mortality

CMV, and there have been occasional reports of cholecystitis,[30] epididymitis,[31] and retinitis.[32] CMV retinitis is rare in SOT recipients and occurs generally late, often in the context of a multiorgan CMV disease.[32] Intrauterine transmission causing congenital CMV infection has been reported in infants of transplant recipients.[33]

In addition to direct effects, CMV has numerous indirect effects because of its ability to modulate the immune system (see **Table 2**). CMV is associated with increased incidence of other infections caused by bacterial pathogens,[34] fungal pathogens,[35] and viruses (ie, Epstein-Barr virus–associated posttransplant lymphoproliferative disease).[36] The increased predisposition to develop these infections is believed to be caused by immune exhaustion during CMV infection.[37] Alternatively (or in addition), CMV infection could be a marker of a globally overimmunosuppressed status (from pharmacologic immunosuppressive therapy), and hence the likelihood of infection with other opportunistic pathogens.[8] CMV infection has been associated with poor allograft survival,[11,38,39] likely because of its influence on acute rejection and chronic allograft injury.[8,40] In this regard, kidney recipients with CMV are more likely to develop chronic allograft nephropathy (or tubulointerstitial fibrosis).[41] Likewise, lung recipients with CMV are at increased risk of bronchiolitis obliterans,[42] whereas heart recipients are at increased risk of accelerated coronary vasculopathy if they developed CMV infection and disease.[43,44]

CMV disease is associated with increased risk of death after SOT.[11,38] Ganciclovir use for prevention and treatment has led to marked reduction in death caused by CMV disease.[45] However, even in the era of effective prevention strategies, the association between CMV disease and death continues. In a cohort of 259 liver recipients, CMV disease that occurred despite antiviral prophylaxis was independently associated with mortality (hazard ratio 14 [95% confidence interval 3.8–54]).[38] In another cohort of 227 high-risk CMV D+/R– liver recipients,[46] CMV infection was associated with an increased risk of death (risk ratio [RR] 2.24) and graft loss or death (RR 2.85). Likewise, CMV disease was associated with an increased risk of death (RR 2.73) and graft loss or death (RR 3.04).[46] A statistically significant association was also observed between tissue-invasive CMV disease and allograft loss or mortality (hazard ratio, 2.85; 95% confidence interval, 1.22–6.67) in a cohort of 176 kidney and pancreas transplant recipients.[11]

RISK FACTORS OF CMV IN SOT

Several factors predispose SOT recipients to develop CMV infection (see **Table 1**). Foremost among the risk factors is having a CMV D+/R– serologic status.[7] Because latent CMV is present in the allograft, its transmission is expected during transplantation. Reactivation of the donor-transmitted latent virus results in primary CMV infection, which could be severe because of lack of preexisting CMV-specific immunity.[47] As discussed, CMV replication is rapid,[48,49] and leads to a high incidence of clinical disease.[7]

The net state of immunosuppression is another major factor that increases the risk of CMV disease. The intensity of the immunosuppressive protocol is influenced by the type of drug, its dose, and duration of use. Lymphocyte-depleting immunosuppressive drugs such as antithymocyte globulin, alemtuzumab, and muromunab-CD3 (OKT3) are specifically associated with increased risk of CMV infection and disease, especially when used for rejection.[50] These drugs severely deplete the number and impair the function of T lymphocytes, which are essential for the control of viruses. High doses of mycophenolate mofetil have also been associated with increased risk of CMV disease.[51] In contrast, the use of mammalian target of rapamycin (mTOR) inhibitors (sirolimus and everolimus) for maintenance immunosuppression has been associated with lower risk of CMV.[52] Several host factors also contribute to the net state of immunosuppression, such as lymphopenia (from any cause), comorbidities, and genetic factors.[53–55] Defects in innate immune recognition and cytokine defects as a result of genetic mutations have been associated with CMV disease.[54,55] For example, polymorphisms in mannose-binding lectin and toll-like receptor 2 genes are associated with increased risk of CMV disease after SOT.[47,55–57]

As discussed, the risk of CMV disease varies by the transplant type, likely in part because of the amount of lymphoid tissue in transplanted allograft (risk is directly related to the amount of lymphoid tissue harboring latent CMV) and intensity of immunosuppression. Allograft rejection is also highly associated with CMV disease.[13] There is a bidirectional relationship between allograft rejection and CMV disease.[8] Although CMV increases the risk of allograft rejection, allograft rejection conversely increases the risk of CMV reactivation.[8] Moreover, the ensuing treatment of acute allograft rejection, especially with lymphocyte-depleting agents or high-dose corticosteroids, further increases the risk of CMV disease by impairing the generation of T lymphocytes necessary for controlling CMV.[8] Coinfections with HHV-6 and HHV-7 have been suggested to increase CMV disease risk in kidney and liver transplant recipients,[58] potentially because of their immunomodulating property.

LABORATORY DIAGNOSIS

Molecular assays that detect and quantify CMV nucleic acid have emerged as the most common method for diagnosis of CMV infection in SOT recipients.[59] Other laboratory methods to confirm CMV are (1) histopathology, (2) culture, (3) serology, and (4) antigenemia (**Table 3**).[59]

Histopathology

Histopathology remains as the gold standard for the diagnosis of tissue-invasive CMV disease. CMV is indicated by an enlargement of the cell and its nucleus and the presence of basophilic cytoplasmic inclusions (known as cytomegalic cells).[59] In situ hybridization and immunohistochemical testing may be needed to confirm the diagnosis.[59] This method entails an invasive procedure to obtain tissue for diagnosis, and there is occasional hesitancy by clinicians to perform these procedures. Accordingly, the use of histopathology to diagnose tissue-invasive CMV disease has declined, especially with the availability of noninvasive or less invasive tests to document CMV in the blood.[29]

Histopathology is recommended in cases in which allograft rejection is a diagnostic consideration. It is not uncommon for the transplanted allograft to be affected by tissue-invasive CMV disease. Clinically, it is difficult to differentiate CMV disease from allograft rejection, and sometimes the 2 conditions coexist, hence, tissue biopsy may be required for diagnosis. Differentiation of these conditions is important to ensure that optimal therapy is provided. Nonresolution of clinical symptoms and laboratory abnormalities despite anti-CMV therapy should raise the suspicion of allograft rejection or the presence of concomitant pathogens. For example, CMV colitis may coexist with another gastrointestinal infection such as *Clostridium difficile*[60] or parasitic infection (eg, *Cryptosporidium parvum*).[61]

Histopathology is needed when CMV disease is suspected but CMV testing in the blood is negative, such as in some cases of gastrointestinal CMV disease.[29] Histopathology may also be needed to document resolution of certain cases of severe gastrointestinal CMV disease.[29] However, repeated histopathology to document clearance of CMV infection in the affected organ, such as the gastrointestinal tract, should not be routinely performed.[29] In 1 study, the risk of CMV relapse did not significantly differ between those who had documented histologic resolution of infection compared with those who did not have documented histologic resolution.[29]

Serology

Serology to detect CMV-immunoglobulin M (IgM) and IgG antibodies is the most common test to document CMV infection in immunocompetent hosts. CMV induces development of IgM early in the course of infection (acute or recent infection) and followed later by IgG antibodies (past or latent infection). However, CMV serology has a limited usefulness for diagnosis of acute CMV disease after transplantation.[14] Because of pharmacologic immunosuppression, SOT recipients have delayed or impaired ability to develop antibody responses.[62]

The main clinical indication of CMV serology testing in transplantation is the pre-transplant screening of donors and transplant candidates.[14] Because CMV-IgG persists for life, it serves as surrogate of previous or latent CMV infection.[14] Knowledge of CMV serology of the donor and recipient assists in stratifying the risk of CMV disease after SOT into high risk (CMV D+/R−), moderate risk (CMV D+/R+ > CMV D−/R+), and low risk (CMV D−/R−).[14]

Viral Culture

Culture is highly specific for the diagnosis of CMV infection.[59] The test can be performed on blood, respiratory secretions (including bronchoalveolar lavage), cerebrospinal fluid (CSF), and tissue biopsy specimens.[59] Virus culture may be performed in urine specimen, but the specificity of urine sample in the diagnosis of CMV in adults is debated, because shedding of the virus may occur even in healthy adults.[14,59] Conversely, urine for CMV culture remains highly useful for diagnosis of CMV infection in pediatric SOT recipients.[14]

Viral culture is limited by its modest sensitivity and slow turnaround time.[59] Conventional tissue culture may take weeks before the virus can be detected. Shell vial centrifugation assay has a more rapid turnaround time, but it remains less sensitive compared with molecular assays.[59] Because of the relatively slower turnaround time and lower sensitivity, viral culture is rarely used to guide contemporary clinical practice. However, it is still needed when phenotypic antiviral drug resistance testing is requested, although genotypic assays are also now the method of choice for this.[63–67]

Antigenemia

CMV antigenemia assay is an assay that detects the pp65 antigen in CMV-infected peripheral blood leukocytes.[59] Because pp65 is secreted during CMV replication, its detection signifies active infection. Polymorphonuclear leukocyte preparations are stained with monoclonal antibodies against pp65 and the number of positive cells is reported. CMV antigenemia has higher sensitivity than virus culture, and is comparable with NAT by polymerase chain reaction (PCR).[59,68]

The severity of CMV infection is estimated by the number of pp65-positive cells. Its detection in a patient with compatible symptoms confirms the diagnosis of CMV disease. CMV antigenemia is used also to detect early CMV replication, and guide the initiation of preemptive therapy.[14] CMV antigenemia is used to guide the efficacy of antiviral treatment.[59] The number of pp65-positive leukocytes is expected to decline during the course of effective antiviral treatment. Its persistence or increase may indicate drug-resistant virus or the need to further reduce immunosuppression.

Table 3
Laboratory methods for the diagnosis of CMV in transplant recipients

Methods	Principle	Sample and Equipment	Turnaround Time	Clinical Usefulness	Advantages	Disadvantages
Serology	Antibody detection (IgG, IgM)	Serology facility	6 h	IgG indicates previous infection IgM implies acute or recent infection	Screening of donors and recipients before transplantation Screening transplant recipients after transplantation to detect seroconversion	Delayed antibody production in transplant recipients (false-negative results) False-positive IgM screening results
Virus culture						
Tube culture	Viral replication	Recovery of PMN within few hours; cell culture facility; light microscopy	2–4 wk	Detection of cytopathic effects	High specificity for infection and disease Phenotypic susceptibility testing	Prolonged processing time Low sensitivity Rapid loss of CMV viability ex vivo (false-negative results)

Shell vial assay	Viral replication	Recovery of PMN within few hours; cell culture facility; immunofluorescence detection	16–48 h	Infectious foci detected by monoclonal antibody directed to immediate early antigen (72 kDa) of CMV	High specificity for CMV infection and disease; More sensitive and rapid than tube cultures	Relatively low sensitivity compared with molecular methods
Antigenemia	pp65 Antigen	Recovery of PMN within 4–6 h; Cytospin; light microscopy or immunofluorescence	6–24 h	Number of CMV-infected cells per total (eg, 2×10^5) cells evaluated; early detection of CMV replication	Rapid diagnosis of CMV; Guide for initiation of preemptive therapy; Guide for treatment responses	Subjective interpretation of results; Requires rapid processing
Nucleic acid detection	DNA or RNA	Plasma, whole blood, leukocytes, other body fluids	4–24 h	Reported as CMV copies per milliliter of sample (should now be standardized to IU/ml of sample); Detection of CMV infection; monitor CMV DNA decline; surrogate marker for antiviral drug resistance	Highly sensitive; Correlation with clinical disease severity; Guides preemptive therapy; Rapid diagnosis of CMV infection and disease; Monitor therapeutic response	Modest positive predictive value for CMV disease; Needs standardization among various assays

Abbreviation: PMN, polymorphonuclear neutrophils.

The disadvantages of CMV antigenemia are its labor-intensive and manual nature of testing, the subjective interpretation of the results, and its limited interlaboratory standardization. The assay also requires the processing of the blood sample within few hours because it is dependent on the life span of leukocytes ex vivo. Because the test relies on leukocytes, antigenemia assay has limited usefulness and may be falsely negative in patients with severe leukopenia.[59]

Molecular Assays

Molecular assays have emerged as the preferred methods for rapid diagnosis of CMV after SOT.[59] The assays detect CMV DNA or RNA in blood and other clinical specimens including CSF, bronchoalveolar lavage fluid, and urine. Several platforms are available for CMV NAT, which until recently lacked standardization.

Detection of CMV RNA indicates CMV replication, highly specific for active CMV infection, and highly correlated with clinical disease.[59] However, CMV RNA detection is not as sensitive as CMV DNA testing.[59] Although it is more sensitive, CMV DNA testing is less specific for active CMV replication because a highly sensitive CMV DNA test may detect latent viral DNA. To increase specificity, laboratories have developed quantitative NAT (QNAT).[59] Active CMV replication is indicated by high or an increasing trend in viral load, whereas low-level viral load may indicate detection of latent viral DNA.[59]

The degree of viral replication, as measured by QNAT, is directly correlated to the severity of clinical disease. Higher viral loads are generally observed in CMV D+/R– compared with CMV R+ SOT recipients. Higher CMV viral loads are associated with symptomatic compared with asymptomatic infection, and with tissue-invasive CMV disease compared with CMV syndrome.[69] In addition to absolute viral load counts, trends (or changes) in viral load (increasing levels) may be monitored to indicate the rate of CMV replication.[16,18,69] Risk of CMV disease is significantly higher in SOT recipients with a faster increase in viral load over time.[16,18]

CMV QNAT using blood sample is highly sensitive for diagnosis of CMV infection and disease.[59,70] In many cases (as discussed earlier), CMV QNAT has obviated obtaining tissue for diagnosis of tissue-invasive CMV disease.[14] For example, the diagnosis of gastrointestinal tissue-invasive CMV disease may be suggested by a positive QNAT in a patient presenting with diarrhea and other symptoms. However, there are occasional patients with very low to undetectable viral load in the blood despite having tissue-invasive CMV disease.[24] These patients with low to undetectable CMV viral load are mostly CMV R+, presenting with very-late-onset (occurring years after transplant) gastrointestinal CMV disease and those with CMV retinitis.[24,29,32] The nondetectable viral load may be caused by CMV disease compartmentalization (occurring only in 1 specific organ without systemic dissemination), or the use of QNAT assay of very low sensitivity.

QNAT is useful for guiding the initiation of preemptive therapy.[59] In addition, QNAT is useful for guiding responses to treatment of CMV infection and disease.[59] Decline in viral load indicates that SOT recipients are responding appropriately to antiviral treatment. In some cases, the viral load may increase during the first 2 weeks of antiviral treatment. Although this may be a natural course in some, its occurrence should suggest the potential for drug-resistant CMV disease.[14]

The major drawback to QNAT was the lack (until recently) of an international reference for assay standardization.[71,72] Studies during the past decade have indicated that various CMV DNA tests are not directly comparable.[73] Because of differences in assay platform, clinical samples, calibrator standards, gene target, and extraction techniques, among others,[71] there was up to a $3-log_{10}$ variation in CMV viral load reports among different CMV QNAT assays.[72] Accordingly, the viral load results of 1 assay cannot be directly extrapolated as equal to that of another assay.[71,74] This lack of assay standardization has limited the generation of widely applicable viral thresholds for preemptive therapy, disease prognostication, and therapeutic monitoring. In 2011, the World Health Organization (WHO) released the first International Reference Standard for the quantification of CMV nucleic acid. Laboratory and commercially developed CMV QNAT assays should now be calibrated to this standard, so that there is uniformity in viral load reporting, thereby facilitating the scientific and medical community to define viral thresholds for various clinical applications.[14]

PREVENTION OF CMV DISEASE

The negative impact of CMV on transplant morbidity and outcomes has made its prevention an essential component in the posttransplant care of SOT recipients. The 2 major strategies for CMV prevention are: (1) antiviral prophylaxis and (2) preemptive therapy. Antiviral prophylaxis entails the administration of an antiviral drug (most commonly valganciclovir) to all at-risk SOT recipients for a defined period after transplantation. Preemptive therapy, on the other hand, is the administration of antiviral drug only in the presence of asymptomatic CMV replication to prevent its progression to CMV disease. Which of the 2 approaches is optimal for CMV prevention is subject to debate, but it is likely influenced by the population at risk, the availability of laboratory assays, and the logistic support in the transplant center. Clinical trials directly comparing the benefits and adverse effects of both approaches are limited to only few randomized trials in kidney recipients.[39,40,75,76] These few studies show that although both are similarly effective for CMV disease prevention, long-term graft survival was superior with antiviral prophylaxis.[39]

There are certain benefits and drawbacks of antiviral prophylaxis and preemptive therapy that may influence which approach is used for CMV prevention (**Table 4**).[47] Antiviral prophylaxis prevents the reactivation not only of CMV but also of other herpes viruses such as herpes simplex viruses 1 and 2, and HHV-6.[6,8,14] It has also been

Table 4
Characteristics of antiviral prophylaxis and preemptive therapy

	Antiviral Prophylaxis	Preemptive Therapy
Efficacy	Highly efficacious for CMV disease prevention Risk of late-onset CMV disease	Prevents CMV disease but not CMV infection
Logistics of use	Needs monitoring of potential adverse effects such as leukopenia	Difficult to coordinate weekly viral load testing and results follow-up Viral load thresholds not standardized
Late-onset CMV disease	Common among CMV D+/R– transplant recipients	Less common
Cost	Higher drug costs	Higher laboratory costs
Toxicity	Greater drug toxicity (leukopenia and bone marrow suppression)	Less drug toxicity (shorter courses of antiviral treatment)
Indirect effects (graft loss, mortality, and opportunistic infections)	Reduction in indirect effects	May not reduce indirect effects (limited data available)
Drug resistance	Yes (but still uncommon)	Yes (but still uncommon)

associated with reduced incidence of infections caused by bacteria and fungi.[6,8,14] Antiviral prophylaxis has been associated with a lower incidence of other major indirect CMV effects, including allograft rejection and allograft loss,[77,78] and improvement in allograft and patient survival.[77,78] The disadvantages of antiviral prophylaxis are the increased antiviral drug cost, higher drug-related toxicity, and a higher incidence of late-onset CMV disease among CMV D+/R− SOT recipients.[13,19–22] In contrast, preemptive therapy is associated with lower antiviral drug costs and fewer adverse drug toxicities. However, the cost saved from lower antiviral drug use is offset by the cost of laboratory testing (QNAT or antigenemia) and the increased logistic coordination that is required. Because of the logistic difficulty of coordinating CMV surveillance testing, preemptive strategy may be a difficult preventive approach for patients residing at considerable distance from the transplant center. The risk of CMV drug resistance has traditionally been associated with antiviral prophylaxis,[64] but recent data indicated an increasing frequency of drug-resistant CMV in patients receiving preemptive therapy.[63–66,79,80]

Antiviral Prophylaxis

The drugs for antiviral prophylaxis are listed in **Table 5**. Valganciclovir is the most common drug for prophylaxis (**Table 6**). Alternatives are oral ganciclovir (limited by poor bioavailability) and intravenous ganciclovir (limited by the need for intravenous access). The efficacy of ganciclovir and valganciclovir prophylaxis has been shown in clinical trials, including a few that directly compared the 2 drugs.[19–22] In a randomized trial of 372 CMV D+/R− kidney, liver, pancreas, and heart recipients, the incidence of CMV disease was comparable between patients who received 3 months of oral ganciclovir and those who received valganciclovir prophylaxis (17.2% valganciclovir compared with 18.4% ganciclovir at 12 months, respectively).[19] In a subgroup analysis of this trial, there was a surprisingly higher rate of CMV disease in liver recipients who received valganciclovir compared with oral ganciclovir prophylaxis. As a result of this finding, the US Food and Drug Administration (FDA) has cautioned against valganciclovir prophylaxis in liver recipients, although many experts still recommend its use in liver recipients.[14,81] A survey of liver transplant centers also reported that valganciclovir is the most common antiviral drug for CMV prevention, despite the FDA caution.[81] The improved bioavailability of valganciclovir and its lower pill burden make it the preferred drug for CMV prophylaxis.[81]

For kidney recipients, valacyclovir is also an effective alternative for CMV prophylaxis. In a randomized placebo-controlled clinical trial, valacyclovir prophylaxis for 3 months significantly prevented CMV disease in modest-risk to high-risk kidney recipients.[21] However, valacyclovir use was associated with neurologic adverse effects and the need for large drug doses. Valacyclovir has not been proved to be an effective drug for the prevention of CMV disease in liver, heart, and lung transplant recipients.[14]

A major consequence of antiviral prophylaxis is late-onset CMV disease, which remains to be significantly associated with allograft failure and mortality after transplantation.[11,38] The potential options for the prevention and management of late-onset CMV disease are: (1) clinical follow-up with early treatment of CMV disease when symptoms occur; (2) virologic surveillance after completion of antiviral prophylaxis, or (3) prolonging antiviral prophylaxis. Regardless of which approach to use, it is important that SOT recipients (especially CMV D+/R−) be advised of the risk of late-onset CMV disease on cessation of antiviral prophylaxis so they seek immediate consultation when signs and symptoms develop. Alternatively, patients who completed prophylaxis may be monitored using pp65 antigenemia or QNAT so that CMV reactivation can be detected early for initiation of antiviral treatment (ie, hybrid

Table 5
Antiviral drugs for CMV prevention and treatment

Drug	Preemptive Therapy and Treatment of CMV Disease	Antiviral Prophylaxis	Comments on Use and Toxicity
Valganciclovir	900 mg by mouth twice daily	900 mg by mouth once daily	Ease of administration Leukopenia
Oral ganciclovir	Not recommended	1 g by mouth 3 times daily	Low oral bioavailability High pill burden Leukopenia Risk of resistance
IV ganciclovir	5 mg/kg IV every 12 h	5 mg/kg IV once daily	IV access Leukopenia
Valacyclovir	Not recommended	2 g by mouth 4 times daily	Kidney transplant recipients only Not recommended for heart, liver, pancreas, lung, intestinal, and composite tissue transplant recipients High pill burden Neurologic adverse effects
Foscarnet	60 mg/kg IV every 8 h (or 90 mg/kg every 12 h) Not recommended for preemptive therapy	Not recommended	Second-line agent for treatment Highly nephrotoxic Treatment of UL97-mutant ganciclovir-resistant CMV
Cidofovir	5 mg/kg once weekly × 2 then every 2 wk thereafter Not recommended for preemptive therapy	Not recommended	Third-line agent Highly nephrotoxic Treatment of UL97-mutant ganciclovir-resistant CMV

Note: CMV Ig has been used by some centers as an adjunct to antiviral prophylaxis, especially in heart and lung transplant recipients. The doses of the antiviral drugs provided are only for adults and should be adjusted based on renal function.
Abbreviation: IV, intravenous.

approach of prophylaxis followed by preemptive therapy).[82,83] The clinical usefulness of this approach is questionable.[82,83] Extending the duration of antiviral prophylaxis has been shown to be effective in further reducing the risk of CMV disease in CMV D+/R− kidney recipients[22] and lung recipients.[84] In a randomized clinical trial that compared 200 versus 100 days of valganciclovir prophylaxis in 318 CMV D+/R− kidney recipients,[22] the incidence of CMV disease was 16.1% versus 36.8% in the 200-day versus 100-day groups, respectively.[22] Similar studies to assess the optimal duration in liver, heart, and pancreas transplant recipients have not been performed, although many centers have already extrapolated these results in the prevention of CMV disease in liver, heart, and pancreas recipients.[14]

Lung recipients are at highest risk of CMV disease among SOT recipients. Studies have shown high incidence of CMV disease with 3 months or short courses of antiviral prophylaxis (less than 6 months).[85] Extending the duration of prophylaxis to at least 6 months was associated with a lower rate of CMV disease.[86] A recent multicenter trial conducted in CMV D+/R− and CMV D+/R+ lung recipients further showed that the incidence of CMV disease and viremia is further reduced in patients who received 12 months of valganciclovir prophylaxis (4% and 10%, respectively) compared with

---

Table 6
Recommendations for the prevention of CMV in SOT recipients

Organ	Risk Category	Recommendation/Options
Heart, kidney, liver, pancreas	D+/R−	Antiviral prophylaxis is preferred Drugs: valganciclovir is preferred (caution in liver recipients[a]); alternative agents are oral ganciclovir and IV ganciclovir; valacyclovir is an alternative agent for kidney recipients; some centers add adjunctive CMV Ig. Duration: 3–6 mo Preemptive therapy is an option but less preferred. Weekly CMV PCR or pp65 antigenemia for 12 wk after transplantation, and if a positive CMV threshold is reached, treat with (1) valganciclovir 900 mg by mouth twice daily, or (2) IV ganciclovir 5 mg/kg IV every 12 h until negative test
	R+	Antiviral prophylaxis Drugs: valganciclovir is preferred (caution in liver recipients[a]); oral ganciclovir and IV ganciclovir are alternative drugs; valacyclovir is an option for kidney recipients Duration: 3 mo Preemptive therapy. Weekly CMV PCR or pp65 antigenemia for 12 wk after transplantation, and if a positive CMV threshold is reached, treat with (1) valganciclovir 900 mg by mouth twice daily, or (2) ganciclovir 5 mg/kg IV every 12 h until negative test
Lung, heart-lung	D+/R−	Antiviral prophylaxis Drugs: valganciclovir or IV ganciclovir Duration: 12 mo Some centers prolong prophylaxis beyond 12 mo Some centers add CMV Ig.
	R+	Antiviral prophylaxis Drugs: valganciclovir or IV ganciclovir Duration: 6–12 mo
Intestinal	D+/R−, R+	Antiviral prophylaxis Drugs: valganciclovir or IV ganciclovir Duration: 3–6 mo.
Composite tissue allograft	D+/R−, R+	Antiviral prophylaxis Drugs: valganciclovir or IV ganciclovir Duration: 3–6 mo

Antiviral prophylaxis should be started as soon as possible, and within 10 days after transplantation.

Preemptive therapy is not recommended for lung, heart-lung, intestinal, and composite tissue allograft transplantation.

Abbreviation: IV, intravenous.

[a] The US FDA has cautioned against valganciclovir prophylaxis in liver recipients because of high rate of tissue-invasive disease compared with oral ganciclovir. However, many experts still recommend its use as prophylaxis in liver recipients.

3 months of valganciclovir prophylaxis (34% and 64%, respectively).[84,87] Many lung transplant centers have extended the duration of antiviral prophylaxis to 1 year after lung transplantation. Others have even observed high rates of CMV disease among CMV D+/R− lung recipients, despite 12 months of antiviral prophylaxis, and have adapted an even longer course of antiviral prophylaxis (eg, some anticipated lifelong)

in CMV D+/R– lung recipients.[88] However, this practice was associated with significant myelotoxicity, which required the temporary or permanent discontinuation of valganciclovir prophylaxis.[88]

In selected patient populations (heart and lung recipients, and intestinal transplant recipients), unselected or CMV-specific Ig preparations have occasionally been used as an adjunct in combination with antiviral drugs.[89,90] A pooled analysis of previous studies suggest that the addition of Ig preparations to antiviral prophylaxis may reduce severe CMV disease and mortality,[91] but this finding has been debated.[92]

Preemptive Therapy

For preemptive therapy, SOT recipients are monitored at regular intervals (usually once weekly for 12 weeks) for evidence of early CMV replication. The 2 laboratory methods that are most commonly used to guide preemptive therapy are CMV QNAT and pp65 antigenemia. Which of these tests is better is debated, and likely affected by numerous factors, including proximity of patients to the transplant center. The duration of monitoring may be extended if the patients remain to be severely immunosuppressed, such as those requiring intensified immunosuppression for recurrent episodes of rejection.[59]

The viral threshold that should trigger antiviral treatment has not been standardized for the 2 assays.[59] Accordingly, site-specific and assay-specific viral load threshold values for initiation of preemptive therapy should be locally validated.[69] The recently released WHO CMV International Reference Standard, to which CMV QNAT assays should be calibrated, should facilitate defining such clinically relevant thresholds.[14]

Once CMV infection is detected above the threshold by pp65 or QNAT, patients should be initiated on treatment doses of valganciclovir or intravenous ganciclovir to prevent the progression of asymptomatic infection into clinical disease (see **Table 6**).[93] In a clinical trial, viral decay kinetics was similar between valganciclovir and intravenous ganciclovir for preemptive treatment of asymptomatic CMV reactivation.[94] Because preemptive therapy should treat low-level asymptomatic viremia, experts recommend oral valganciclovir as preferable compared with intravenous ganciclovir for logistic issues.[14] Antiviral therapy should be continued until CMV DNAemia or antigenemia is no longer detectable, and many experts recommend treating until 2 consecutive negative weekly pp65 antigenemia or QNAT tests are attained.[14]

Experts have cautioned against preemptive therapy among the high-risk CMV D+/R– SOT recipients, which are characterized by a very rapid rate of viral replication.[14] There is a potential failure of once-weekly surveillance in detecting CMV replication if the rate of replication is very rapid, and this may result in the development of CMV disease during the period between testing.[16] Despite this concern, preemptive therapy has been shown to be effective for preventing CMV disease even in this population.[76] Nonetheless, there are more experts who prefer antiviral prophylaxis for the highest-risk SOT recipients such as D+/R– and lung transplant recipients.[14]

In addition to laboratory monitoring, another trigger for preemptive therapy is treatment with lymphocyte-depleting immunosuppressive agents, which is a major risk factor for CMV disease.[14,50,95,96] Use of intravenous ganciclovir in patients receiving these drugs was associated with lower incidence of CMV disease.[95,96] Guidelines recommend that antiviral drug, usually valganciclovir, should be given for 1 to 3 months to patients receiving antilymphocyte antibody therapy either as induction or for the treatment of rejection.[14] Alternatively, if these patients are not given antiviral drug, they should be monitored for CMV replication using CMV QNAT or pp65 antigenemia, and preemptively treated on detection of CMV viremia.[14]

TREATMENT OF CMV DISEASE

The drugs used for the treatment of CMV disease are listed in **Table 5**. All 3 are nucleoside analogues that inhibit CMV replication by serving as competitive substrates for viral *UL54*-encoded enzyme DNA polymerase. Among them, the first line for therapy is intravenous ganciclovir and oral valganciclovir.[45] Oral ganciclovir, on the other hand, should not be used for treatment, because it has poor bioavailability and it is unable to reach sufficient systemic concentrations to be effective for treatment.[14]

Intravenous ganciclovir has been the mainstay for the treatment of CMV disease,[14] and its efficacy has been shown in numerous clinical trials.[45,97,98] Valganciclovir achieves blood levels comparable with intravenous ganciclovir, and has been used for the treatment of mild to moderate CMV disease.[45] In a randomized controlled trial conducted in 321 SOT recipients with mild to moderate CMV disease,[45] the clinical and virologic efficacy of 3 weeks of oral valganciclovir treatment was comparable with intravenous ganciclovir. Almost half of the patients receiving valganciclovir or intravenous ganciclovir remained viremic at 3 weeks (and they may benefit from extended duration of treatment).[45] Because this study was conducted in patients with mild to moderate CMV disease, experts recommend that valganciclovir should be used only for CMV disease of mild to moderate severity.[14] For patients with severe disease, the initial treatment should be intravenous ganciclovir.[14] Intravenous ganciclovir is also the drug of choice for the treatment of CMV disease characterized by high initial viral load, and for patients with impaired or questionable gastrointestinal absorption.[14] For patients initiated on intravenous ganciclovir, it is reasonable to move to oral valganciclovir on resolution of clinical symptoms and once good control of viremia is attained.[14]

Cidofovir and foscarnet are highly active against CMV, but they are less preferred agents for treatment because of the high risk of nephrotoxicity.[14] In some cases, especially those with CMV pneumonia and lung recipients with severe life-threatening CMV disease, intravenous Ig or CMV Ig may be used as an adjunct to antiviral treatment.[14] As in other cases of opportunistic infection, cautious reduction in the degree of immunosuppression is highly recommended as a component of treatment of CMV disease.[14]

The duration of antiviral therapy should be individualized based on clinical and virologic responses.[45,97,98] Three criteria should be met before discontinuation of antiviral treatment.[14] First, the clinical symptoms should have resolved. Second, the viral load should have declined to an undetectable level (or lower than the validated threshold). Virologic response is monitored by once-weekly CMV QNAT or pp65 antigenemia. The efficacy of antiviral treatment is correlated with a decline in viral load over time. Third, treatment should be given for a minimum duration of 2 weeks.

Treatment should be continued for all patients with CMV disease until the viral load has declined to an undetectable level (or lower than the validated threshold for CMV QNAT or pp65 antigenemia).[14] This recommendation is aimed at reducing the risk of CMV disease relapse, which has been observed at higher rates in patients with persistent viremia at the end of therapy.[97–99] Because the assays used for monitoring are not standardized (yet), the duration of antiviral treatment is dependent on assay sensitivity. A more prolonged treatment course is anticipated for patients monitored by an ultrasensitive assay.[70,100] In 1 recent study that compared outcomes of CMV QNAT using the more-sensitive whole blood sample and the less-sensitive plasma, there was no increased risk of CMV relapse in patients with negative plasma but with low-positive whole blood assay.[100] These data suggest that the lowest limit of clinically relevant viremia for the optimal discontinuation of antiviral treatment needs to be defined.[14] However, absence of viremia does not guarantee no relapse, because CMV relapse may still occur even in patients with viral load reduced to undetectable levels.[29]

After completion of full-dose antiviral treatment, a 1-month to 3-month course of secondary prophylaxis may be considered for selected patients.[14] This practice is aimed at reducing the risk of clinical relapse, which has been observed in 15% of patients with CMV disease, and the risk of virologic recurrence, which has been reported in 35% of patients.[14] However, the data to support this practice are limited, and thus it should not be uniformly practiced. Some recommend that it should be considered for SOT recipients with severe immunosuppression and those still lacking CMV-specific immunity.[14] Alternatively, if secondary antiviral prophylaxis is not desired, high-risk patients should be monitored clinically and by CMV surveillance after discontinuation of treatment.[14]

DRUG-RESISTANT CMV INFECTION AND DISEASE

Drug-resistant CMV is an emerging infection in SOT recipients.[64] Although still uncommon, infection with drug-resistant virus is associated with significant morbidity and it is potentially fatal.[64] Drug-resistant CMV should be suspected if viral load fails to decline or increases despite antiviral therapy.[14] This infection is more common in patients who have been exposed to antiviral drugs for a prolonged period, either as antiviral prophylaxis or preemptive therapy.[14] Infection with drug-resistant CMV is more common in lung transplant recipients, and almost all cases have been reported among CMV D+/R− patients (**Table 7**).[14]

Ganciclovir resistance is the most commonly observed phenotype for drug-resistant CMV.[101] Cross-resistance or isolated resistance to cidofovir or foscarnet occurs less commonly. The mechanism of antiviral drug resistance involves mutations in key viral genes that are needed for drug activation (*UL97*) or viral replication (*UL54*). To attain antiviral activity, ganciclovir has to undergo triphosphorylation into ganciclovir triphosphate, a process that is initiated by a viral kinase encoded by the CMV gene *UL97*.[101] Mutations in *UL97* (**Table 8**) impairs ganciclovir phosphorylation, resulting in a lack of active drug.[101] Subsequent phosphorylation by cellular enzymes leads to the active ganciclovir triphosphate, which competitively inhibits CMV DNA polymerase encoded by the viral gene *UL54*. Mutations in *UL54* therefore confer ganciclovir resistance.[67,101] Like ganciclovir, foscarnet and cidofovir act to inhibit CMV DNA

Table 7	
Definite and possible risk factors for drug-resistant CMV in SOT recipients	
Host factors	Lack of CMV-specific immunity (ie, CMV donor positive/recipient negative) Lung transplant recipients Kidney-pancreas transplant recipients
Viral factors	High degree of viral replication (ie, high viral load) Recurrent episodes of CMV disease
Drug factors	Prolonged antiviral drug administration: antiviral prophylaxis > preemptive therapy Suboptimal tissue-plasma antiviral drug concentration (oral ganciclovir, minidose valganciclovir)
Immunosuppression factors	Receipt of potent immunosuppression (lymphocyte-depleting agents) Allograft rejection

Table 8 Seven most common CMV UL97 gene mutations conferring ganciclovir resistance	
UL97 Mutation	**Ganciclovir Ratio[a]**
M460I	5
M460V	8
H520Q	10
C592G	3
A594V	8
L595S	9
C603W	8

[a] Ganciclovir ratio: IC_{50} (half maximal inhibitory concentration) of mutant/IC_{50} of wild type.

polymerase, and hence, mutations in *UL54* may confer cross-resistance to these drugs. Unlike ganciclovir, foscarnet and cidofovir do not rely on *UL97*, and hence remain active for CMV with isolated *UL97* mutation. Depending on the genetic mutation involved, resistance to ganciclovir by CMV *UL97* mutants may confer a low-level or high-level resistance.[67] Combined mutations (*UL97* and *UL54*) generally confer high-level resistance to ganciclovir.[101] Isolated *UL54* mutation (in the absence of *UL97* mutation) very rarely occurs.[67] In our center, we have seen only a single case of CMV with isolated *UL54* mutation, whereas all 8 other cases involved isolated *UL97* or less commonly, combined *UL97* and *UL54* mutation.

The incidence of ganciclovir-resistant CMV remains low.[67] In our center, only a total of 9 drug-resistant CMV diseases have been treated during a span of a decade, out of the total of 3444 transplants performed (incidence of 0.26%). In previous studies conducted among higher-risk CMV D+/R– SOT patients, the incidence was 1.9% in those who received 3 months of oral ganciclovir prophylaxis.[102] The incidence of ganciclovir resistance may increase with prolonged antiviral drug administration, although this was not observed in the trial that compared 3 and 6 months of valganciclovir prophylaxis.[63] Previous reports have implicated prolonged antiviral prophylaxis, but recent data have shown increasing frequency of drug-resistant CMV in patients receiving preemptive therapy.[80] The incidence of drug-resistant CMV may be higher in patients with higher intensity of immunosuppression and history of recurrent rejection episodes.[103] Previous studies have also identified pancreas and lung transplant recipients to be at a higher risk of resistance.[66,104] Most cases have occurred in CMV D+/R– recipients.[103] All 9 cases of drug-resistant CMV disease in our center have occurred in CMV D+/R– recipients.

Treatment of ganciclovir-resistant CMV is limited. Reduction in immunosuppression is an essential component of treatment.[14] Reducing the immunosuppression allows patients to develop and augment CMV-specific immunity, which is important in the control of infection. The choice of antiviral therapy against drug-resistant CMV should be guided by genotypic analysis.[14] Most ganciclovir-resistant CMV isolates have isolated *UL97* mutations and remain susceptible to foscarnet and cidofovir. The first-line empirical antiviral treatment is foscarnet.[67] In some cases, the *UL97* mutation confers only low-level ganciclovir resistance, and experts believe that this may be overcome by increasing the dose of ganciclovir (ie, switching to intravenous formulation or increasing the dose by 50%–100%).[14] In some situations, foscarnet has been combined with ganciclovir for treatment of proven isolated *UL97* mutant infection.[64,105–107] The major adverse effect of foscarnet is nephrotoxicity, which is common and has led to renal failure and allograft loss among kidney recipients.[64,105–107] Cidofovir is the alternative for treatment, although it is also highly nephrotoxic.[64,105–107] CMV Igs have been used as an adjunct to antiviral therapy.[14]

Treatment of drug-resistant CMV with mutations in *UL54*-encoded CMV DNA polymerase is more limited.[14] Because ganciclovir, foscarnet, and cidofovir act by competitively inhibiting *UL54*-encoded CMV DNA polymerase, mutations in the *UL54* may result in resistance to any or all of these drugs depending on the site of the mutation.[67] If all 3 drugs are not active based on genotypic analysis, the treatment may involve 1 of several investigational drugs (eg, letermovir [AIC246], maribavir, CMX001)[108–111] or the use of other drugs that have been approved for other indications (eg, leflunomide, artesunate).[112,113] Data on the efficacy of these drugs are anecdotal, experimental, or based on single case reports or series. Consideration may also be given to switching immunosuppression to one containing sirolimus and other mTOR inhibitors, because these drugs have been associated with a lower risk of CMV disease.[14] Adoptive transfer of CMV-specific T cells has been used in some cases, but this approach remains investigational and can be performed only in select centers.[14,114]

FUTURE DIRECTIONS

Several exciting developments in CMV after SOT deserve brief discussion. There are several antiviral drugs in various stages of clinical development. Letermovir (AIC246), which inhibits CMV replication through a specific mechanism that targets viral terminase,[108–110] is undergoing clinical trials in transplant recipients. It has been used on a compassionate basis in a lung transplant recipient with CMV disease that was resistant to treatment with ganciclovir, foscarnet, and cidofovir.[110] An oral formulation of cidofovir, CMX001, is being investigated for the treatment of various double-stranded DNA viruses, including CMV, and it has been available on a compassionate basis for the treatment of ganciclovir-resistant CMV disease.[111] Another drug in clinical development is cyclopropravir, which is a DNA polymerase inhibitor with anti-CMV activity.[115] However, the clinical development of maribavir is uncertain because of disappointing results in clinical trials conducted in bone marrow transplant and liver transplant populations, although it has been used for the treatment of few cases of drug-resistant CMV disease.[116]

Several vaccines are being developed for prevention of CMV in transplant recipients.[114,117,118] In a clinical trial that used CMV glycoprotein B with MF59 adjuvant, a significant humoral response was elicited in liver and kidney transplant candidates and recipients.[118] Assays of CMV-specific T-cell function are in various stages of development or are in use in some countries.[119,120] Patients with detectable CMV-specific T lymphocyte and function are less likely to develop CMV infection and disease after transplantation.[119,120] Optimization and standardization of these assays and their translation in clinical practice supplement the current methods aimed at reducing the impact of CMV infection and disease on the outcome of transplantation.

REFERENCES

1. Beam E, Razonable RR. Cytomegalovirus in solid organ transplantation: epidemiology, prevention, and treatment. Curr Infect Dis Rep 2012;14(6):633–41.
2. Bate SL, Dollard SC, Cannon MJ. Cytomegalovirus seroprevalence in the United States: the national health and nutrition examination surveys, 1988-2004. Clin Infect Dis 2010;50(11):1439–47.
3. Cannon MJ, Schmid DS, Hyde TB. Review of cytomegalovirus seroprevalence and demographic characteristics associated with infection. Rev Med Virol 2010;20(4):202–13.

4. Watkins RR, Lemonovich TL, Razonable RR. Immune response to CMV in solid organ transplant recipients: current concepts and future directions. Expert Rev Clin Immunol 2012;8(4):383–93.

5. Dunn HS, Haney DJ, Ghanekar SA, et al. Dynamics of CD4 and CD8 T cell responses to cytomegalovirus in healthy human donors. J Infect Dis 2002; 186(1):15–22.

6. Razonable RR. Epidemiology of cytomegalovirus disease in solid organ and hematopoietic stem cell transplant recipients. Am J Health Syst Pharm 2005; 62(8 Suppl 1):S7–13.

7. Manuel O, Pang XL, Humar A, et al. An assessment of donor-to-recipient transmission patterns of human cytomegalovirus by analysis of viral genomic variants. J Infect Dis 2009;199(11):1621–8.

8. Razonable R. Direct and indirect effects of cytomegalovirus: can we prevent them? Enferm Infecc Microbiol Clin 2010;28(1):1–5.

9. Arthurs SK, Eid AJ, Deziel PJ, et al. The impact of invasive fungal diseases on survival after lung transplantation. Clin Transplant 2010;24(3):341–8.

10. Arthurs SK, Eid AJ, Pedersen RA, et al. Delayed-onset primary cytomegalovirus disease after liver transplantation. Liver Transpl 2007;13(12):1703–9.

11. Arthurs SK, Eid AJ, Pedersen RA, et al. Delayed-onset primary cytomegalovirus disease and the risk of allograft failure and mortality after kidney transplantation. Clin Infect Dis 2008;46(6):840–6.

12. Asberg A, Jardine AG, Bignamini AA, et al. Effects of the intensity of immunosuppressive therapy on outcome of treatment for CMV disease in organ transplant recipients. Am J Transplant 2010;10(8):1881–8.

13. Razonable RR, Rivero A, Rodriguez A, et al. Allograft rejection predicts the occurrence of late-onset cytomegalovirus (CMV) disease among CMV-mismatched solid organ transplant patients receiving prophylaxis with oral ganciclovir. J Infect Dis 2001;184(11):1461–4.

14. Razonable R, Humar A. Cytomegalovirus in solid organ transplant recipients. Am J Transplant 2013;13(Suppl 4):93–106.

15. Chou SW. Acquisition of donor strains of cytomegalovirus by renal-transplant recipients. N Engl J Med 1986;314(22):1418–23.

16. Emery VC, Hassan-Walker AF, Burroughs AK, et al. Human cytomegalovirus (HCMV) replication dynamics in HCMV-naive and -experienced immunocompromised hosts. J Infect Dis 2002;185(12):1723–8.

17. Emery VC, Manuel O, Asberg A, et al. Differential decay kinetics of human cytomegalovirus glycoprotein B genotypes following antiviral chemotherapy. J Clin Virol 2012;54(1):56–60.

18. Emery VC, Sabin CA, Cope AV, et al. Application of viral-load kinetics to identify patients who develop cytomegalovirus disease after transplantation. Lancet 2000;355(9220):2032–6.

19. Paya C, Humar A, Dominguez E, et al. Efficacy and safety of valganciclovir vs. oral ganciclovir for prevention of cytomegalovirus disease in solid organ transplant recipients. Am J Transplant 2004;4(4):611–20.

20. Gane E, Saliba F, Valdecasas GJ, et al. Randomised trial of efficacy and safety of oral ganciclovir in the prevention of cytomegalovirus disease in liver-transplant recipients. The Oral Ganciclovir International Transplantation Study Group [corrected]. Lancet 1997;350(9093):1729–33.

21. Lowance D, Neumayer HH, Legendre CM, et al. Valacyclovir for the prevention of cytomegalovirus disease after renal transplantation. International Valacyclovir

Cytomegalovirus Prophylaxis Transplantation Study Group. N Engl J Med 1999; 340(19):1462–70.

22. Humar A, Lebranchu Y, Vincenti F, et al. The efficacy and safety of 200 days valganciclovir cytomegalovirus prophylaxis in high-risk kidney transplant recipients. Am J Transplant 2010;10(5):1228–37.

23. Humar A, Limaye AP, Blumberg EA, et al. Extended valganciclovir prophylaxis in D+/R- kidney transplant recipients is associated with long-term reduction in cytomegalovirus disease: two-year results of the IMPACT study. Transplantation 2010;90(12):1427–31.

24. Cummins NW, Deziel PJ, Abraham RS, et al. Deficiency of cytomegalovirus (CMV)-specific CD8+ T cells in patients presenting with late-onset CMV disease several years after transplantation. Transpl Infect Dis 2009;11(1):20–7.

25. Slifkin M, Tempesti P, Poutsiaka DD, et al. Late and atypical cytomegalovirus disease in solid-organ transplant recipients. Clin Infect Dis 2001;33(7): E62–8.

26. Razonable RR, Burak KW, van Cruijsen H, et al. The pathogenesis of hepatitis C virus is influenced by cytomegalovirus. Clin Infect Dis 2002;35(8):974–81.

27. Humar A, Michaels M. American Society of Transplantation recommendations for screening, monitoring and reporting of infectious complications in immunosuppression trials in recipients of organ transplantation. Am J Transplant 2006;6(2):262–74.

28. Ljungman P, Griffiths P, Paya C. Definitions of cytomegalovirus infection and disease in transplant recipients. Clin Infect Dis 2002;34(8):1094–7.

29. Eid AJ, Arthurs SK, Deziel PJ, et al. Clinical predictors of relapse after treatment of primary gastrointestinal cytomegalovirus disease in solid organ transplant recipients. Am J Transplant 2010;10(1):157–61.

30. Drage M, Reid A, Callaghan CJ, et al. Acute cytomegalovirus cholecystitis following renal transplantation. Am J Transplant 2009;9(5):1249–52.

31. Kini U, Nirmala V. Post-transplantation epididymitis associated with cytomegalovirus. Indian J Pathol Microbiol 1996;39(2):151–3.

32. Eid AJ, Bakri SJ, Kijpittayarit S, et al. Clinical features and outcomes of cytomegalovirus retinitis after transplantation. Transpl Infect Dis 2008;10(1):13–8.

33. Laifer SA, Ehrlich GD, Huff DS, et al. Congenital cytomegalovirus infection in offspring of liver transplant recipients. Clin Infect Dis 1995;20(1):52–5.

34. Munoz-Price LS, Slifkin M, Ruthazer R, et al. The clinical impact of ganciclovir prophylaxis on the occurrence of bacteremia in orthotopic liver transplant recipients. Clin Infect Dis 2004;39(9):1293–9.

35. George MJ, Snydman DR, Werner BG, et al. The independent role of cytomegalovirus as a risk factor for invasive fungal disease in orthotopic liver transplant recipients. Boston Center for Liver Transplantation CMVIG-Study Group. Cytogam, Medimmune, Inc. Gaithersburg, Maryland. Am J Med 1997;103(2): 106–13.

36. Walker RC, Marshall WF, Strickler JG, et al. Pretransplantation assessment of the risk of lymphoproliferative disorder. Clin Infect Dis 1995;20(5):1346–53.

37. Antoine P, Olislagers V, Huygens A, et al. Functional exhaustion of CD4+ t lymphocytes during primary cytomegalovirus infection. J Immunol 2012;189(5): 2665–72.

38. Limaye AP, Bakthavatsalam R, Kim HW, et al. Late-onset cytomegalovirus disease in liver transplant recipients despite antiviral prophylaxis. Transplantation 2004;78(9):1390–6.

39. Kliem V, Fricke L, Wollbrink T, et al. Improvement in long-term renal graft survival due to CMV prophylaxis with oral ganciclovir: results of a randomized clinical trial. Am J Transplant 2008;8(5):975–83.

40. Reischig T, Jindra P, Hes O, et al. Valacyclovir prophylaxis versus preemptive valganciclovir therapy to prevent cytomegalovirus disease after renal transplantation. Am J Transplant 2008;8(1):69–77.

41. Helantera I, Lautenschlager I, Koskinen P. The risk of cytomegalovirus recurrence after kidney transplantation. Transpl Int 2011;24(12):1170–8.

42. Zamora MR. Controversies in lung transplantation: management of cytomegalovirus infections. J Heart Lung Transplant 2002;21(8):841–9.

43. Potena L, Valantine HA. Cytomegalovirus-associated allograft rejection in heart transplant patients. Curr Opin Infect Dis 2007;20(4):425–31.

44. Valantine H. Cardiac allograft vasculopathy after heart transplantation: risk factors and management. J Heart Lung Transplant 2004;23(Suppl 5):S187–93.

45. Asberg A, Humar A, Rollag H, et al. Oral valganciclovir is noninferior to intravenous ganciclovir for the treatment of cytomegalovirus disease in solid organ transplant recipients. Am J Transplant 2007;7(9):2106–13.

46. Bosch W, Heckman MG, Diehl NN, et al. Association of cytomegalovirus infection and disease with death and graft loss after liver transplant in high-risk recipients. Am J Transplant 2011;11(10):2181–9.

47. Eid AJ, Razonable RR. New developments in the management of cytomegalovirus infection after solid organ transplantation. Drugs 2010;70(8):965–81.

48. Atabani SF, Smith C, Atkinson C, et al. Cytomegalovirus replication kinetics in solid organ transplant recipients managed by preemptive therapy. Am J Transplant 2012;12(9):2457–64.

49. Emery VC, Cope AV, Bowen EF, et al. The dynamics of human cytomegalovirus replication in vivo. J Exp Med 1999;190(2):177–82.

50. Portela D, Patel R, Larson-Keller JJ, et al. OKT3 treatment for allograft rejection is a risk factor for cytomegalovirus disease in liver transplantation. J Infect Dis 1995;171(4):1014–8.

51. Sarmiento JM, Dockrell DH, Schwab TR, et al. Mycophenolate mofetil increases cytomegalovirus invasive organ disease in renal transplant patients. Clin Transplant 2000;14(2):136–8.

52. Brennan DC, Legendre C, Patel D, et al. Cytomegalovirus incidence between everolimus versus mycophenolate in de novo renal transplants: pooled analysis of three clinical trials. Am J Transplant 2011;11(11):2453–62.

53. Corona-Nakamura AL, Monteon-Ramos FJ, Troyo-Sanroman R, et al. Incidence and predictive factors for cytomegalovirus infection in renal transplant recipients. Transplant Proc 2009;41(6):2412–5.

54. Kijpittayarit S, Eid AJ, Brown RA, et al. Relationship between toll-like receptor 2 polymorphism and cytomegalovirus disease after liver transplantation. Clin Infect Dis 2007;44(10):1315–20.

55. Kang SH, Abdel-Massih RC, Brown RA, et al. Homozygosity for the toll-like receptor 2 R753Q single-nucleotide polymorphism is a risk factor for cytomegalovirus disease after liver transplantation. J Infect Dis 2012;205(4):639–46.

56. de Rooij BJ, van der Beek MT, van Hoek B, et al. Mannose-binding lectin and ficolin-2 gene polymorphisms predispose to cytomegalovirus (re)infection after orthotopic liver transplantation. J Hepatol 2011;55(4):800–7.

57. Kwakkel-van Erp JM, Paantjens AW, van Kessel DA, et al. Mannose-binding lectin deficiency linked to cytomegalovirus (CMV) reactivation and survival in lung transplantation. Clin Exp Immunol 2011;165(3):410–6.

58. Humar A, Asberg A, Kumar D, et al. An assessment of herpesvirus co-infections in patients with CMV disease: correlation with clinical and virologic outcomes. Am J Transplant 2009;9(2):374–81.
59. Razonable RR, Paya CV, Smith TF. Role of the laboratory in diagnosis and management of cytomegalovirus infection in hematopoietic stem cell and solid-organ transplant recipients. J Clin Microbiol 2002;40(3):746–52.
60. Florescu DF, Mindru C, Chambers HE, et al. *Clostridium difficile* and cytomegalovirus colitis co-infection: search for the hidden 'bug'. Transpl Infect Dis 2011; 13(4):411–5.
61. Arslan H, Inci EK, Azap OK, et al. Etiologic agents of diarrhea in solid organ recipients. Transpl Infect Dis 2007;9(4):270–5.
62. Humar A, Mazzulli T, Moussa G, et al. Clinical utility of cytomegalovirus (CMV) serology testing in high-risk CMV D+/R- transplant recipients. Am J Transplant 2005;5(5):1065–70.
63. Boivin G, Goyette N, Farhan M, et al. Incidence of cytomegalovirus UL97 and UL54 amino acid substitutions detected after 100 or 200 days of valganciclovir prophylaxis. J Clin Virol 2012;53(3):208–13.
64. Eid AJ, Arthurs SK, Deziel PJ, et al. Emergence of drug-resistant cytomegalovirus in the era of valganciclovir prophylaxis: therapeutic implications and outcomes. Clin Transplant 2008;22(2):162–70.
65. Limaye AP, Corey L, Koelle DM, et al. Emergence of ganciclovir-resistant cytomegalovirus disease among recipients of solid-organ transplants. Lancet 2000; 356(9230):645–9.
66. Limaye AP, Raghu G, Koelle DM, et al. High incidence of ganciclovir-resistant cytomegalovirus infection among lung transplant recipients receiving preemptive therapy. J Infect Dis 2002;185(1):20–7.
67. Lurain NS, Chou S. Antiviral drug resistance of human cytomegalovirus. Clin Microbiol Rev 2010;23(4):689–712.
68. Caliendo AM, St George K, Kao SY, et al. Comparison of quantitative cytomegalovirus (CMV) PCR in plasma and CMV antigenemia assay: clinical utility of the prototype AMPLICOR CMV MONITOR test in transplant recipients. J Clin Microbiol 2000;38(6):2122–7.
69. Humar A, Gregson D, Caliendo AM, et al. Clinical utility of quantitative cytomegalovirus viral load determination for predicting cytomegalovirus disease in liver transplant recipients. Transplantation 1999;68(9):1305–11.
70. Razonable RR, Brown RA, Wilson J, et al. The clinical use of various blood compartments for cytomegalovirus (CMV) DNA quantitation in transplant recipients with CMV disease. Transplantation 2002;73(6):968–73.
71. Hayden RT, Yan X, Wick MT, et al. Factors contributing to variability of quantitative viral PCR results in proficiency testing samples: a multivariate analysis. J Clin Microbiol 2012;50(2):337–45.
72. Pang XL, Fox JD, Fenton JM, et al. Interlaboratory comparison of cytomegalovirus viral load assays. Am J Transplant 2009;9(2):258–68.
73. Razonable RR, Brown RA, Espy MJ, et al. Comparative quantitation of cytomegalovirus (CMV) DNA in solid organ transplant recipients with CMV infection by using two high-throughput automated systems. J Clin Microbiol 2001;39(12):4472–6.
74. Pang XL, Chui L, Fenton J, et al. Comparison of LightCycler-based PCR, COBAS amplicor CMV monitor, and pp65 antigenemia assays for quantitative measurement of cytomegalovirus viral load in peripheral blood specimens from patients after solid organ transplantation. J Clin Microbiol 2003;41(7): 3167–74.

75. Khoury JA, Storch GA, Bohl DL, et al. Prophylactic versus preemptive oral valganciclovir for the management of cytomegalovirus infection in adult renal transplant recipients. Am J Transplant 2006;6(9):2134–43.
76. Witzke O, Hauser IA, Bartels M, et al. Valganciclovir prophylaxis versus preemptive therapy in cytomegalovirus-positive renal allograft recipients: 1-year results of a randomized clinical trial. Transplantation 2012;93(1):61–8.
77. Kalil AC, Levitsky J, Lyden E, et al. Meta-analysis: the efficacy of strategies to prevent organ disease by cytomegalovirus in solid organ transplant recipients. Ann Intern Med 2005;143(12):870–80.
78. Small LN, Lau J, Snydman DR. Preventing post-organ transplantation cytomegalovirus disease with ganciclovir: a meta-analysis comparing prophylactic and preemptive therapies. Clin Infect Dis 2006;43(7):869–80.
79. Boivin G, Goyette N, Rollag H, et al. Cytomegalovirus resistance in solid organ transplant recipients treated with intravenous ganciclovir or oral valganciclovir. Antivir Ther 2009;14(5):697–704.
80. Myhre HA, Haug Dorenberg D, Kristiansen KI, et al. Incidence and outcomes of ganciclovir-resistant cytomegalovirus infections in 1244 kidney transplant recipients. Transplantation 2011;92(2):217–23.
81. Levitsky J, Singh N, Wagener MM, et al. A survey of CMV prevention strategies after liver transplantation. Am J Transplant 2008;8(1):158–61.
82. Humar A, Paya C, Pescovitz MD, et al. Clinical utility of cytomegalovirus viral load testing for predicting CMV disease in D+/R- solid organ transplant recipients. Am J Transplant 2004;4(4):644–9.
83. Lisboa LF, Preiksaitis JK, Humar A, et al. Clinical utility of molecular surveillance for cytomegalovirus after antiviral prophylaxis in high-risk solid organ transplant recipients. Transplantation 2011;92(9):1063–8.
84. Palmer SM, Limaye AP, Banks M, et al. Extended valganciclovir prophylaxis to prevent cytomegalovirus after lung transplantation: a randomized, controlled trial. Ann Intern Med 2010;152(12):761–9.
85. Humar A, Kumar D, Preiksaitis J, et al. A trial of valganciclovir prophylaxis for cytomegalovirus prevention in lung transplant recipients. Am J Transplant 2005;5(6):1462–8.
86. Zamora MR, Nicolls MR, Hodges TN, et al. Following universal prophylaxis with intravenous ganciclovir and cytomegalovirus immune globulin, valganciclovir is safe and effective for prevention of CMV infection following lung transplantation. Am J Transplant 2004;4(10):1635–42.
87. Finlen Copeland CA, Davis WA, Snyder LD, et al. Long-term efficacy and safety of 12 months of valganciclovir prophylaxis compared with 3 months after lung transplantation: a single-center, long-term follow-up analysis from a randomized, controlled cytomegalovirus prevention trial. J Heart Lung Transplant 2011;30(9):990–6.
88. Wiita AP, Roubinian N, Khan Y, et al. Cytomegalovirus disease and infection in lung transplant recipients in the setting of planned indefinite valganciclovir prophylaxis. Transpl Infect Dis 2012;14(3):248–58.
89. Snydman DR, Falagas ME, Avery R, et al. Use of combination cytomegalovirus immune globulin plus ganciclovir for prophylaxis in CMV-seronegative liver transplant recipients of a CMV-seropositive donor organ: a multicenter, open-label study. Transplant Proc 2001;33(4):2571–5.
90. Snydman DR, Werner BG, Dougherty NN, et al. Cytomegalovirus immune globulin prophylaxis in liver transplantation. A randomized, double-blind, placebo-controlled trial. Ann Intern Med 1993;119(10):984–91.

91. Bonaros N, Mayer B, Schachner T, et al. CMV-hyperimmune globulin for preventing cytomegalovirus infection and disease in solid organ transplant recipients: a meta-analysis. Clin Transplant 2008;22(1):89–97.
92. Hodson EM, Jones CA, Strippoli GF, et al. Immunoglobulins, vaccines or interferon for preventing cytomegalovirus disease in solid organ transplant recipients. Cochrane Database Syst Rev 2007;(2):CD005129.
93. Razonable RR, van Cruijsen H, Brown RA, et al. Dynamics of cytomegalovirus replication during preemptive therapy with oral ganciclovir. J Infect Dis 2003; 187(11):1801–8.
94. Mattes FM, Hainsworth EG, Hassan-Walker AF, et al. Kinetics of cytomegalovirus load decrease in solid-organ transplant recipients after preemptive therapy with valganciclovir. J Infect Dis 2005;191(1):89–92.
95. Conti DJ, Freed BM, Singh TP, et al. Preemptive ganciclovir therapy in cytomegalovirus-seropositive renal transplants recipients. Arch Surg 1995; 130(11):1217–21 [discussion: 21–2].
96. Hibberd PL, Tolkoff-Rubin NE, Conti D, et al. Preemptive ganciclovir therapy to prevent cytomegalovirus disease in cytomegalovirus antibody-positive renal transplant recipients. A randomized controlled trial. Ann Intern Med 1995; 123(1):18–26.
97. Humar A, Kumar D, Boivin G, et al. Cytomegalovirus (CMV) virus load kinetics to predict recurrent disease in solid-organ transplant patients with CMV disease. J Infect Dis 2002;186(6):829–33.
98. Sia IG, Wilson JA, Groettum CM, et al. Cytomegalovirus (CMV) DNA load predicts relapsing CMV infection after solid organ transplantation. J Infect Dis 2000;181(2):717–20.
99. Asberg A, Humar A, Jardine AG, et al. Long-term outcomes of CMV disease treatment with valganciclovir versus IV ganciclovir in solid organ transplant recipients. Am J Transplant 2009;9(5):1205–13.
100. Lisboa LF, Asberg A, Kumar D, et al. The clinical utility of whole blood versus plasma cytomegalovirus viral load assays for monitoring therapeutic response. Transplantation 2011;91(2):231–6.
101. Razonable RR. Antiviral drugs for viruses other than human immunodeficiency virus. Mayo Clin Proc 2011;86(10):1009–26.
102. Boivin G, Goyette N, Gilbert C, et al. Absence of cytomegalovirus-resistance mutations after valganciclovir prophylaxis, in a prospective multicenter study of solid-organ transplant recipients. J Infect Dis 2004;189(9):1615–8.
103. Razonable RR, Paya CV. Herpesvirus infections in transplant recipients: current challenges in the clinical management of cytomegalovirus and Epstein-Barr virus infections. Herpes 2003;10(3):60–5.
104. Bhorade SM, Lurain NS, Jordan A, et al. Emergence of ganciclovir-resistant cytomegalovirus in lung transplant recipients. J Heart Lung Transplant 2002; 21(12):1274–82.
105. Klintmalm G, Lonnqvist B, Oberg B, et al. Intravenous foscarnet for the treatment of severe cytomegalovirus infection in allograft recipients. Scand J Infect Dis 1985;17(2):157–63.
106. Locke TJ, Odom NJ, Tapson JS, et al. Successful treatment with trisodium phosphonoformate for primary cytomegalovirus infection after heart transplantation. J Heart Transplant 1987;6(2):120–2.
107. Mylonakis E, Kallas WM, Fishman JA. Combination antiviral therapy for ganciclovir-resistant cytomegalovirus infection in solid-organ transplant recipients. Clin Infect Dis 2002;34(10):1337–41.

108. Marschall M, Stamminger T, Urban A, et al. In vitro evaluation of the activities of the novel anticytomegalovirus compound AIC246 (letermovir) against herpesviruses and other human pathogenic viruses. Antimicrob Agents Chemother 2012;56(2):1135–7.
109. Goldner T, Hewlett G, Ettischer N, et al. The novel anticytomegalovirus compound AIC246 (letermovir) inhibits human cytomegalovirus replication through a specific antiviral mechanism that involves the viral terminase. J Virol 2011; 85(20):10884–93.
110. Kaul DR, Stoelben S, Cober E, et al. First report of successful treatment of multidrug-resistant cytomegalovirus disease with the novel anti-CMV compound AIC246. Am J Transplant 2011;11(5):1079–84.
111. Price NB, Prichard MN. Progress in the development of new therapies for herpesvirus infections. Curr Opin Virol 2011;1(6):548–54.
112. Avery RK, Mossad SB, Poggio E, et al. Utility of leflunomide in the treatment of complex cytomegalovirus syndromes. Transplantation 2010;90(4):419–26.
113. Wolf DG, Shimoni A, Resnick IB, et al. Human cytomegalovirus kinetics following institution of artesunate after hematopoietic stem cell transplantation. Antiviral Res 2011;90(3):183–6.
114. Razonable RR. Immune-based therapies for cytomegalovirus infection. Immunotherapy 2010;2(1):117–30.
115. Chou S, Marousek G, Bowlin TL. Cyclopropavir susceptibility of cytomegalovirus DNA polymerase mutants selected after antiviral drug exposure. Antimicrob Agents Chemother 2012;56(1):197–201.
116. Avery RK, Marty FM, Strasfeld L, et al. Oral maribavir for treatment of refractory or resistant cytomegalovirus infections in transplant recipients. Transpl Infect Dis 2010;12(6):489–96.
117. La Rosa C, Longmate J, Lacey SF, et al. Clinical evaluation of safety and immunogenicity of PADRE-cytomegalovirus (CMV) and tetanus-CMV fusion peptide vaccines with or without PF03512676 adjuvant. J Infect Dis 2012;205(8): 1294–304.
118. Griffiths PD, Stanton A, McCarrell E, et al. Cytomegalovirus glycoprotein-B vaccine with MF59 adjuvant in transplant recipients: a phase 2 randomised placebo-controlled trial. Lancet 2011;377(9773):1256–63.
119. Manuel O, Husain S, Kumar D, et al. Assessment of cytomegalovirus specific cell-mediated immunity for the prediction of cytomegalovirus disease in high-risk solid-organ transplant recipients: a multicenter cohort study. Clin Infect Dis 2013;56(6):817–24.
120. Lisboa LF, Kumar D, Wilson LE, et al. Clinical utility of cytomegalovirus cell-mediated immunity in transplant recipients with cytomegalovirus viremia. Transplantation 2012;93(2):195–200.

Impact of Multidrug-Resistant Organisms on Patients Considered for Lung Transplantation

Shmuel Shoham, MD*, Pali D. Shah, MD

KEYWORDS

- Lung transplant • Multidrug-resistant organism • Microbiology • Epidemiology

KEY POINTS

- In prospective transplant recipients, the most important multidrug-resistant (MDR) organisms are *Pseudomonas aeruginosa*, and species of *Burkholderia, Acinetobacter*, nontuberculous mycobacteria, and *Scedosporium*.
- Carriage of MDR organisms before transplant can predict the development of difficult-to-treat infections after lung transplantation.
- Identification of colonization and infection with MDR organisms is important to help guide antimicrobial decisions before and after transplant, and to determine suitability for lung transplantation.
- Development of personalized antimicrobial regimens for lung transplant recipients depends on an understanding of the epidemiology, microbiology, and clinical implications of these organisms.

INTRODUCTION

The long-term success of lung transplantation is limited by the development of infections and chronic rejection, otherwise known as bronchiolitis obliterans syndrome (BOS).[1] Infection with multidrug-resistant (MDR) organisms is particularly problematic in patients with cystic fibrosis (CF), which is the third most common indication for lung transplant. Understanding the clinical impact and management options for these pathogens is critical for optimizing posttransplant outcomes and maximizing the benefit of a limited supply of donor organs.

Patients with CF are increasingly colonized and infected with MDR bacteria and fungi before transplant.[1,2] Although *Pseudomonas aeruginosa* remains the predominant pathogen in patients with CF undergoing lung transplant evaluation, the prevalence of other species such as *Stenotrophomonas maltophila*, *Achromobacter xylosoxidans*,

Transplant and Oncology Infectious Diseases Program, Johns Hopkins University School of Medicine, 1830 East Monument Street, Room 450-D, Baltimore, MD 21205, USA
* Corresponding author.
E-mail address: sshoham1@jhmi.edu

Infect Dis Clin N Am 27 (2013) 343–358
http://dx.doi.org/10.1016/j.idc.2013.02.006
0891-5520/13/$ – see front matter © 2013 Elsevier Inc. All rights reserved.

id.theclinics.com

Pandorea, and *Ralstonia* has also increased over the past decade.[3–5] Outcomes in CF have greatly improved with the introduction of inhaled tobramycin and oral azithromycin, but the increasing use of these and other broad-spectrum antimicrobials has also led to changes in CF sputum microbiology.[6,7] Antibiotic use has led to a loss of diversity in respiratory flora and increases in antimicrobial resistance.[6,8,9] With regard to MDR pathogens, few data are available to guide specific therapy and predict the posttransplant outcomes for pathogens other than *P aeruginosa* (**Table 1**).[10]

SPECIFIC ORGANISMS
Pseudomonas aeruginosa

Microbiology and ecology
P aeruginosa is an opportunistic gram-negative aerobic bacillus found commonly in indoor and outdoor freshwater environments.[11] Displaying a multitude of virulence factors, *P aeruginosa* often manifests in 1 of 2 distinct phenotypes, a tissue-invasive pathogen causing acute pneumonia and sepsis or as a chronic colonizer in damaged airways, such as in CF.[12,13] Although *P aeruginosa* has a variety of virulence factors that may predispose this organism to severe acute infections, genome analysis of *P aeruginosa* strains in chronically infected recipients with CF has demonstrated that strains tend to display a different set of characteristics that allow the organism to persist as a chronic colonizer. These factors include

- Hyper mutability[14]
- Downregulation of virulence factors including toxin production, flagellum, and lipopolysaccharide O chains[15]
- Mucoid phenotype, characterized by production of alginate biofilm
- Evasion from and inhibition of phagocytosis[15,16]
- Multiple mechanisms of antibiotic resistance

Table 1
Commonly used antimicrobials for MDR pathogens

Organism	1st Line Antimicrobials	Contraindication to Transplant
MDR. *P aeruginosa*	Carbapenem, piperacillin/tazobactam, cefepime +/− an aminoglycoside or quinolone	Rare
Pan resistant *P aeruginosa*	Any of above +/− colistin	
B cenocepacia	Ceftazidime, tetracyclines, trimethoprim-sulfamethoxazole, carbapenem	Probable
B gladioli	Piperacillin, aminoglycosides, carbapenem, ciprofloxacin	Possible
A baumannii	Carbapenem, colistin, tigecycline, ampicillin/sulbactam	Possible
M abscessus	Clarithromycin + amikacin	Possible
	2nd line: Clarithromycin + imipenem or cefoxitin	
M avium complex	Clarithromycin, ethambutol, rifampin	Rare
S apiospermum	Voriconazole +/− echinocandin	Possible
S prolificans	Voriconazole +/− echinocandin +/− terbinafine	Possible
A terreus	Voriconazole +/− echinocandin	Rare

Data from.[62,112,113]

Epidemiology

Among patients being considered for lung transplantation, most pseudomonal infections are seen in chronic suppurative lung diseases, with a prevalence of *P aeruginosa* in up to 80% of patients with CF and bronchiectatic lung diseases.[17] Pretransplant colonization is a significant risk factor for infection after transplant, increasing the risk of infection by an odds ratio of 4.7.[18,19] *Pseudomonas* is the most common cause of pneumonia in the first month after transplant and accounts for one-third of posttransplant pneumonias.[20,21] This organism is particularly problematic in patients with CF.[22] Posttransplant airway colonization with *P aeruginosa* has also been associated with BOS, which is the primary cause of mortality in lung transplant recipients. It is not clear whether the risk of BOS is seen only in patients with de novo infection or whether this extends to patients who were colonized before transplant.[23,24] The posttransplant survival of patients colonized with pan-resistant *P aeruginosa* before transplant is similar to those with sensitive bacteria at 1 year (88% vs 96%), but worse at 3 years (63.2% vs 90.7%).[25] However, the average mortality with pan-resistant bacteria is comparable with that of the entire lung transplant population and thus patients should not be denied transplant candidacy because of pan-resistant *P aeruginosa*.[10]

MDR *P aeruginosa*, defined as resistance to greater than 3 or more classes of antibiotics, is common in patients with CF, with prevalence rates ranging from 10% to 45%.[26-28] Cutting-edge sequencing techniques have provided new insights into the longitudinal effects of antibiotic treatment on the bacterial ecosystem in these patients.[8,9] Findings from these recent studies by Zhao and colleagues[8] and Fodor and colleagues[9] suggest that use of antibiotics seemed to be the primary driver of the loss of diversity in respiratory flora, as opposed to age or lung function. A comparison between 1996 and 2008 demonstrated increased resistance to tobramycin in *P aeruginosa* isolates (11.8% vs 30.4%, $P<.001$), and increased carbapenem-resistant, aztreonam-resistant, and MDR *P aeruginosa* in patients who were exposed to intravenous carbapenems.[6]

Pretransplant management

CF Foundation guidelines recommend chronic use of inhaled antibiotics, such as tobramycin or aztreonam, reserving systemic antibiotics for symptomatic exacerbations. Antibiotics are typically selected based on local susceptibility testing; typical classes of antibiotics with antipseudomonal activity include extended spectrum cephalosporins, β-lactam/anti-β-lactamase, carbapenems, quinolones, and aminoglycosides. The increase in MDR *P aeruginosa* over the past 2 decades had led to interest in assessment of synergy with antibiotics, using either the checkerboard dilution assay or the multiple combination bactericidal assay (MCBT).[29,30] Synergy is defined as those combinations with demonstrable bactericidal activity. In studies from 1990 to 2006, combinations containing meropenem had the most bactericidal activity, showing in vitro efficacy in greater than 60% of strains.[29] Studies of the clinical efficacy of synergy testing have shown mixed results. In a randomized trial of patients with CF with respiratory exacerbations, antibiotic therapy guided by MCBT therapy did not improve the time interval between exacerbations, lung function, or end-of-treatment bacterial density before transplant.[31]

Posttransplant treatment

Most centers treat recipients with a history of *P aeruginosa* with 2-drug antipseudomonal therapy for 2 to 3 weeks postoperatively to reduce the risk of pneumonia and allograft colonization, based on previous susceptibilities.[32-34] However, most centers avoid systemic colistin and aminoglycosides if possible because of cumulative nephrotoxicity when combined with calcineurin inhibitors for immunosuppression. Synergy testing may be beneficial in patients with CF with MDR *P aeruginosa* who are undergoing lung transplant, based on lower rates of septicemia and pleural infections seen in a retrospective study. Inhaled tobramycin and colistin are components of successful eradication strategies for de novo *P aeruginosa* in pediatric patients with CF, and may have a role in preventing colonization of the new allograft after transplant. However, the efficacy of these agents for posttransplant eradication has not been well studied. Surgical debridement of the sinuses after transplant has also been associated with reduced incidence of bacterial pneumonia and BOS.

Burkholderia Species

Microbiology and ecology

Burkholderia species are gram-negative bacteria found ubiquitously in the soil and moist environment. Members of this genus include *Burkholderia cepacia* complex, *gladioli* and *mallei*, and *pseudomallei*. Previously believed to represent 1 species, advances in genetics have shown that the *B cepacia* complex (BCC) comprises several phylogenetically similar but distinct species, including *B multivorans* and *B cenocepacia*. The latter has recently been further subdivided into epidemic (transmissible) and nonepidemic strains. Because patient-to-patient transmission of *Burkholderia* species has been consistently documented, the CF Foundation has recommended segregation of patients infected with BCC from each other and from other patients. Recent subclassification of *Burkholderia* species has shown strain-specific differences in the virulence of these pathogens, in the pretransplant and posttransplant settings.

Epidemiology

Although BCC are generally not pathogenic in healthy hosts, *Burkholderia* species colonize the respiratory tract in 15% to 22% of patients with CF. Although early eradication strategies have been used in the CF population, most patients who acquire these organisms develop chronic infection.[35] Chronic infection with BCC, defined as the isolation of a species on 2 or more occasions over a minimum of 6 months, has been associated with an accelerated decline in lung function and increased mortality in recipients with CF.[36] Unfortunately, pretransplant colonization with *B cenocepacia* has been associated with the highest risk for posttransplant mortality (relative risk 8.43, *P*<.005) and most lung transplant centers have denied transplantation to candidates infected with this species.[37–39] More recently, it has been appreciated that infection with transmissible strains of *B cenocepacia* may not be as hazardous as infection with the nontransmissible strains.[37] Further studies are needed to determine if patient selection criteria or other factors also played a role in the observed mortality differences. Pretransplant colonization with *B gladioli* has also been associated with increased mortality in lung transplant recipients (hazard ratio 2.23, *P* = .04) and complications that include mediastinal abscesses, pleural infection, and chest wall infection.[37,40–42] There is currently insufficient data to determine whether the increased posttransplant mortality is primarily attributable to chronic and MDR infection or also extends to those transiently infected with *B gladioli* before transplant. Many transplant centers currently consider *B gladioli* to be a relative contraindication to lung transplant. Given the strain and species, and the specific virulence of the various members of the BCC, programs should refer specimens to reference laboratories with DNA fingerprinting capacity, if needed to determine the exact species and strain.

Treatment

Treatment of most acute exacerbations with *Burkholderia* species include trimethoprim sulfamethoxazole as the drug of choice as well as typical antipseudomonal antibiotics, such as ceftazidime and meropenem.[40,43] As a result of multiple resistance mechanisms, including an efflux pump, chronic infection with BCC is associated with an 80% prevalence of MDR, defined as resistance to 3 or more classes of antibiotics.[40,44] In this setting, some experts recommend synergy testing to determine optimal antibiotic combinations, although its efficacy is uncertain.[45] There are limited data about the optimal treatment approach after transplant, although most centers recommend prolonged combination antibiotic therapy given the high risk of fatal infection after transplant.

Acinetobacter baumannii

Microbiology

Acinetobacter is a gram-negative coccobacillus found in a broad variety of environments. Historically, a pathogen of humid climates, *Acinetobacter* species have become increasingly prevalent as causes of nosocomial infections.[46,47] *A baumannii* can be particularly problematic due to some of the following virulence factors:

- Ability to survive dry environmental conditions for weeks[48]
- Wide range of resistance mechanisms[49,50]
- Enhanced adherence to bronchial epithelium using fimbriae[51]
- Production of a polysaccharide capsule that can delay phagocytosis[52]

In the United States, transmission is typically traced to common source contamination in nosocomial settings, such as respiratory equipment in intensive care units, but community infection has been reported in other continents.

Epidemiology

Most of the nosocomial *A baumannii* infections occur in the setting of outbreaks; however, prolonged colonization can contribute to the endemicity of this pathogen after an outbreak. In 1 multicenter study, the prevalence of *Acinetobacter* in intensive care patients approximated 3%, predominantly as outbreaks.[53] Furthermore, the rapid acquisition of multiple mechanisms of resistance has led to the emergence of strains that are pan resistant.[54]

Peritransplant management

Treatment of *Acinetobacter* infections is based on local susceptibility patterns, but typical antibiotic choices include third-generation or fourth-generation cephalosporins, carbapenems, and β-lactams/anti-β-lactamase combinations. Colistin may be of benefit with resistant strains. In the pretransplant setting, *Acinetobacter* infections may become more prevalent as more centers become willing to transplant candidates who are on mechanical ventilatory or extracorporeal life support. Although there are currently no published reports describing the incidence or effect of pretransplant *Acinetobacter* infections on posttransplant outcomes, the concern for fatal posttransplant infection likely prevents many from being considered for transplantation. Infections with MDR *A baumannii* in lung transplant recipients can have devastating outcomes. In 1 series of 6 patients infected with carbapenem-resistant *A baumannii* during a hospital outbreak, the organism was persistently recovered from the respiratory tract in 4 of 6 recipients despite aggressive treatment and all 4 died as a result of this infection.[55] In another report that included 16 solid-organ transplant recipients with *A baumannii* that was resistant to all antimicrobials except tigecycline and colistin, patients who were initially treated with colistin monotherapy demonstrated 91% mortality.[56] However, following a new protocol to determine the local mechanism of resistance (OXA-23 gene) and subsequent synergy testing, an initial treatment regimen of carbapenem and colistin resulted in a 60% survival rate in subsequent patients infected with *A baumannii*. Further studies are needed to determine the circumstances under which patients with pretransplant *A baumannii* infection can undergo lung transplantation with acceptable posttransplant outcomes.

Nontuberculous Mycobacteria

Infections with nontuberculous mycobacteria (NTM) are fairly prevalent in patients with several pretransplant chronic lung processes including adult-onset bronchiectasis and CF. Overall, there is no difference in posttransplant mortality between patients with or without positive NTM cultures, however the rate of NTM disease is highest in patients with *Mycobacterium abscessus*.[57] Key points about NTM and lung transplant candidates are[57–61]

- Prevalence estimates of carriage are 3% to 13% in pretransplant patients and 10% to 22% after transplant.
- Many patients (~40%) who have pretransplant NTM continue to have positive cultures after transplant.
- *M abscessus* is considered a relative contraindication to transplant because of its virulence and intrinsic resistance to antimicrobial agents.

M abscessus

Microbiology

M abscessus, a rapidly growing mycobacterium (ie demonstrating visible growth on solid media within 7 days) is increasingly recognized as an important human pathogen.[62] This bacteria is found in water and soil and is capable of colonizing skin surfaces, the gastrointestinal tract, and the respiratory tract of humans. It is one of the most resistant organisms to antimicrobial agents, the mechanisms of which are the focus of increasing research. Natural and acquired resistance mechanisms include

- The presence of a waxy impermeable cell wall
- Antibiotic-modifying enzymes
- Target-modifying enzymes that confer resistance to macrolides
- Efflux pumps

The complete genome sequence became available in 2009, allowing for further classification of substrains and the discovery that *M abscessus* shares several characteristics with slow-growing mycobacteria.

Epidemiology

Before transplant, the most frequently isolated species are *Mycobacterium avium* complex (41%) followed by *M abscessus* (7%). *M abscessus* can cause skin infections in nosocomial settings, bronchopulmonary infections in patients with chronic lung diseases, and disseminated infections in immunocompromised hosts. There are few data on the clinical outcome of *M abscessus* infections in transplant recipients. Chernenko and colleagues[60] conducted a follow-up survey of 62 centers to determine the incidence and clinical outcomes of *M abscessus* infections before and after lung transplant.[61] Seventeen of 5200 transplant recipients were infected with *M abscessus* after transplant; of these, only 2 were infected with *M abscessus* before transplant, suggesting that pretransplant infection with *M abscessus* may have been a contraindication to transplant at many centers.

Peritransplant treatment

Treatment is recommended in patients who have progressive disease, or who may need lung transplantation in the future. *M abscessus* infections are intrinsically resistant to most standard antibiotics and antituberculous agents. Typical modal minimum inhibitory concentrations are less than tissue/serum levels only for clarithromycin, aminoglycosides, cefoxitin, and tigecycline, with some strain-specific variability in susceptibility patterns. Most recommendations are to use a multidrug regimen including clarithromycin, aminoglycoside, and a third agent for 24 months, but the efficacy of the multidrug approach is mixed. The success rates of sputum conversion and maintenance of negative cultures depend significantly on resistance profiles, ranging from 60% for macrolide-sensitive organisms to less than 20% in macrolide-resistant strains. Although *Mycobacterium avium* complex is more frequently recovered from respiratory samples, the isolation of the species rarely meets the American Thoracic Society (ATS) definition of clinical disease and may not require treatment.[58] In those cases that meet the ATS criteria, standard treatment approaches include clarithromycin, ethambutol, and rifampin for a minimum of 12 months.[62]

Scedosporium Species

Scedosporium colonization is common in patients with advanced CF, and infections are a problem in lung transplant recipients.[63] Among North American lung transplant recipients, *Scedosporium* species are the second most common cause of filamentous fungal infection, following only aspergillosis.[64,65] *Scedosporium* colonization is a risk factor for invasive disease after lung transplant.[65] Patients who are colonized with *Scedosporium* before transplant can develop infections with the same strain after the transplant.[66] Identifying patients who are carrying *Scedosporium* before transplant is crucial in that it gives clinicians a chance to try to modify the risk for posttransplant infection. Such information can also be used to inform decisions regarding the suitability of the patient for lung transplant.

Ecology and microbiology of Scedosporium
Clinically relevant species include *S prolificans*, *S apiospermum*, and the closely related *Pseudallescheria boydii*. Recent work has identified *S aurantiacum* as a new species within the *P boydii* complex.[67] Because the nomenclature has evolved in recent years, references to these fungi in the literature can be confusing. For example, *S apiospermum*, *P boydii* and *S aurantiacum* have previously been reported as 1 species.

Scedosporium species are found in soil, water, and air. Their abundance is related to increasing nitrogen concentrations and decreasing pH within a range of 6.1 to 7.5. Human activity, including intense fertilization and hydrocarbon waste, supports growth of *Scedosporium* species in the environment. Some of the highest concentrations of *Scedosporium* species can be found at industrial sites, near gas stations, in urban parks, and within agricultural areas.[68]

Geographic locale affects the epidemiology and microbiology of *Scedosporium* carriage in at-risk patients.

- *Scedosporium* colonization and infection are particularly prevalent in Australia.
- Environmental sampling in Australia has revealed an abundance of *S aurantiacum* and *S prolificans* in locations of high human activity.[69]

In 1 Australian medical center, molecular epidemiology analysis showed a single common type isolated in multiple patients suggesting a shared exposure source.[70] In general, however, exposure tends to be spread out over diverse regions, and in most studies a point source cannot be identified.[71,72]

Epidemiology of Scedosporium carriage
Presence of *Scedosporium* species can be a common finding in the respiratory tract and sinuses of patients with CF, bronchiectasis, and even interstitial lung disease.[70,73–75]

- Patients with late-stage CF are at particularly high risk for carriage.
- After *Aspergillus*, *Scedosporium* species are typically the most commonly isolated filamentous fungi in patients with CF.
- Carriage rates have been reported to be in the 3% to 10% range.[63,76,77]

The intersection of environmental exposure and host factors affects the epidemiology of colonization and infection. In CF, the conditions created by viscous secretions, airway abnormalities, and the impact of chronic and recurrent bacterial colonization and infection favor carriage of these fungi. In 1 study, patients with *Scedosporium* colonization were significantly less likely to be colonized with mucoid strains of *P aeruginosa*, whereas colonization rates were higher in those who had received previous therapy with antistaphylococcal penicillins.[78]

Accurate detection of respiratory tract colonization with *Scedosporium* and identification to the species level can be challenging. Because treatment regimens differ by infecting species, identifying *Scedosporium* to the species level is crucial. Molecular techniques can assist in this task. Additional techniques that are in development include use of mass spectroscopy and assays that detect a siderophore that is specific for *S apiospermum*.[79,80]

- When using standard culture media, *Scedosporium* carriage can be underestimated because of overgrowth by faster-growing bacteria and fungi (eg, *P aeruginosa* and *Aspergillus* species).
- Specialized semiselective mycologic isolation medium such as SceSel can increase yield.[81,82] Such media should be used in addition to standard fungal culture techniques when evaluating patients.[77]
- Once the fungus is grown in culture, a species-specific multiplex polymerase chain reaction (PCR) can differentiate between clinically relevant species.[83]
- Application of PCR directly to sputum is another approach that can be used to detect occult organisms to the species level.[84]

The natural history of *Scedosporium* carriage is variable. Colonization may be transient or persist in the bronchial passages or sinuses for years.[85] Once persistent colonization is established, it becomes difficult to eradicate.[86,87] Patients tend to become exclusively colonized with 1 species (eg, *S prolificans, S aurantiacum* or *S apiospermum*), but may carry multiple strains of that species.[88]

Clinical manifestations and treatment before transplant

Clinical manifestations of *Scedosporium* in patients with CF (before transplant) include[63,86]

- Asymptomatic carriage; this is the most common presentation.
- Mycetoma, which tends to occur in preexisting lung cavities and is sometimes referred to as a fungus ball.
- Allergic bronchopulmonary disease, which is a syndrome much like allergic bronchopulmonary aspergillosis.
- Invasive disease is uncommon, but may occur in patients with CF. Can be limited to the lung or present as disseminated infection.[89]

Evaluation of a patient with CF with findings suggestive of invasive infection, mycetoma, or allergic bronchopulmonary disease should include a search for *Scedosporium*.

Scedosporium species are difficult to treat with antifungal agents. Based on in vitro data and clinical experience, treatment options for *S apiospermum* (and the related *P boydii*) and for *S aurantiacum* are[90,91]

- Voriconazole, which is probably the best choice
- Combination therapy with an echinocandin and either voriconazole or amphotericin B (AmB)

S prolificans can be resistant to multiple antifungal agents, including voriconazole and AmB. Treatment options for invasive infection with S prolificans include[92–96]

- Surgical management
- Micafungin combined with voriconazole or AmB
- Voriconazole combined with terbinafine has also been effective in vitro and in clinical S prolificans infections

The role of posaconazole for any of the Scedosporium species is unclear at this time, but may be an option for those that are intolerant or not responding to voriconazole.[97] Susceptibility testing, which generally requires sending the isolate to a reference laboratory, is an important element in constructing an antifungal regimen for such infections.

Treatment considerations in patients with chronic lung disease who are carrying Scedosporium depend on the species, the clinical scenario, and the prospects for lung transplant. The decision to treat is generally straightforward in patients with invasive disease. The approach to asymptomatic colonization is a more difficult decision point. Patients who are colonized with Scedosporium before transplantation may progress to disseminated infection after lung transplant. Therefore, an effort should be made to control the fungus in such patients.[85] Voriconazole is usually the drug of choice in this situation, but breakthrough infections have developed with this and other agents (eg, AmB and itraconazole).[66,97] Moreover, eradication of Scedosporium may not be possible, requiring consideration of indefinite fungal prophylaxis after transplant.

Infections after lung transplant
The clinical manifestations of Scedosporium infection after lung transplant are diverse and range from asymptomatic colonization to severe invasive disease.[97–100] In 1 study, proven (including disseminated) infection was diagnosed in 36% of lung recipients from whom Scedosporium was recovered.[101]

- Infection in lung transplant recipients generally originates in the lungs and sinuses, which are also the typical sites of pretransplant colonization.
- An important aspect of Scedosporium infections in lung transplant recipients is a tendency toward disseminated infection with clinical manifestations that include fungemia, brain abscess, endocarditis, cutaneous involvement, spondylodiscitis, and endophthalmitis.[65,97,100,102]
- Once disseminated infection develops, the disease is nearly always fatal despite use of multiple antifungal agents and surgical excision.

Treatment options for invasive scedosporiosis after lung transplant are generally unsatisfactory.[75] Response to therapy depends on the extent of infection and the infecting organism. Disseminated infection with any of the Scedosporium species is nearly always associated with mortality. Infections caused by S prolificans are extraordinarily difficult to treat and tend to have poorer responses to antifungal therapy than those caused by S apiospermum.[103] The ideal treatment regimens for infection with the various Scedosporium species are not known. Treatment failures are common and, when successful, antifungal therapy generally needs to be given for months or longer. Relapses are common and lifelong therapy may be required.

The general approach to Scedosporium infection after transplant is

- *S apiospermum* and *S aurantiacum*: voriconazole ± echinocandin
- *S prolificans*: surgical therapy and adjunctive voriconazole ± an echinocandin ± terbinafine

Aspergillus terreus

Aspergillosis is the most common fungal infection in lung transplant recipients.[104] A small but significant proportion of cases are caused by *Aspergullus terreus*. Exposure to this difficult-to-treat fungus is via inhalation of airborne conidia from environmental sources. Colonization or infection in a patient with chronic lung disease before transplant can be particularly problematic. *A terreus* has been identified in outdoor air, home tapwater, and compost.[105–107] After transplant, *A terreus* infection can progress rapidly and is associated with a high mortality rate.[108] *A terreus* tends to be resistant to AmB. Prophylactic use of aerosolized AmB, which is a common practice in lung transplant programs, is a risk factor for infection with this fungus.[109–113] *A terreus* is generally susceptible to voriconazole and this is the drug of choice for invasive disease.

SUMMARY

Advances in supportive care, including broad use of antimicrobial agents, are prolonging the lives of patients with advanced lung disease. A byproduct of these advances has been an increasing prevalence of carriage and infection with MDR organisms. When such infections occur after transplant, the results can be disastrous. In this regard, infections with highly resistant strains of *P aeruginosa*, *Burkholderia*, *Acinetobacter*, nontuberculous mycobacteria, *Scedosporium*, and *A terreus* can be particularly problematic. An understanding of the epidemiology, diagnosis, and treatment of these infections is important when evaluating a pretransplant candidate.

REFERENCES

1. Christie JD, Edwards LB, Kucheryavaya AY, et al. The Registry of the International Society for Heart and Lung Transplantation: twenty-eighth adult lung and heart-lung transplant report–2011. J Heart Lung Transplant 2011;30(10): 1104–22.
2. Liou TG, Woo MS, Cahill BC. Lung transplantation for cystic fibrosis. Curr Opin Pulm Med 2006;12(6):459–63.
3. Wine JJ. The genesis of cystic fibrosis lung disease. J Clin Invest 1999;103(3): 309–12.
4. Mayer-Hamblett N, Rosenfeld M, Emerson J, et al. Developing cystic fibrosis lung transplant referral criteria using predictors of 2-year mortality. Am J Respir Crit Care Med 2002;166(12 Pt 1):1550–5.
5. Emerson J, Rosenfeld M, McNamara S, et al. *Pseudomonas aeruginosa* and other predictors of mortality and morbidity in young children with cystic fibrosis. Pediatr Pulmonol 2002;34(2):91–100.
6. Emerson J, McNamara S, Buccat AM, et al. Changes in cystic fibrosis sputum microbiology in the United States between 1995 and 2008. Pediatr Pulmonol 2010;45(4):363–70.
7. Knudsen PK, Olesen HV, Hoiby N, et al. Differences in prevalence and treatment of *Pseudomonas aeruginosa* in cystic fibrosis centres in Denmark, Norway and Sweden. J Cyst Fibros 2009;8(2):135–42.
8. Zhao J, Schloss PD, Kalikin LM, et al. Decade-long bacterial community dynamics in cystic fibrosis airways. Proc Natl Acad Sci U S A 2012;109(15):5809–14.

9. Fodor AA, Klem ER, Gilpin DF, et al. The adult cystic fibrosis airway microbiota is stable over time and infection type, and highly resilient to antibiotic treatment of exacerbations. PLoS One 2012;7(9):e45001.

10. Orens JB, Estenne M, Arcasoy S, et al. International guidelines for the selection of lung transplant candidates: 2006 update–a consensus report from the Pulmonary Scientific Council of the International Society for Heart and Lung Transplantation. J Heart Lung Transplant 2006;25(7):745–55.

11. Favero MS, Carson LA, Bond WW, et al. Pseudomonas aeruginosa: growth in distilled water from hospitals. Science 1971;173(3999):836–8.

12. Bodey GP, Jadeja L, Elting L. *Pseudomonas bacteremia*. Retrospective analysis of 410 episodes. Arch Intern Med 1985;145(9):1621–9.

13. Kosorok MR, Jalaluddin M, Farrell PM, et al. Comprehensive analysis of risk factors for acquisition of *Pseudomonas aeruginosa* in young children with cystic fibrosis. Pediatr Pulmonol 1998;26(2):81–8.

14. Oliver A, Canton R, Campo P, et al. High frequency of hypermutable *Pseudomonas aeruginosa* in cystic fibrosis lung infection. Science 2000;288(5469):1251–4.

15. Smith EE, Buckley DG, Wu Z, et al. Genetic adaptation by *Pseudomonas aeruginosa* to the airways of cystic fibrosis patients. Proc Natl Acad Sci U S A 2006;103(22):8487–92.

16. Li Z, Kosorok MR, Farrell PM, et al. Longitudinal development of mucoid *Pseudomonas aeruginosa* infection and lung disease progression in children with cystic fibrosis. JAMA 2005;293(5):581–8.

17. Doring G, Conway SP, Heijerman HG, et al. Antibiotic therapy against *Pseudomonas aeruginosa* in cystic fibrosis: a European consensus. Eur Respir J 2000;16(4):749–67.

18. Bonvillain RW, Valentine VG, Lombard G, et al. Post-operative infections in cystic fibrosis and non-cystic fibrosis patients after lung transplantation. J Heart Lung Transplant 2007;26(9):890–7.

19. Palmer SM, Alexander BD, Sanders LL, et al. Significance of blood stream infection after lung transplantation: analysis in 176 consecutive patients. Transplantation 2000;69(11):2360–6.

20. Aguilar-Guisado M, Givalda J, Ussetti P, et al. Pneumonia after lung transplantation in the RESITRA cohort: a multicenter prospective study. Am J Transplant 2007;7(8):1989–96.

21. Campos S, Caramori M, Teixeira R, et al. Bacterial and fungal pneumonias after lung transplantation. Transplant Proc 2008;40(3):822–4.

22. Valentine VG, Bonvillain RW, Gupta MR, et al. Infections in lung allograft recipients: ganciclovir era. J Heart Lung Transplant 2008;27(5):528–35.

23. Vos R, Vanaudenaerde BM, Geudens N, et al. Pseudomonal airway colonisation: risk factor for bronchiolitis obliterans syndrome after lung transplantation? Eur Respir J 2008;31(5):1037–45.

24. Botha P, Archer L, Anderson RL, et al. *Pseudomonas aeruginosa* colonization of the allograft after lung transplantation and the risk of bronchiolitis obliterans syndrome. Transplantation 2008;85(5):771–4.

25. Hadjiliadis D, Steele MP, Chaparro C, et al. Survival of lung transplant patients with cystic fibrosis harboring panresistant bacteria other than *Burkholderia cepacia*, compared with patients harboring sensitive bacteria. J Heart Lung Transplant 2007;26(8):834–8.

26. Lechtzin N, John M, Irizarry R, et al. Outcomes of adults with cystic fibrosis infected with antibiotic-resistant *Pseudomonas aeruginosa*. Respiration 2006; 73(1):27–33.

27. Lambiase A, Raia V, Del Pezzo M, et al. Microbiology of airway disease in a cohort of patients with cystic fibrosis. BMC Infect Dis 2006;6:4.
28. Johnson C, Butler SM, Konstan MW, et al. Factors influencing outcomes in cystic fibrosis: a center-based analysis. Chest 2003;123(1):20–7.
29. Saiman L. Clinical utility of synergy testing for multidrug-resistant *Pseudomonas aeruginosa* isolated from patients with cystic fibrosis: 'the motion for'. Paediatr Respir Rev 2007;8(3):249–55.
30. Lang BJ, Aaron SD, Ferris W, et al. Multiple combination bactericidal antibiotic testing for patients with cystic fibrosis infected with multiresistant strains of *Pseudomonas aeruginosa*. Am J Respir Crit Care Med 2000;162(6):2241–5.
31. Aaron SD, Vandemheen KL, Ferris W, et al. Combination antibiotic susceptibility testing to treat exacerbations of cystic fibrosis associated with multiresistant bacteria: a randomised, double-blind, controlled clinical trial. Lancet 2005; 366(9484):463–71.
32. Flume PA, O'Sullivan BP, Robinson KA, et al. Cystic fibrosis pulmonary guidelines: chronic medications for maintenance of lung health. Am J Respir Crit Care Med 2007;176(10):957–69.
33. Bauldoff GS, Nunley DR, Manzetti JD, et al. Use of aerosolized colistin sodium in cystic fibrosis patients awaiting lung transplantation. Transplantation 1997; 64(5):748–52.
34. Flume PA, Mogayzel PJ Jr, Robinson KA, et al. Cystic fibrosis pulmonary guidelines: treatment of pulmonary exacerbations. Am J Respir Crit Care Med 2009; 180(9):802–8.
35. Horsley A, Webb K, Bright-Thomas R, et al. Can early *Burkholderia cepacia* complex infection in cystic fibrosis be eradicated with antibiotic therapy? Front Cell Infect Microbiol 2011;1:18.
36. Kalish LA, Waltz DA, Dovey M, et al. Impact of *Burkholderia dolosa* on lung function and survival in cystic fibrosis. Am J Respir Crit Care Med 2006;173(4):421–5.
37. Murray S, Charbeneau J, Marshall BC, et al. Impact of *Burkholderia* infection on lung transplantation in cystic fibrosis. Am J Respir Crit Care Med 2008;178(4): 363–71.
38. De Soyza A, McDowell A, Archer L, et al. *Burkholderia cepacia* complex genomovars and pulmonary transplantation outcomes in patients with cystic fibrosis. Lancet 2001;358(9295):1780–1.
39. Alexander BD, Petzold EW, Reller LB, et al. Survival after lung transplantation of cystic fibrosis patients infected with *Burkholderia cepacia* complex. Am J Transplant 2008;8(5):1025–30.
40. Kennedy MP, Coakley RD, Donaldson SH, et al. *Burkholderia gladioli*: five year experience in a cystic fibrosis and lung transplantation center. J Cyst Fibros 2007;6(4):267–73.
41. Church AC, Sivasothy P, Parmer J, et al. Mediastinal abscess after lung transplantation secondary to *Burkholderia gladioli* infection. J Heart Lung Transplant 2009;28(5):511–4.
42. Kanj SS, Tapson V, Davis RD, et al. Infections in patients with cystic fibrosis following lung transplantation. Chest 1997;112(4):924–30.
43. Avgeri SG, Matthaiou DK, Dimopoulos G, et al. Therapeutic options for *Burkholderia cepacia* infections beyond co-trimoxazole: a systematic review of the clinical evidence. Int J Antimicrob Agents 2009;33(5):394–404.
44. Nair BM, Joachimiak LA, Chattopadhyay S, et al. Conservation of a novel protein associated with an antibiotic efflux operon in *Burkholderia cenocepacia*. FEMS Microbiol Lett 2005;245(2):337–44.

45. Lipuma JJ. Update on the *Burkholderia cepacia* complex. Curr Opin Pulm Med 2005;11(6):528–33.
46. Urban C, Segal-Maurer S, Rahal JJ. Considerations in control and treatment of nosocomial infections due to multidrug-resistant *Acinetobacter baumannii*. Clin Infect Dis 2003;36(10):1268–74.
47. Fournier PE, Richet H. The epidemiology and control of *Acinetobacter baumannii* in health care facilities. Clin Infect Dis 2006;42(5):692–9.
48. Wendt C, Dietze B, Dietz E, et al. Survival of *Acinetobacter baumannii* on dry surfaces. J Clin Microbiol 1997;35(6):1394–7.
49. Boucher HW, Talbot GH, Bradley JS, et al. Bad bugs, no drugs: no ESKAPE! An update from the Infectious Diseases Society of America. Clin Infect Dis 2009; 48(1):1–12.
50. Mak JK, Kim MJ, Pham J, et al. Antibiotic resistance determinants in nosocomial strains of multidrug-resistant *Acinetobacter baumannii*. J Antimicrob Chemother 2009;63(1):47–54.
51. Lee JC, Koerten H, van den Broek P, et al. Adherence of *Acinetobacter baumannii* strains to human bronchial epithelial cells. Res Microbiol 2006;157(4):360–6.
52. Kaplan N, Rosenberg E, Jann B, et al. Structural studies of the capsular polysaccharide of *Acinetobacter calcoaceticus* BD4. Eur J Biochem 1985;152(2): 453–8.
53. Chatellier D, Burucoa C, Pinsard M, et al. Prevalence of *Acinetobacter baumannii* carriage in patients of 53 French intensive care units on a given day. Med Mal Infect 2007;37(2):112–7 [in French].
54. Lolans K, Rice TW, Munoz-Price LS, et al. Multicity outbreak of carbapenem-resistant *Acinetobacter baumannii* isolates producing the carbapenemase OXA-40. Antimicrob Agents Chemother 2006;50(9):2941–5.
55. Nunley DR, Bauldoff GS, Mangino JE, et al. Mortality associated with *Acinetobacter baumannii* infections experienced by lung transplant recipients. Lung 2010; 188(5):381–5.
56. Shields RK, Kwak EJ, Potoski BA, et al. High mortality rates among solid organ transplant recipients infected with extensively drug-resistant *Acinetobacter baumannii*: using in vitro antibiotic combination testing to identify the combination of a carbapenem and colistin as an effective treatment regimen. Diagn Microbiol Infect Dis 2011;70(2):246–52.
57. Chalermskulrat W, Sood N, Neuringer IP, et al. Non-tuberculous mycobacteria in end stage cystic fibrosis: implications for lung transplantation. Thorax 2006; 61(6):507–13.
58. Knoll BM, Kappagoda S, Gill RR, et al. Non-tuberculous mycobacterial infection among lung transplant recipients: a 15-year cohort study. Transpl Infect Dis 2012;14(5):452–60.
59. Fowler SJ, French J, Screaton NJ, et al. Nontuberculous mycobacteria in bronchiectasis: prevalence and patient characteristics. Eur Respir J 2006;28(6):1204–10.
60. Chernenko SM, Humar A, Hutcheon M, et al. *Mycobacterium abscessus* infections in lung transplant recipients: the international experience. J Heart Lung Transplant 2006;25(12):1447–55.
61. Sanguinetti M, Ardito F, Fiscarelli E, et al. Fatal pulmonary infection due to multidrug-resistant *Mycobacterium abscessus* in a patient with cystic fibrosis. J Clin Microbiol 2001;39(2):816–9.
62. Griffith DE, Aksamit T, Brown-Elliott BA, et al. An official ATS/IDSA statement: diagnosis, treatment, and prevention of nontuberculous mycobacterial diseases. Am J Respir Crit Care Med 2007;175(4):367–416.

63. Paugam A, Baixench MT, Demazes-Dufeu N, et al. Characteristics and consequences of airway colonization by filamentous fungi in 201 adult patients with cystic fibrosis in France. Med Mycol 2010;48(Suppl 1):S32–6.

64. Park BJ, Pappas PG, Wannemuehler KA, et al. Invasive non-*Aspergillus* mold infections in transplant recipients, United States, 2001-2006. Emerg Infect Dis 2011;17(10):1855–64.

65. Morio F, Horeau-Langlard D, Gay-Andrieu F, et al. Disseminated *Scedosporium/Pseudallescheria* infection after double-lung transplantation in patients with cystic fibrosis. J Clin Microbiol 2010;48(5):1978–82.

66. Symoens F, Knoop C, Schrooyen M, et al. Disseminated *Scedosporium apiospermum* infection in a cystic fibrosis patient after double-lung transplantation. J Heart Lung Transplant 2006;25(5):603–7.

67. Alastruey-Izquierdo A, Cuenca-Estrella M, Monzon A, et al. Prevalence and susceptibility testing of new species of *Pseudallescheria* and *Scedosporium* in a collection of clinical mold isolates. Antimicrob Agents Chemother 2007;51(2): 748–51.

68. Kaltseis J, Rainer J, De Hoog GS. Ecology of *Pseudallescheria* and *Scedosporium* species in human-dominated and natural environments and their distribution in clinical samples. Med Mycol 2009;47(4):398–405.

69. Harun A, Gilgado F, Chen SC, et al. Abundance of *Pseudallescheria/Scedosporium* species in the Australian urban environment suggests a possible source for scedosporiosis including the colonization of airways in cystic fibrosis. Med Mycol 2010; 48(Suppl 1):S70–6.

70. Williamson EC, Speers D, Arthur IH, et al. Molecular epidemiology of *Scedosporium apiospermum* infection determined by PCR amplification of ribosomal intergenic spacer sequences in patients with chronic lung disease. J Clin Microbiol 2001;39(1):47–50.

71. Delhaes L, Harun A, Chen SC, et al. Molecular typing of Australian *Scedosporium* isolates showing genetic variability and numerous *S. aurantiacum*. Emerg Infect Dis 2008;14(2):282–90.

72. San Millan R, Quindos G, Garaizar J, et al. Characterization of *Scedosporium prolificans* clinical isolates by randomly amplified polymorphic DNA analysis. J Clin Microbiol 1997;35(9):2270–4.

73. Cooley L, Spelman D, Thursky K, et al. Infection with *Scedosporium apiospermum* and *S. prolificans*, Australia. Emerg Infect Dis 2007;13(8):1170–7.

74. Castiglioni B, Sutton DA, Rinaldi MG, et al. *Pseudallescheria boydii* (Anamorph *Scedosporium apiospermum*). Infection in solid organ transplant recipients in a tertiary medical center and review of the literature. Medicine (Baltimore) 2002; 81(5):333–48.

75. Rodriguez-Tudela JL, Berenguer J, Guarro J, et al. Epidemiology and outcome of *Scedosporium prolificans* infection, a review of 162 cases. Med Mycol 2009; 47(4):359–70.

76. Cimon B, Carrere J, Vinatier JF, et al. Clinical significance of *Scedosporium apiospermum* in patients with cystic fibrosis. Eur J Clin Microbiol Infect Dis 2000;19(1):53–6.

77. Blyth CC, Harun A, Middleton PG, et al. Detection of occult *Scedosporium* species in respiratory tract specimens from patients with cystic fibrosis by use of selective media. J Clin Microbiol 2010;48(1):314–6.

78. Blyth CC, Middleton PG, Harun A, et al. Clinical associations and prevalence of *Scedosporium* spp. in Australian cystic fibrosis patients: identification of novel risk factors? Med Mycol 2010;48(Suppl 1):S37–44.

79. Coulibaly O, Marinach-Patrice C, Cassagne C, et al. *Pseudallescheria/Scedosporium* complex species identification by matrix-assisted laser desorption ionization time-of-flight mass spectrometry. Med Mycol 2011;49(6): 621–6.

80. Bertrand S, Bouchara JP, Venier MC, et al. N(alpha)-Methyl coprogen B, a potential marker of the airway colonization by *Scedosporium apiospermum* in patients with cystic fibrosis. Med Mycol 2010;48(Suppl 1):S98–107.

81. Horre R, Marklein G, Siekmeier R, et al. Selective isolation of *Pseudallescheria* and *Scedosporium* species from respiratory tract specimens of cystic fibrosis patients. Respiration 2009;77(3):320–4.

82. Borman AM, Palmer MD, Delhaes L, et al. Lack of standardization in the procedures for mycological examination of sputum samples from CF patients: a possible cause for variations in the prevalence of filamentous fungi. Med Mycol 2010;48(Suppl 1):S88–97.

83. Harun A, Blyth CC, Gilgado F, et al. Development and validation of a multiplex PCR for detection of *Scedosporium* spp. in respiratory tract specimens from patients with cystic fibrosis. J Clin Microbiol 2011;49(4):1508–12.

84. Lu Q, van den Ende AH, de Hoog GS, et al. Reverse line blot hybridisation screening of *Pseudallescheria/Scedosporium* species in patients with cystic fibrosis. Mycoses 2011;54(Suppl 3):5–11.

85. Tintelnot K, Just-Nubling G, Horre R, et al. A review of German *Scedosporium prolificans* cases from 1993 to 2007. Med Mycol 2009;47(4):351–8.

86. Borghi E, Iatta R, Manca A, et al. Chronic airway colonization by *Scedosporium apiospermum* with a fatal outcome in a patient with cystic fibrosis. Med Mycol 2010;48(Suppl 1):S108–13.

87. Defontaine A, Zouhair R, Cimon B, et al. Genotyping study of *Scedosporium apiospermum* isolates from patients with cystic fibrosis. J Clin Microbiol 2002; 40(6):2108–14.

88. Lackner M, Rezusta A, Villuendas MC, et al. Infection and colonisation due to *Scedosporium* in Northern Spain. An in vitro antifungal susceptibility and molecular epidemiology study of 60 isolates. Mycoses 2011;54(Suppl 3): 12–21.

89. Guignard S, Hubert D, Dupont B, et al. Multifocal *Scedosporium apiospermum* spondylitis in a cystic fibrosis patient. J Cyst Fibros 2008;7(1):89–91.

90. Lackner M, de Hoog GS, Verweij PE, et al. Species-specific antifungal susceptibility patterns of *Scedosporium* and *Pseudallescheria* species. Antimicrob Agents Chemother 2012;56(5):2635–42.

91. Cortez KJ, Roilides E, Quiroz-Telles F, et al. Infections caused by *Scedosporium* spp. Clin Microbiol Rev 2008;21(1):157–97.

92. Rodriguez MM, Calvo E, Serena C, et al. Effects of double and triple combinations of antifungal drugs in a murine model of disseminated infection by *Scedosporium prolificans*. Antimicrob Agents Chemother 2009;53(5):2153–5.

93. Heyn K, Tredup A, Salvenmoser S, et al. Effect of voriconazole combined with micafungin against *Candida*, *Aspergillus*, and *Scedosporium* spp. and *Fusarium solani*. Antimicrob Agents Chemother 2005;49(12):5157–9.

94. Yustes C, Guarro J. In vitro synergistic interaction between amphotericin B and micafungin against *Scedosporium* spp. Antimicrob Agents Chemother 2005; 49(8):3498–500.

95. Meletiadis J, Mouton JW, Meis JF, et al. In vitro drug interaction modeling of combinations of azoles with terbinafine against clinical *Scedosporium prolificans* isolates. Antimicrob Agents Chemother 2003;47(1):106–17.

96. Howden BP, Slavin MA, Schwarer AP, et al. Successful control of disseminated *Scedosporium prolificans* infection with a combination of voriconazole and terbinafine. Eur J Clin Microbiol Infect Dis 2003;22(2):111–3.

97. Sahi H, Avery RK, Minai OA, et al. *Scedosporium apiospermum* (*Pseudoallescheria boydii*) infection in lung transplant recipients. J Heart Lung Transplant 2007;26(4):350–6.

98. Vagefi MR, Kim ET, Alvarado RG, et al. Bilateral endogenous *Scedosporium prolificans* endophthalmitis after lung transplantation. Am J Ophthalmol 2005;139(2): 370–3.

99. Raj R, Frost AE. *Scedosporium apiospermum* fungemia in a lung transplant recipient. Chest 2002;121(5):1714–6.

100. Rabodonirina M, Paulus S, Thevenet F, et al. Disseminated *Scedosporium prolificans* (*S. inflatum*) infection after single-lung transplantation. Clin Infect Dis 1994;19(1):138–42.

101. Heath CH, Slavin MA, Sorrell TC, et al. Population-based surveillance for scedosporiosis in Australia: epidemiology, disease manifestations and emergence of *Scedosporium aurantiacum* infection. Clin Microbiol Infect 2009;15(7):689–93.

102. Miraldi F, Anile M, Ruberto F, et al. *Scedosporium apiospermum* atrial mycetomas after lung transplantation for cystic fibrosis. Transpl Infect Dis 2012;14(2):188–91.

103. Troke P, Aguirrebengoa K, Arteaga C, et al. Treatment of scedosporiosis with voriconazole: clinical experience with 107 patients. Antimicrob Agents Chemother 2008;52(5):1743–50.

104. Neofytos D, Fishman JA, Horn D, et al. Epidemiology and outcome of invasive fungal infections in solid organ transplant recipients. Transpl Infect Dis 2010; 12(3):220–9.

105. Mortensen KL, Mellado E, Lass-Florl C, et al. Environmental study of azole-resistant *Aspergillus fumigatus* and other aspergilli in Austria, Denmark, and Spain. Antimicrob Agents Chemother 2010;54(11):4545–9.

106. Blum G, Perkhofer S, Grif K, et al. A 1-year *Aspergillus terreus* surveillance study at the University Hospital of Innsbruck: molecular typing of environmental and clinical isolates. Clin Microbiol Infect 2008;14(12):1146–51.

107. Vesper SJ, Haugland RA, Rogers ME, et al. Opportunistic *Aspergillus* pathogens measured in home and hospital tap water by quantitative PCR (QPCR). J Water Health 2007;5(3):427–31.

108. Lass-Florl C, Griff K, Mayr A, et al. Epidemiology and outcome of infections due to *Aspergillus terreus*: 10-year single centre experience. Br J Haematol 2005; 131(2):201–7.

109. Steinbach WJ, Marr KA, Anaissie EJ, et al. Clinical epidemiology of 960 patients with invasive aspergillosis from the PATH Alliance registry. J Infect 2012;65(5):453–64.

110. Ruping MJ, Gerlach S, Fischer G, et al. Environmental and clinical epidemiology of *Aspergillus terreus*: data from a prospective surveillance study. J Hosp Infect 2011;78(3):226–30.

111. Caston JJ, Linares MJ, Gallego C, et al. Risk factors for pulmonary *Aspergillus terreus* infection in patients with positive culture for filamentous fungi. Chest 2007;131(1):230–6.

112. Zhou J, Chen Y, Tabibi S, et al. Antimicrobial susceptibility and synergy studies of *Burkholderia cepacia* complex isolated from patients with cystic fibrosis. Antimicrob Agents Chemother 2007;51(3):1085–8.

113. Segonds C, Clavel-Batut P, Thouverez M, et al. Microbiological and epidemiological features of clinical respiratory isolates of *Burkholderia gladioli*. J Clin Microbiol 2009;47(5):1510–6.

Infections in Intestinal and Multivisceral Transplant Recipients

Joseph G. Timpone Jr, MD*, Raffaele Girlanda, MD,
Lauren Rudolph, BA, Thomas M. Fishbein, MD

KEYWORDS

- Infection • Intestinal and multivisceral • Transplantation • Intestinal failure
- Short bowel syndrome

KEY POINTS

- Patients with intestinal failure and short bowel syndrome experience multiple complications related to their disease, predisposing them to recurrent infections before transplantation.
- Intestinal and multivisceral transplant recipients tend to be at greatest risk for developing health care–associated infections immediately after transplantation, although this risk continues indefinitely.
- The most common types of infection in the immediate posttransplant period are often due to multidrug-resistant organisms and *Candida* species, and often cause intra-abdominal and bloodstream infections.
- Opportunistic viral and fungal infections tend to affect intestinal and multivisceral recipients later in the posttransplant time period.
- Viral allograft enteritis due to cytomegalovirus, Epstein-Barr virus, adenovirus, rotavirus, and norovirus are common complications in intestinal and multivisceral transplant recipients.
- Intestinal and multivisceral transplant recipients may be at higher risk for infectious disease complications because of the technically difficult intra-abdominal surgical procedure and the need for higher levels of immunosuppression in comparison with other solid organ transplant recipients.

INTRODUCTION

Intestinal and multivisceral transplantation (IMVTx) represents the most recent development in abdominal organ transplantation. It began as an experimental procedure,

The authors have nothing to disclose.
Division of Infectious Diseases, Department of Medicine, MedStar Georgetown University Hospital, 3800 Reservoir Road Northwest, 5PHC, Washington, DC 20007, USA
* Corresponding author.
E-mail address: timponej@gunet.georgetown.edu

Infect Dis Clin N Am 27 (2013) 359–377
http://dx.doi.org/10.1016/j.idc.2013.02.012
0891-5520/13/$ – see front matter © 2013 Elsevier Inc. All rights reserved.

with about 2200 transplants performed worldwide since 1985 according to the 2009 Intestinal Transplant Registry report.[1] However, this number only recently increased, reaching 200 transplants per year in the last 4 years. Unlike liver or kidney transplants that are performed in virtually every transplant program, IMVTx is performed in only a few specialized centers. As of 2009, only 8 centers worldwide had performed 100 IMVTx or more.

Today, IMVTx has become an effective treatment for patients with irreversible intestinal failure and life-threatening complications from parenteral nutrition (PN).[2] The indication for IMVTx as recognized by the Centers for Medicare and Medicaid services[3] is irreversible intestinal failure defined as: (1) the loss of nutritional autonomy of the gut associated with life-threatening complications of PN including liver failure, (2) loss of central venous access secondary to thrombosis, (3) systemic sepsis from line infection requiring hospitalization, and (4) frequent episodes of dehydration. The most common cause of intestinal failure is short bowel syndrome (SBS), which has multiple causes including complications from prior abdominal surgery, complications from Crohn disease, intra-abdominal trauma caused by gunshot injuries, mesenteric vascular thrombosis/ischemia, radiation enteritis, recurrent intestinal obstruction, necrotizing enterocolitis, intestinal atresia, intestinal volvulus, and congenital short small bowel. Other causes of intestinal failure include motility disorders, malabsorption (mucosal defects), and neoplasms of the mesentery.

Three types of transplants are available for the patient with intestinal failure. First, an isolated intestinal transplant may be performed, whereby the small intestine (jejunoileum) is transplanted alone with systemic drainage to the vena cava. The second type of transplant is a composite liver and intestinal transplant that typically includes the duodenum and an intact biliary system and portal circulation, whereby the native foregut is preserved. The third type is a multivisceral transplant involving the liver, stomach, duodenum, pancreas, and small intestine, whereby the foregut is removed and a new stomach is transplanted. This third type of transplant sometimes includes the colon, kidney, or both. In addition, the inclusion of the colon with the isolated intestinal and the intestinal-liver transplant has become an acceptable surgical technique, and is often performed at the authors' center. The combined small intestinal–liver transplant is indicated in patients who develop liver failure as a result of chronic use of PN.

Infectious complications are of major concern for the IMVTx patient. According to several studies, infection continues to be an important cause of morbidity and mortality in patients receiving IMVTx.[2,4,5] In one series, although infection was the attributable cause of mortality in 17.8% of intestinal transplant recipients, of all patients who had expired, infection was documented in 76.2%.[5] Furthermore, in one large retrospective series, infection was the second most common cause associated with allograft loss after rejection.[4] It is estimated that nearly 90% of patients who have undergone IMVTx develop a bacterial infection by their follow-up at 6 months,[5] and approximately 61% develop a bloodstream infection during their first 6 months after transplantation.[6] Within the first postoperative month alone, infection rates have been shown to occur in 58% to 80% of patients who have undergone IMVTx.[5,7,8]

This high risk of infection begins during the pretransplant period, persists throughout the perioperative and postoperative periods, and remains an important threat during the years of follow-up in patients who have undergone successful IMVTx. The risk factors that predispose IMVTx recipients to infection as well as the infectious complications associated with intestinal failure that precede transplantation makes this a very unique and challenging patient population that requires a multidisciplinary approach. The different types of infections that commonly affect this patient population can be organized temporally. In this article the clinical course of IMVTx is divided into 3 time periods: pretransplantation, immediate posttransplantation, and "later" posttransplantation. The associated infections and risk factors for infection are discussed according to this timeline.

PRETRANSPLANTATION

Patients with intestinal failure and SBS being considered for IMVTx are at particular risk of infection during the pretransplant period. Several factors are responsible, including multiple hospitalizations, intra-abdominal anatomic abnormalities, the use of PN, and the immunosuppression associated with malnutrition. These risk factors are summarized in **Table 1** and are discussed in detail here.

Of note, intestinal failure is associated with numerous comorbidities that can result in multiple hospital admissions, prolonged lengths of stay, and many surgical procedures. Both repeat and prolonged hospital stays increase patients' exposure to health care–associated pathogens, ultimately leading to health care–acquired infections. Multiple surgical procedures, such as resection of ischemic bowel in the setting of mesenteric thrombosis, or resection and repair of intra-abdominal fistulas experienced in Crohn disease, often result in intra-abdominal abnormalities predisposed to infection. In addition, patients with intestinal failure frequently develop spontaneous intra-abdominal abscesses from perforations associated with their diseased bowel.

Furthermore, enterocutaneous fistulas, common in these patients, may serve as a source of abdominal sepsis and colonization with enteric bacteria as well as streptococcal and staphylococcal species. It is estimated that 80% of deaths associated with enterocutaneous fistulas are due to abdominal sepsis.[9–11] Enterocutaneous fistulas may be associated with peritonitis and discrete intra-abdominal abscesses as well. A high index of suspicion for intra-abdominal infections is appropriate when caring for a patient with intestinal failure and an enterocutaneous fistula, because approximately 50% of patients with enterocutaneous fistulas will have an intra-abdominal abscess present on abdominal imaging.[12] Patients with enterocutaneous fistulas complicated by intra-abdominal infection require appropriate antibiotic treatment, often of an extended duration, owing to either recurrences or failure to adequately drain the abscess cavity. The need for prolonged antibiotic therapy and the associated prolonged hospital stay can place these patients at risk for colonization and infection with multidrug-resistant organisms.[13–15]

PN is an important treatment for patients with intestinal failure and SBS, but the presence of intravascular catheters for nutritional support place the patient at risk

Table 1	
Risk factors for infection in intestinal and multivisceral transplantation	
Pretransplantation	**Posttransplantation**
Intra-abdominal anatomic abnormalities	Donor intestinal allograft with dense microbial burden
Multiple hospitalizations	
Prolonged hospital stays	Complicated surgical procedures in IMVTx
Multiple intra-abdominal surgical procedures	Multiple hospitalizations
	Prolonged hospital stays
Parenteral nutrition	Intensive immunosuppression
Immunosuppression secondary to malnutrition	High rates of allograft rejection
	Mucosal injury with rejection associated with bacterial translocation

Abbreviation: IMVTx, intestinal and multivisceral transplant.

for central line–associated bloodstream infections (CLABSIs). One study identified PN use in intestinal failure as the most significant risk factor for the development of CLAB-SIs.[16] An observational study noted that patients receiving chronic PN had an 80.9% risk of developing a CLABSI, 78.9% of whom had more than 1 CLABSI, with 23.8% of these episodes being polymicrobial.[17]

More specifically, CLABSIs are common in young patients with SBS. According to a study by Mohammed and colleagues,[18] CLABSIs occurred in 66% of children on home PN within the first 6 months of hospital discharge. In the same study, the highest incidence occurred within the first month and the most common infections were poly-microbial followed by gram-positive, gram-negative, and fungal causes, respectively. Moreover, the use of PN in the neonatal patient population with SBS has been asso-ciated with a relatively rapid development of cholestasis, which has been observed as a complication of infection and sepsis.[19,20]

Most patients with CLABSIs present with fevers or with a clinical picture of sepsis. However, one study reported that 33% of patients with SBS and liver disease on PN had occult bacteremia just before their intestinal transplantation. This patient group had more postoperative days of mechanical ventilation and a more prolonged length of stay in comparison with patients who did not have occult bacteremia at the time of transplantation.[21]

There are no large studies specifically addressing the microbiological causes of CLABSIs in patients on chronic PN who are awaiting IMVTx. These patients require frequent hospitalizations and likely experience CLABSIs caused by pathogens similar to those in other patient populations such as staphylococci, enterococci, Candida species, and gram-negative bacilli. Although CLABSIs have not been formally studied in this population, a major study of CLABSIs in hospitalized patients revealed that gram-positive organisms accounted for 65%, gram-negative bacilli accounted for 25%, and fungi accounted for 9.5%.[22] Although colonization by skin flora (staphylo-cocci and streptococci) is the most likely source of CLABSIs in patients on chronic PN who are awaiting IMVTx, these patients may be at increased risk for enteric path-ogens such as gram-negative bacilli, enterococci, and vancomycin-resistant entero-cocci, because of alterations in the integrity of their gastrointestinal tract.

The use of PN also places patients at risk for infection by way of contaminated infu-sates. Several studies have reported contaminated infusates as a source of infection. Gram-negative organisms such as Serratia and Pseudomonas species have been associated with infusate contaminations.[23,24] Candida parapsilosis fungemia has also been associated with contaminated PN infusate.[25–27] Overall, patients with intes-tinal failure and SBS have numerous risk factors associated with invasive candidiasis and candidemia, which include the use of PN, the risk of contaminated infusate, the chronic use of central vascular catheters, the use of broad-spectrum antibiotics, and multiple intra-abdominal surgical procedures.[28–30] Candidemia has been associ-ated with mortality rates as high as 47% in adults and 29% in children.[29] Although Candida albicans remains the most common isolate, nonalbicans species such as Candida glabrata have been reported more recently.[30,31] It appears that PN places pa-tients with SBS at an increased risk for fungemia attributable to all Candida species. Furthermore, the use of PN has been associated with Candida chorioretinitis and endophthalmitis in other patient populations.[32–34]

Lastly, malnutrition is common in patients with intestinal failure and may contribute to a patient's net state of immunosuppression, ultimately resulting in an increased risk of infection. Malnutrition is associated with T-lymphocyte depletion and their response to mitogens, failure of B cells to respond appropriately to antigen presentation, and decreased function of neutrophils.[35] The fasting state has been associated with a decrease in circulating CD4$^+$ T-helper lymphocytes and an attenuated interleukin-2 response to mitogen stimulation.[36]

Chronic liver disease secondary to chronic PN may also contribute to the level of immunosuppression in this patient population. In addition to placing patients at risk for CLABSIs as already mentioned, the chronic use of PN places patients at risk for liver disease. It is estimated that 50% of patients on chronic PN will develop liver disease within 5 to 7 years.[37] Chronic liver disease can further contribute to the level of immunosuppression in this patient population, being associated with defects in humoral immunity and neutrophil dysfunction. These patients often have decreased capacity for the opsonization of foreign antigens because of hypocomplementemia.[38] Neutrophil chemotaxis and adherence is also depressed in patients with liver disease.[39] In cirrhotic patients, the sinusoidal macrophages or Kupffer cells, which play an important role in the clearance of bacteria and foreign antigens, may be bypassed because of portosystemic shunting.[40]

In summary, Patients with intestinal failure have a very complicated pretransplant course that is often associated with multiple intra-abdominal surgeries, and prolonged and recurrent hospitalizations that place them at a very high risk for hospital-acquired infections caused by multidrug-resistant organisms. The reliance on PN for nutritional support results in an ongoing risk for CLABSIs. Patients with intestinal failure and SBS being considered for IMVTx may experience secondary immunodeficiency attributable to nutritional status or PN-induced chronic liver disease. All of these factors make this patient population vulnerable to high rates of morbidity caused by infections.

POSTTRANSPLANTATION

As in other solid organ transplant recipients, the risk of infection continues after IMVTx because of the high level of immunosuppression as well as the unique nature of the intestinal allograft (**Table 2**). Unlike other transplants that are sterile, the intestine is transplanted with a large content of intraluminal commensal microbes. In the past the intestinal graft was decontaminated at the time of procurement by flushing the lumen with antimicrobial decontamination solution. This procedure is no longer performed at the authors' center, given the potential chemical damage to the graft mucosa from such solutions and recognition of the important role of the intraluminal flora.

The intestine is a highly immunogenic graft because it is heavily populated with a large number of immune cells. However, it also carries a high risk of infection, given its rich composition of microbes. In addition, there is the potential for bacterial translocation associated with damaged intestinal mucosa in the setting of acute rejection. Furthermore, higher levels of immunosuppression are necessary to treat and prevent rejection in this patient population, which also experiences relatively higher rates of acute cellular rejection in comparison with other types of abdominal organ transplant recipients. Induction therapy with the T-cell–depleting agents such as thymoglobulin and alemtuzumab, or the interleukin-2 receptor blockers basiliximab and daclizumab, are routinely used. Maintenance immunosuppression includes tacrolimus, sirolimus, mycophenolate, and prednisone. During the posttransplant period, tacrolimus is maintained at a higher level than in other solid organ transplant recipients. This particular combination of circumstances results in a drastically elevated risk for the development of infection. To complicate matters, alterations of the intraluminal flora of the graft have been recently associated with an increased risk of rejection, although the exact cause-and-effect relationship remains to be clarified.[41]

Table 2		
Types of infections encountered in intestinal and multivisceral transplantation		
Pre-IMVTx (Months to Years Before IMVTx)	Immediate Post-IMVTx (<6 wk After IMVTx)	"Later" Post-IMVTx (>6 wk After IMVTx)
Bacterial/Fungal Infections Intra-abdominal abscess Peritonitis CLABSIs Enteric gram-negative rods Staphylococci Enterococci (VRE) Candida Health care–associated infections	Bacterial/Fungal Infections (health care–associated infections) Intra-abdominal infections (abscess, peritonitis) CLABSIs HCAP Surgical-site infection UTI Etiology Gram-negative enterics Enterococci/VRE Staphylococci Candida species Aspergillus	Bacterial/Fungal Infections (health care–associated infections) Viral infections of the intestinal allograft CMV EBV-associated PTLD Adenovirus Rotavirus Norovirus Sepsis Miscellaneous (PCP, Toxoplasma, Nocardia, molds, Isospora, cryptosporidium, etc)

Abbreviations: CLABSI, central line–associated bloodstream infection; CMV, cytomegalovirus; EBV, Epstein-Barr virus; HCAP, health care–acquired pneumonia; IMVTx, intestinal and multivisceral transplant; PCP, Pneumocystis pneumonia; PTLD, posttransplant lymphoproliferative disorder; UTI, urinary tract infection; VRE, vancomycin-resistant enterococci.

In addition to intensive immunosuppressive regimens and numerous rejection episodes after transplantation, the patient population is additionally unique for several reasons. IMVTx recipients often encounter multiple postoperative complications and experience relatively high rates of repeat surgeries. Both prolonged postoperative hospital courses and recurrent hospitalizations are common occurrences in the posttransplant period. All of these factors, which predispose such patients to infection, are also responsible for variability in the timeline of infections seen after IMVTx.

The timeline of posttransplant infections in IMVTx recipients is not well delineated in comparison with the traditional timeline of posttransplant infections in other solid organ transplant patient populations. There is only one published prospective study that defines a timeline for the development of various types of infections. In this small cohort of IMVTx recipients, it was noted that the median time from the day of transplant to the development of bacterial infections was 11 days, for viral infections (cytomegalovirus [CMV] and Epstein-Barr virus [EBV]) 91 days, and for fungal infections 181 days.[7]

The authors propose a posttransplantation timeline based on risk for infection. In their experience the mean length of stay for adult patients who have undergone IMVTx is 35 days; this increases to 42 days in patients who develop 1 or more infections. For patients who develop multiple infections (>2), the length of stay increases to 71 days.[8] The median duration for length of stay in the hospital after IMVTx in patients with at least 1 infection is 42 days (6 weeks), and for this reason the authors divide the posttransplant time period into 2 categories. The time from day zero to 6 weeks after IMTVx is defined as "immediate posttransplantation," when patients are at greatest risk for hospital-associated infections. The period after 6 weeks is termed "later posttransplantation" and correlates with an elevated risk of opportunistic infections. Although the risk of health care–associated infections is highest during the immediate posttransplant period when IMVTx recipients are in the hospital, it has been the authors' experience that this risk continues during the later posttransplant period. In fact, it seems that these patients are always at risk for health care–associated infections. A visual representation of this concept is depicted in **Fig. 1**. The risk of hospital-associated infections is always present because these patients are often readmitted to the hospital for complications such as acute kidney injury and dehydration. In fact, the risk of infection continues indefinitely after transplantation because of the relatively high levels of immunosuppression required, coupled with the need for recurrent hospitalizations.

Immediate Posttransplantation

Health care–associated infections

The most common infections seen during the immediate posttransplant period include bloodstream, intra-abdominal, respiratory tract, surgical site, and urinary tract infections. These health care–associated infections, roughly occurring within 6 weeks after IMVTx, are predominately caused by bacteria and *Candida* species. Specifically, bacterial infections occur in at least 58% of IMVTx recipients within the first 4 weeks after transplantation, then increase to approximately 80% by 8 weeks after transplantation.[5,8] The incidence of bacterial infections decreases to 3% per month after 6 months from the time of transplantation.[5] Initial bacterial infections occur very early in the postoperative period, with a mean or median time to first infection of 9 to 11 days.[5,7,8]

Bloodstream infections Most common of the health care–associated infections are bloodstream infections and sepsis, which represent between 26% and 59% of bacterial infections during the immediate posttransplant period.[5,7,8] The 6-month cumulative incidence in adult and pediatric patients who had undergone IMVTx at the

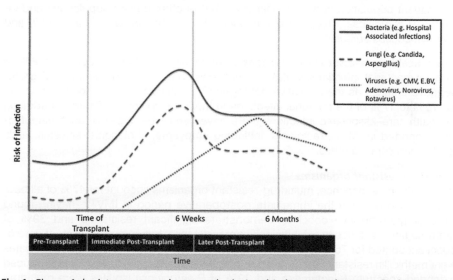

Fig. 1. Figure 1 depicts a proposed temporal relationship between the type of infection during the pre-transplantation period, the immediate post-operative transplantation period, and the "later" post-transplantation period in patients who have undergone small intestinal and/or multi-visceral transplantation. Note that these patients are at risk for bacterial and fungal infections in the pre-transplantation period, and this risk increases during the immediate post-operative period (within 6 weeks of transplantation). Although the risk of bacterial and fungal infection decreases after 6 weeks, there is still a potential for these types of infections. Opportunistic viral infections develop usually after the first 4 weeks post-transplantation with a peak incidence that occurs during month 1 through month 6 post-transplantation.

authors' center was noted to be 61%, and was more common in patients who received a liver as part of their transplantation.[6] Pediatric transplant recipients were more likely to develop a bloodstream infection than were adult patients.[6] The predominant causative organisms associated with bloodstream infections are gram-positive cocci, accounting for 59% to 66% of the isolates, followed by gram-negative enterics, accounting for 34% to 41% of the isolates, and *Candida* species, accounting for approximately 3% of the isolates.[5,6] Note that one study reported *Enterococcus* species, including vancomycin-resistant *Enterococcus faecium*, were the most common gram-positive isolate identified.[6]

Intra-abdominal infections Intra-abdominal abscesses, infected intra-abdominal fluid collections, and peritonitis are also common during the immediate postoperative period. These intra-abdominal infections account for approximately 13% to 37% of bacterial infections within the immediate postoperative period.[5,7,8] One study noted a high mortality rate associated with the presence of an intra-abdominal abscess and a positive peritoneal culture within the first month of diagnosis in IMVTx recipients.[5] Collectively, enteric pathogens including *Pseudomonas aeruginosa*, *Enterococcus* species (including vancomycin-resistant enterococci), *Enterobacter cloacae*, *Escherichia coli*, and *Candida* species are most commonly reported.[5,8]

Respiratory tract infections Health care–associated pneumonia (HCAP) and other respiratory tract infections account for 14% to 17% of bacterial infections in IMVTx recipients.[5,7,8] It has been reported that 39.5% of HCAPs occur within the first 2 months after transplantation, with a median onset of 36.5 days.[5] The microbiology of HCAPs in this patient population does not differ from that of other patient populations and includes *P aeruginosa*, *Klebsiella pneumoniae*, *E coli*, *Acinetobacter baumannii*, and *Staphylococcus aureus*.[5,8]

Other health care–associated infections Surgical-site infections account for 9% to 17% of bacterial infections in IMVTx recipients, with a high percentage of gram-negative enterics as the causative pathogens.[5,8] Urinary tract infections accounted for 15% to 17% of the bacterial infections in IMVTx recipients.[7,8] Finally, in addition to health care–associated infections there have been other types of bacterial infections reported in IMVTx recipients, including empyema, cholangitis, sinusitis, otitis media, and septic arthritis.[5]

Multidrug-resistant organisms

In the authors' experience, multidrug-resistant organisms account for 47% of all bacterial infections within the immediate postoperative period in IMVTx, having found 71% of gram-positive cocci to demonstrate significant resistance and 39% of gram-negative enterics to exhibit significant resistance. Vancomycin-resistant enterococci accounted for 75% of all enterococcal isolates, and 100% of *S aureus* isolates were methicillin resistant. Thirty-one percent of *Klebsiella* and *E coli* isolates produced extended-spectrum β-lactamase and 39% of *P aeruginosa* isolates were multidrug resistant.[8] Therefore, clinicians ought to consider empiric coverage for multidrug-resistant organisms based on local antimicrobial resistance patterns when an infection is suspected in an IMVTx recipient during the immediate posttransplant period.

"Later" Posttransplantation

Viral infections
Most viral infections that occur more than 6 weeks after transplantation in IMVTx recipients cause viral enteritis. CMV, EBV, adenovirus, norovirus, and rotavirus all

have the ability to cause intestinal allograft viral enteritis. Adenovirus, norovirus, and rotavirus present in a relatively similar manner, whereas CMV and EBV have additional important manifestations.

Intestinal allograft viral enteritis Overall, bacterial and viral infections target the intestinal graft, with an incidence of up to 39% after IMVTx.[42] Two-thirds of allograft infections are secondary to viral enteritis, which include the double-stranded DNA viruses of the herpesvirus family CMV and EBV, as well as another DNA virus, adenovirus, and the enterotropic RNA viruses norovirus and rotavirus. The morbidity and mortality associated with the herpesviruses is more significant than with the enterotropic RNA viruses.

Most causes of viral enteritis affect the pediatric population with greater frequency, although adult recipients are not excluded from infection.[43] The severity of infection in intestinal allograft viral enteritis is related to the intensity of immunosuppression. Mild infection occurs in the setting of low immunosuppression, whereas more severe disease is associated with heavy immunosuppression. For example, adenovirus can cause multisystem involvement with significant mortality of up to 20% after heavy immunosuppression.[44] Note that management of viral enteritis involves reduction of maintenance immunosuppression levels.

Viral enteritis may be clinically indistinguishable from intestinal graft rejection, and it is critical to differentiate between these 2 entities. Intestinal viruses must be ruled out because the treatment of viral infections requires decreasing the level of immunosuppression, whereas the treatment of allograft rejection requires increased levels of immunosuppression, often with pulse corticosteroids and possibly with T-cell–depleting agents. Treatment of rejection can result in viral dissemination (as in the setting of adenovirus enteritis) whereas reduction of immunosuppressive therapy for treatment of viral enteritis may promote graft rejection. Furthermore, it is important to identify the correct pathogen causing infection because the treatments differ. Endoscopy and biopsy will help to distinguish viral enteritis from rejection. Endoscopic features of rejection include a coarse mucosal surface with focal erosions. On biopsy, rejection is characterized by crypt apoptosis with nuclear fragmentation, but usually, unlike in viral infections, the surface epithelium is preserved.

Adenovirus Adenovirus is a DNA virus that can be transmitted from the donor within the intestinal allograft. Like EBV, it may remain latent in lymphoid tissue, thus exposing the recipient to the risk of reactivation after transplantation. Adenovirus infection is more common in infants than in young children and adults, with an incidence reported between 20% and 50% in pediatric intestinal transplant series.[45,46] In a recent study of IMTVx patients infected with adenovirus, 36% of the cases were diagnosed in the first month, 32% in the following 5 months, 16% between 6 and 12 months, and 16% more than 1 year after transplantation.[47] The main manifestation of adenoviral enteritis is usually osmotic diarrhea, infrequently accompanied by fever and rarely by gastrointestinal bleeding. Histologically the main features of adenoviral enteritis are apoptosis (as in rejection), villous injury (usually more prominent than in rejection), and cytopathic nuclear inclusions, the latter being a key component in differentiating adenoviral infection from rejection.[47,48] The diagnosis of adenovirus is confirmed by serum and tissue DNA polymerase chain reaction (PCR) and immunohistochemistry. Adenovirus predominantly affects the intestinal allograft, although in the setting of heavy immunosuppression it can disseminate to the lungs, liver, and pancreas.[44] Treatment of adenovirus includes supportive care, reduction in immunosuppression, and the use of the antiviral agent cidofovir.[49]

Rotavirus Rotavirus enteritis presents with sudden watery osmotic diarrhea causing significant dehydration, requiring intravenous fluid resuscitation and often temporary PN. As in the case of adenovirus, it has a predilection to affect pediatric small intestinal transplant recipients.[43] Endoscopic findings include mild erythema, villous atrophy and edema, villous blunting, mixed inflammatory infiltrate, superficial epithelial disarray, and goblet-cell depletion. A diagnosis of rotavirus is confirmed by culture and immunostaining, and treatment is supportive care. Up to 69% of patients will develop allograft rejection after rotavirus infection, possibly resulting from immune activation and decreased absorption of the immunosuppressive medications.[43]

Norovirus Norovirus can cause protracted diarrhea and severe dehydration in pediatric IMVTx recipients.[50,51] It has also been observed to result in prolonged viral shedding (up to 80 days).[51] Given the absence of established monitoring strategies, the incidence of norovirus infection is not known in the IMVTx population. The timing of infection varies between 17 days and 1 year posttransplant in the limited published series.[51] Histologically norovirus enteritis shows apoptosis involving both villous enterocytes and crypts, making it more challenging to differentiate from rejection based solely on biopsy. Diagnosis is confirmed by reverse transcription–PCR of biopsy material and intestinal fluid.[50] Although often protracted, the infection is usually self-limited, with restoration of normal graft function and limited morbidity unless superimposed infections such as adenovirus or CMV occur. Management is with supportive care, including nutritional support and reduction of immunosuppression.

Cytomegalovirus Among the most common viral infections after transplantation, CMV is a major cause of morbidity in IMVTx recipients. The heavy immunosuppressive regimens used in these patients, including high tacrolimus levels, place them at high risk for CMV disease. The authors' center observed an 18.8% incidence of CMV infection in 88 adult and pediatric IMVTx recipients from 2003 to 2008.[52] A recent study of pediatric IMVTx patients reported an 18% incidence of CMV infection after transplantation and a 7% incidence of invasive CMV disease.[53] The majority of invasive CMV disease involves the intestinal allograft, and recurrences reported are between 50% and 86%.[53,54] When the indirect immunomodulatory effects and the associated increased risk of other infections are considered in addition to the direct cytopathic effects of the virus, CMV disease significantly affects survival, with an 11-fold increase in mortality.

Donor and recipient CMV serologic status is an important predictor of posttransplant CMV infection.[55] The highest risk for development of invasive CMV, recurrent CMV, and ganciclovir-resistant CMV is in CMV seronegative recipients of a CMV seropositive donor (D+/R−). However, a seropositive recipient is still at risk for CMV reactivation regardless of donor status. Although not an absolute contraindication to transplantation, D+/R− status is an indication for more intensive monitoring and more stringent preventive strategies after transplantation. Practices for IMVTx are center specific and some programs such as the authors' now exclude CMV D+/R− transplantation. In fact, CMV disease in D+/R− takes much longer to resolve histologically and, in addition to involving the graft, also frequently involves the native gastrointestinal tract.[54] It is established practice that seronegative recipients receive CMV-negative blood products during the transplant procedure and postoperatively.

Manifestations of CMV infection in IMVTx recipients range from asymptomatic detectable CMV DNA, to a viral syndrome including fever, myalgia, leukopenia, and elevated transaminases, to target-organ involvement. In addition to systemic symptoms, CMV enteritis manifests with increased ileostomy output or diarrhea and gastrointestinal bleeding.[53,54] The intestinal allograft is affected more than the native gastrointestinal tract in CMV enteritis. Endoscopic findings of CMV allograft enteritis vary between mild superficial ulceration and severe mucosal damage with the potential for bowel perforation, especially following T-cell depletion therapy for acute rejection. Histologically CMV enteritis demonstrates mucosal injury with crypt and villus loss associated with plasma cell and lymphocyte infiltrate, as well as the presence of CMV inclusion bodies. Although serum CMV PCR monitoring has dramatically improved the early diagnosis of CMV in solid organ transplant recipients, 48% of patients with histologic CMV involvement of the intestinal allograft had undetectable CMV PCR in the blood.[56]

Prophylaxis with intravenous ganciclovir is generally recommended for all IMVTx recipients to prevent infection with CMV and other herpesviruses. The optimal duration of prophylaxis is not uniformly established, and varies between 3 months to indefinitely. As in other types of transplantation, late-onset CMV disease is a potential problem, occurring in 15% to 30% of cases after discontinuation of prophylaxis.[55] Treatment of CMV infection includes oral valganciclovir or intravenous ganciclovir, although given potential issues with decreased drug exposure due to intestinal allograft enteritis, the authors have routinely used intravenous ganciclovir in this setting. Although there are no clear data to support its use in CMV allograft enteritis, CMV hyperimmune globulin is often administered in addition to ganciclovir.

Epstein-Barr virus In addition to causing viral enteritis, clinical manifestations of EBV infection occurring after IMVTx include infectious mononucleosis, hepatitis, pneumonitis, leukopenia, thrombocytopenia, hemolytic anemia, and hemophagocytosis. It may progress to a posttransplant lymphoproliferative disorder (PTLD) caused by inadequate anti-EBV cytotoxic T cells. It can also result in EBV-induced lymphoma from EBV-driven proliferation. EBV-related PTLD is a feared complication among all solid organ transplant recipients; however, IMVTx recipients are at the highest risk for development of PTLD.[57] Recently, the incidence of PTLD in IMVTx recipients has decreased to 5% to 10% from 30% in the early era of IMVTx, secondary to routine quantitative EBV DNA PCR monitoring.[58] In fact, patients with undetectable or low viral loads for the first 6 months after IMVTx are unlikely to develop PTLD regardless of their pretransplant EBV serologic status.[59] The main risk factors for PTLD include primary EBV infection after transplantation and the net state of immunosuppression.[57,60] CMV infection affects the net state of immunosuppression and is known to be a risk factor for PTLD.[57] In regard of EBV serologic status, D+/R− extends the greatest risk for developing posttransplant infection and PTLD, although EBV-seropositive recipients remain at significant risk.[58] The development of PTLD most commonly occurs within the first year after transplantation, but cases have been described as late as 10 years after transplantation.[61]

Manifestations of PTLD are multiple, and include subcutaneous hard and immobile nodules, generalized lymphadenopathy, snoring in children caused by adenoidal hypertrophy, mouth breathing with ulcerating palatine tonsils, pneumonia with lung and/or mediastinal masses, diarrhea secondary to diffuse small-bowel mucosal infiltration, gastrointestinal bleeding in cases of multiple ulcerating lesions, and abdominal pain with or without bowel obstruction.[58] PTLD of the intestinal graft may be discovered incidentally during routine surveillance endoscopy for rejection or following symptoms of mass, abdominal pain, partial obstruction, feeding intolerance in children, fever, and gastrointestinal bleeding.[58] Prophylaxis with ganciclovir does not affect EBV-driven B-cell proliferation but may reduce the number of EBV-infected cells, thus reducing the risk of PTLD, especially in EBV D+/R− mismatch.[61] Although the management of PTLD is beyond the scope of this article, treatment approaches include reduction in immunosuppression, intravenous ganciclovir, CMV hyperimmune globulin, and rituximab.[61,62]

Fungal infections
The increased availability of diverse and potent immunosuppressive drugs has improved outcomes of IMVTx but with an increased risk of opportunistic infections, including fungal infections. Typically fungal infections are health care acquired. *Candida* and *Aspergillus* are the 2 predominant fungal species affecting IMVTx recipients, with a reported incidence of approximately 25%.[63,64]

Candida In general, *C albicans* accounts for approximately 50% of all infections with *Candida* species, and nonalbicans *Candida* collectively account for the other 50%. However, in the IMVTx recipient, 63% of *Candida* infections are due to nonalbicans *Candida*, and *C albicans* accounts for only 37%.[63] Risk factors for *Candida* infection in IMVTx recipients include the presence of central vascular catheters, use of PN, exposure to broad-spectrum antibiotics, use of immunosuppression for induction and rejection episodes, anastomotic leaks or intra-abdominal collections, the need for multiple abdominal surgical procedures, and the presence of a multivisceral graft.

Clinical manifestations of *Candida* infection in this patient population predominantly involve the bloodstream and the abdominal cavity. In one series candidemia accounted for 66%, and *Candida* intra-abdominal infections accounted for 29% of all yeast infections.[63] Other sites of infection include the urinary tract and respiratory tract. The authors have observed an endovascular infection caused by *C albicans* at a mesenteric anastomotic site in an IMVTx recipient. In other patient populations, candidemia has been associated with a mortality rate of up to 40%,[65] especially if empiric antifungal treatment is delayed until positive blood cultures are documented.[66]

As in other solid organ transplant recipients, *Candida* species are the most common invasive fungal infections to occur in IMVTx recipients.[28,67] *Candida* infections usually occur during the first 3 months after transplantation in solid organ recipients. It can occur later in IMVTx recipients, as it may be associated with intensification of immunosuppression for the treatment of rejection episodes. In a study of pediatric IMVTx recipients, nearly 80% of candidemia episodes occurred around 6 months after transplantation, with a median occurrence time of 163 days posttransplantation.[63] At the same center it was noted that approximately 70% of pediatric IMVTx recipients developed fungemia within 1 year of transplantation.[63] The incidence of invasive candidiasis in IMVTx recipients may be up to 28%.[7,68] The diagnosis of invasive candidiasis depends on the demonstration of *Candida* in sterile body sites, although culture methods, especially blood cultures, often have limited sensitivity (70%).[28]

Many centers use antifungal prophylaxis, usually with fluconazole, in the immediate postoperative period. The duration of fluconazole prophylaxis for *Candida* infection is variable and may be up to 4 weeks after transplantation, but it is prolonged further in the presence of ongoing intestinal mucosal injury or in the setting of rejection episodes. Detailed management guidelines are provided elsewhere[28]; however, for candidemia, central vascular catheter removal is indicated and treatment with antifungal therapy for at least 2 weeks after clearance of blood cultures is warranted. As the authors' center uses fluconazole prophylaxis postoperatively, empiric treatment with an echinocandin is usually initiated in the setting of suspected fungemia due to *Candida* species.

Aspergillus In the immunosuppressed patient, *Aspergillus* species may invade the lungs and spread to other organs, including the sinuses, brain, gastrointestinal tract, skin, and rarely, the bones. Particularly in IMVTx recipients, the most common site of infection is the lung. These patients may present with fever, cough, chest pain, and shortness of breath. Angioinvasion results in tissue necrosis, which may ultimately lead to cavitation and/or hemoptysis. Dissemination to the central nervous system also appears to be common in this patient population.[69]

Invasive aspergillosis represents only 1% to 3% of invasive fungal infections in IMVTx recipients, but is associated with significant morbidity and mortality of up to 60% to 90%.[69–71] There are no case-control studies that determine risk factors for invasive aspergillosis in the IMVTx population. However, comparisons can be made with solid organ transplant recipients and, most appropriately, liver transplant recipients, as many IMVTx procedures include livers. Factors associated with increased risk of invasive aspergillosis in liver transplant recipients include retransplantation, renal failure requiring renal replacement therapy, CMV infection, and prolonged stay in an intensive care unit.[72–77] The most important risk factor for the development of aspergillosis in solid organ transplant recipients is the net state of immunosuppression secondary to the intensity of the immunosuppressive therapies used, and coinfection with immunomodulatory viruses such as CMV. A definitive diagnosis of invasive aspergillosis can be difficult to make without confirmed histopathology demonstrating tissue invasion. At present, there are no established guidelines for the prophylaxis of invasive aspergillosis in IMVTx recipients, and because there are no large case series involving the IMVTx patient population, clinicians should use guidelines that are established for other solid organ transplant recipients.[70] Although voriconazole appears to be the recommended treatment, caution must be exercised with immunosuppressive drugs such as tacrolimus because of the significant drug interactions.

Miscellaneous infections

Although bacteria, fungi, and viruses are the predominant causes of infection, there have been isolated case reports of other infections in IMVTx. Other typical opportunistic infections that are commonly seen in other solid organ transplant recipients (in the absence of trimethoprim-sulfamethoxazole prophylaxis) are relatively rare in IMVTx recipients. Only a few cases of *Pneumocystis jiroveci* and disseminated toxoplasmosis have been reported.[78–80] The authors have encountered one case of pulmonary nocardiosis with dissemination to the central nervous system, and another case has also been reported in the literature.[81] Although viral allograft enteritis is the most common gastrointestinal infection, there have been isolated reported cases of infections caused by *Cryptosporidium* and *Isospora belli*.[82,83] Other uncommon fungal infections include a single case each of cryptococcal meningitis, sinusitis due to *Trichoderma longibrachiatum*, and esophagitis due to *Cladophialophora bantiana*.[84–86] Of note, to date there have been no reports of infections attributable to *Mycobacterium tuberculosis*, nontuberculous mycobacteria, or endemic mycoses reported in IMVTx recipients.

Antimicrobial Prophylaxis in the Perioperative and Postoperative Transplant Periods

Although protocols are often center specific, antimicrobial prophylaxis against bacterial, fungal, viral, and protozoal pathogens follows many of the same principles as in other solid organ transplantations. Perioperative prophylaxis for bacterial infections includes agents with activity against enteric gram-negative bacilli and anaerobes such as ampicillin/sulbactam, as well as piperacillin/tazobactam. The duration of surgical prophylaxis varies from 3 days to approximately 7 days, and is often center specific. It may be reasonable to maintain antibiotic prophylaxis until surveillance enteroscopy demonstrates integrity of the intestinal allograft.

Antifungal prophylaxis with azole therapy such as fluconazole, as well as a lipid preparation of amphotericin B, has been used by most centers. The duration of antifungal prophylaxis is also center specific. The authors often maintain fluconazole prophylaxis until allograft function has been documented by enteroscopy. The discontinuation of azole prophylaxis must be closely coordinated with the transplant team, owing to significant drug interactions with tacrolimus.

All IMVTx recipients receive intravenous ganciclovir at an induction dosage of 5 mg/kg every 12 hours to prevent infection with CMV and other herpesviruses. At the authors' center, patients are usually maintained at this induction dose for at least 2 weeks and then are switched to maintenance dosing with oral valganciclovir. In addition, CMV hyperimmune globulin is administered weekly for 4 weeks after transplantation.

Although *Pneumocystis* pneumonia has been rarely reported in IMVTx recipients, prophylaxis for *Pneumocystis jiroveci* with trimethoprim-sulfamethoxazole is also initiated postoperatively and is maintained for at least 6 months after transplantation. It is not unreasonable to consider lifelong prophylaxis because of the high level of immunosuppression that these patients undergo. Trimethoprim-sulfamethoxazole may also provide prophylaxis against *Toxoplasma gondii*, *Listeria monocytogenes*, and some *Nocardia* species.

SUMMARY

IMVTx has evolved to become an effective treatment option for patients with irreversible intestinal failure, although the infectious disease challenges remain significant. Patients with intestinal failure resulting from short bowel syndrome have a very complicated medical course because of the nature of their underlying illness, which results in a marked risk for infectious disease complications that predate the time of intestinal transplantation. The complicated nature of this intra-abdominal procedure coupled with the need for intensive immunosuppression places this patient population at a significant lifelong risk for infections caused by bacterial and opportunistic pathogens. In addition, because of the high rates of intestinal allograft rejection, this patient population often experiences intermittent increases in the level of immunosuppression, which will clearly place them at risk for viral and fungal pathogens. Ultimately, the balance between effective immunosuppression and prophylaxis of infections remains a major challenge in the management of IMVTx recipients. Clinicians caring for these patients should have a high index of suspicion for these infectious disease complications.

REFERENCES

1. Intestinal Transplant Association. Intestinal transplant registry report. 2009. Available at: http://www.intestinaltransplant.org/itr/.
2. Fishbein TM. Intestinal transplantation. N Engl J Med 2009;361(10):998–1008.
3. Centers for Medicare & Medicaid Services. Centers for medicare & medicaid services. 2012. Available at: http://www.cms.gov/. Accessed August 16, 2012.
4. Abu-Elmagd KM, Costa G, Bond GJ, et al. Evolution of the immunosuppressive strategies for the intestinal and multivisceral recipients with special reference to allograft immunity and achievement of partial tolerance. Transpl Int 2009;22(1): 96–109.
5. Loinaz C, Kato T, Nishida S, et al. Bacterial infections after intestine and multivisceral transplantation. The experience of the University of Miami (1994-2001). Hepatogastroenterology 2006;53(68):234–42.
6. Akhter K, Timpone J, Matsumoto C, et al. Six-month incidence of bloodstream infections in intestinal transplant patients. Transpl Infect Dis 2012;14(3):242–7.

 7. Guaraldi G, Cocchi S, Codeluppi M, et al. Outcome, incidence, and timing of infectious complications in small bowel and multivisceral organ transplantation patients. Transplantation 2005;80(12):1742–8.
 8. Primeggia J, Timpone J, Karacki P, et al. Infection among small bowel and multivisceral transplant recipients in the 30-day post-operative period. Transpl Infect Dis, in press.
 9. Kaushal M, Carlson GL. Management of enterocutaneous fistulas. Clin Colon Rectal Surg 2004;17(2):79–88.
10. Soeters PB, Ebeid AM, Fischer JE. Review of 404 patients with gastrointestinal fistulas. Impact of parenteral nutrition. Ann Surg 1979;190(2):189–202.
11. McLauchlan GJ, Anderson ID, Grant IS, et al. Outcome of patients with abdominal sepsis treated in an intensive care unit. Br J Surg 1995;82(4):524–9.
12. Thomas HA. Radiologic investigation and treatment of gastrointestinal fistulas. Surg Clin North Am 1996;76(5):1081–94.
13. Paterson DL. The epidemiological profile of infections with multidrug-resistant *Pseudomonas aeruginosa* and *Acinetobacter* species. Clin Infect Dis 2006; 43(Suppl 2):S43–8.
14. Jacobson KL, Cohen SH, Inciardi JF, et al. The relationship between antecedent antibiotic use and resistance to extended-spectrum cephalosporins in group I beta-lactamase-producing organisms. Clin Infect Dis 1995;21(5):1107–13.
15. Fraimow HS, Tsigrelis C. Antimicrobial resistance in the intensive care unit: mechanisms, epidemiology, and management of specific resistant pathogens. Crit Care Clin 2011;27(1):163–205. http://dx.doi.org/10.1016/j.ccc.2010.11.002.
16. Ishizuka M, Nagata H, Takagi K, et al. Total parenteral nutrition is a major risk factor for central venous catheter-related bloodstream infection in colorectal cancer patients receiving postoperative chemotherapy. Eur Surg Res 2008;41(4):341–5.
17. Marra AR, Opilla M, Edmond MB, et al. Epidemiology of bloodstream infections in patients receiving long-term total parenteral nutrition. J Clin Gastroenterol 2007;41(1):19–28.
18. Mohammed A, Grant FK, Zhao VM, et al. Characterization of posthospital bloodstream infections in children requiring home parenteral nutrition. J Parenter Eternal Nutr 2011;35(5):581–7.
19. Sondheimer JM, Asturias E, Cadnapaphornchai M. Infection and cholestasis in neonates with intestinal resection and long-term parenteral nutrition. J Pediatr Gastroenterol Nutr 1998;27(2):131–7.
20. Beath SV, Davies P, Papadopoulou A, et al. Parenteral nutrition-related cholestasis in postsurgical neonates: multivariate analysis of risk factors. J Pediatr Surg 1996;31(4):604–6.
21. Matsumoto C, Kaufman S, Fennelly E, et al. Impact of positive preoperative surveillance blood cultures from chronic indwelling catheters in cadaveric intestinal transplant recipients. Transplant Proc 2006;38(6):1676–7.
22. Wisplinghoff H, Bischoff T, Tallent SM, et al. Nosocomial bloodstream infections in US hospitals: analysis of 24,179 cases from a prospective nationwide surveillance study. Clin Infect Dis 2004;39(3):309–17.
23. Ostrowsky BE, Whitener C, Bredenberg HK, et al. Serratia marcescens bacteremia traced to an infused narcotic. N Engl J Med 2002;346(20):1529–37.
24. Centers for Disease Control and Prevention (CDC): Morbidity and Mortality Weekly Report. *Pseudomonas* bloodstream infections associated with a heparin/saline flush—Missouri, New York, Texas, and Michigan, 2004-2005. 2005. Available at: http://www.cdc.gov/mmwr/preview/mmwrhtml/mm5411a1.htm. Accessed August 3, 2012.

25. Maki DG. Infections due to infusion therapy. In: Jarvis WR, editor. Bennett and Brachman's hospital infections. 5th edition. Philadelphia: Lippincott Williams & Wilkins; 2007. p. 611–48.
26. Plouffe JF, Brown DG, Silva J Jr, et al. Nosocomial outbreak of *Candida parapsilosis* fungemia related to intravenous infusions. Arch Intern Med 1977;137(12):1686–9.
27. Solomon SL, Khabbaz RF, Parker RH, et al. An outbreak of *Candida parapsilosis* bloodstream infections in patients receiving parenteral nutrition. J Infect Dis 1984;149(1):98–102.
28. Pappas PG, Kauffman CA, Andes D, et al. Clinical practice guidelines for the management of candidiasis: 2009 update by the Infectious Diseases Society of America. Clin Infect Dis 2009;48(5):503–35.
29. Pappas PG, Rex JH, Lee J, et al. A prospective observational study of candidemia: epidemiology, therapy, and influences on mortality in hospitalized adult and pediatric patients. Clin Infect Dis 2003;37(5):634–43.
30. Tortorano AM, Peman J, Bernhardt H, et al. Epidemiology of candidaemia in Europe: results of 28-month European Confederation of Medical Mycology (ECMM) hospital-based surveillance study. Eur J Clin Microbiol Infect Dis 2004;23(4):317–22.
31. Trick WE, Fridkin SK, Edwards JR, et al, National Nosocomial Infections Surveillance System, Hospitals. Secular trend of hospital-acquired candidemia among intensive care unit patients in the United States during 1989-1999. Clin Infect Dis 2002;35(5):627–30.
32. Curry CR, Quie PG. Fungal septicemia in patients receiving parenteral hyperalimentation. N Engl J Med 1971;285(22):1221–5.
33. Henderson DK, Edwards JE Jr, Montgomerie JZ. Hematogenous *Candida* endophthalmitis in patients receiving parenteral hyperalimentation fluids. J Infect Dis 1981;143(5):655–61.
34. Montgomerie JZ, Edwards JE Jr. Association of infection due to *Candida albicans* with intravenous hyperalimentation. J Infect Dis 1978;137(2):197–201.
35. Santos JI. Nutrition, infection, and immunocompetence. Infect Dis Clin North Am 1994;8(1):243–67.
36. Savendahl L, Underwood LE. Decreased interleukin-2 production from cultured peripheral blood mononuclear cells in human acute starvation. J Clin Endocrinol Metab 1997;82(4):1177–80.
37. Garg M, Jones RM, Vaughan RB, et al. Intestinal transplantation: current status and future directions. J Gastroenterol Hepatol 2011;26(8):1221–8.
38. Carbone J, Micheloud D, Salcedo M, et al. Humoral and cellular immune monitoring might be useful to identify liver transplant recipients at risk for development of infection. Transpl Infect Dis 2008;10(6):396–402.
39. Altin M, Rajkovic IA, Hughes RD, et al. Neutrophil adherence in chronic liver disease and fulminant hepatic failure. Gut 1983;24(8):746–50.
40. Seki S, Habu Y, Kawamura T, et al. The liver as a crucial organ in the first line of host defense: the roles of Kupffer cells, natural killer (NK) cells and NK1.1 Ag+ T cells in T helper 1 immune responses. Immunol Rev 2000;174:35–46.
41. Oh PL, Martinez I, Sun Y, et al. Characterization of the ileal microbiota in rejecting and nonrejecting recipients of small bowel transplants. Am J Transplant 2012;12(3):753–62.
42. Ziring D, Tran R, Edelstein S, et al. Infectious enteritis after intestinal transplantation: incidence, timing, and outcome. Transplantation 2005;79(6):702–9.

43. Adeyi OA, Costa G, Abu-Elmagd KM, et al. Rotavirus infection in adult small intestine allografts: a clinicopathological study of a cohort of 23 patients. Am J Transplant 2010;10(12):2683–9.

44. Pinchoff RJ, Kaufman SS, Magid MS, et al. Adenovirus infection in pediatric small bowel transplantation recipients. Transplantation 2003;76(1):183–9.

45. McLaughlin GE, Delis S, Kashimawo L, et al. Adenovirus infection in pediatric liver and intestinal transplant recipients: utility of DNA detection by PCR. Am J Transplant 2003;3(2):224–8.

46. Berho M, Torroella M, Viciana A, et al. Adenovirus enterocolitis in human small bowel transplants. Pediatr Transplant 1998;2(4):277–82.

47. Adeyi OA, Randhawa PA, Nalesnik MA, et al. Posttransplant adenoviral enteropathy in patients with small bowel transplantation. Arch Pathol Lab Med 2008; 132(4):703–5.

48. Kaufman SS, Magid MS, Tschernia A, et al. Discrimination between acute rejection and adenoviral enteritis in intestinal transplant recipients. Transplant Proc 2002;34(3):943–5.

49. Ison MG, Green M, AST Infectious Diseases Community of Practice. Adenovirus in solid organ transplant recipients. Am J Transplant 2009;9(Suppl 4):S161–5.

50. Kaufman SS, Chatterjee NK, Fuschino ME, et al. Calicivirus enteritis in an intestinal transplant recipient. Am J Transplant 2003;3(6):764–8.

51. Kaufman SS, Chatterjee NK, Fuschino ME, et al. Characteristics of human calicivirus enteritis in intestinal transplant recipients. J Pediatr Gastroenterol Nutr 2005;40(3):328–33.

52. Yimen M, Goldstein D, Timpone J, et al. Cytomegalovirus resistance in intestinal transplant recipients. Abstract presented at American Transplant Congress. Philadelphia (PA); April 30, 2011.

53. Florescu DF, Langnas AN, Grant W, et al. Incidence, risk factors, and outcomes associated with cytomegalovirus disease in small bowel transplant recipients. Pediatr Transplant 2012;16(3):294–301.

54. Bueno J, Green M, Kocoshis S, et al. Cytomegalovirus infection after intestinal transplantation in children. Clin Infect Dis 1997;25(5):1078–83.

55. Kotton CN, Kumar D, Caliendo AM, et al. International consensus guidelines on the management of cytomegalovirus in solid organ transplantation. Transplantation 2010;89(7):779–95.

56. Manez R, Kusne S, Green M, et al. Incidence and risk factors associated with the development of cytomegalovirus disease after intestinal transplantation. Transplantation 1995;59(7):1010–4.

57. Allen U, Preiksaitis J, AST Infectious Diseases Community of Practice. Epstein-Barr virus and posttransplant lymphoproliferative disorder in solid organ transplant recipients. Am J Transplant 2009;9(Suppl 4):S87–96.

58. Kaufman S. Small intestinal transplantation. In: Kleinman RE, Walker WA, editors. Walker's pediatric gastrointestinal disease: physiology, diagnosis, management. Hamilton (Ontario), Lewiston (NY): BC Decker; 2008. p. 621.

59. Green M, Bueno J, Rowe D, et al. Predictive negative value of persistent low Epstein-Barr virus viral load after intestinal transplantation in children. Transplantation 2000;70(4):593–6.

60. Opelz G, Dohler B. Lymphomas after solid organ transplantation: a collaborative transplant study report. Am J Transplant 2004;4(2):222–30.

61. Gross TG. Management of posttransplant lymphoproliferative disease. In: Langnas AN, editor. Intestinal failure: diagnosis, management and transplantation. Oxford (UK): Blackwell Pub; 2008.

62. Oertel SH, Verschuuren E, Reinke P, et al. Effect of anti-CD 20 antibody rituximab in patients with post-transplant lymphoproliferative disorder (PTLD). Am J Transplant 2005;5(12):2901–6.

63. Florescu DF, Islam MK, Mercer DF, et al. Incidence and outcome of fungal infections in pediatric small bowel transplant recipients. Transpl Infect Dis 2010; 12(6):497–504.

64. Singh N. Antifungal prophylaxis for solid organ transplant recipients: seeking clarity amidst controversy. Clin Infect Dis 2000;31(2):545–53.

65. Sauvat F, Dupic L, Caldari D, et al. Factors influencing outcome after intestinal transplantation in children. Transplant Proc 2006;38(6):1689–91.

66. Morrell M, Fraser VJ, Kollef MH. Delaying the empiric treatment of candida bloodstream infection until positive blood culture results are obtained: a potential risk factor for hospital mortality. Antimicrobial Agents Chemother 2005;49(9): 3640–5.

67. Pappas PG, Alexander BD, Andes DR, et al. Invasive fungal infections among organ transplant recipients: results of the Transplant-Associated Infection Surveillance Network (TRANSNET). Clin Infect Dis 2010;50(8):1101–11.

68. Kusne S, Furukawa H, Abu-Elmagd K, et al. Infectious complications after small bowel transplantation in adults: an update. Transplant Proc 1996;28(5):2761–2.

69. Kohler S, Gerlach U, Guckelberger O, et al. Successful treatment of invasive sphenoidal, pulmonary and intracerebral aspergillosis after multivisceral transplantation. Transpl Int 2009;22(5):589–91.

70. Singh N, Husain S, AST Infectious Diseases Community of Practice. Invasive aspergillosis in solid organ transplant recipients. Am J Transplant 2009; 9(Suppl 4):S180–91.

71. Vianna R, Misra V, Fridell JA, et al. Survival after disseminated invasive aspergillosis in a multivisceral transplant recipient. Transplant Proc 2007;39(1):305–7.

72. Singh N, Avery RK, Munoz P, et al. Trends in risk profiles for and mortality associated with invasive aspergillosis among liver transplant recipients. Clin Infect Dis 2003;36(1):46–52.

73. Gavalda J, Len O, San Juan R, RESITRA (Spanish Network for Research on Infection in Transplantation). Risk factors for invasive aspergillosis in solid-organ transplant recipients: a case-control study. Clin Infect Dis 2005;41(1): 52–9.

74. Kusne S, Torre-Cisneros J, Manez R, et al. Factors associated with invasive lung aspergillosis and the significance of positive *Aspergillus* culture after liver transplant. J Infect Dis 1992;166(6):1379–83.

75. Osawa M, Ito Y, Hirai T, et al. Risk factors for invasive aspergillosis in living donor liver transplant recipients. Liver Transpl 2007;13(4):566–70.

76. George MJ, Snydman DR, Werner BG, et al. The independent role of cytomegalovirus as a risk factor for invasive fungal disease in orthotopic liver transplant recipients. Boston Center for Liver Transplantation CMVIG-study group. Cytogam, MedImmune, Inc. Gaithersburg, Maryland. Am J Med 1997;103(2): 106–13.

77. Collins LA, Samore MH, Roberts MS, et al. Risk factors for invasive fungal infections complicating orthotopic liver transplantation. J Infect Dis 1994;170(3): 644–52.

78. Reyes J, Todo S, Green M, et al. Graft-versus-host disease after liver and small bowel transplantation in a child. Clin Transplant 1997;11(5 Pt 1):345–8.

79. Uemoto S, Fujimoto Y, Inomata Y, et al. Living-related small bowel transplantation: the first case in Japan. Pediatr Transplant 1998;2(1):40–4.

80. Campbell AL, Goldberg CL, Magid MS, et al. First case of toxoplasmosis following small bowel transplantation and systematic review of tissue-invasive toxoplasmosis following noncardiac solid organ transplantation. Transplantation 2006;81(3):408–17.
81. Qu L, Strollo DC, Bond G, et al. Nocardia prostatitis in a small intestine transplant recipient. Transpl Infect Dis 2003;5(2):94–7.
82. Gerber DA, Green M, Jaffe R, et al. Cryptosporidial infections after solid organ transplantation in children. Pediatr Transplant 2000;4(1):50–5.
83. Gruz F, Fuxman C, Errea A, et al. *Isospora belli* infection after isolated intestinal transplant. Transpl Infect Dis 2010;12(1):69–72.
84. Wu G, Vilchez RA, Eidelman B, et al. Cryptococcal meningitis: an analysis among 5,521 consecutive organ transplant recipients. Transpl Infect Dis 2002; 4(4):183–8.
85. Furukawa H, Kusne S, Sutton DA, et al. Acute invasive sinusitis due to *Trichoderma longibrachiatum* in a liver and small bowel transplant recipient. Clin Infect Dis 1998;26(2):487–9.
86. Singh N, Chang FY, Gayowski T, et al. Infections due to dematiaceous fungi in organ transplant recipients: case report and review. Clin Infect Dis 1997; 24(3):369–74.

Infections in Composite Tissue Allograft Recipients

Sarah P. Hammond, MD

KEYWORDS

- Composite tissue allotransplantation • Facial transplantation • Hand transplantation
- Posttransplant infection • Cytomegalovirus

KEY POINTS

- Serious bacterial infection caused by pneumonia or surgical site infection is a common complication after facial composite tissue allotransplantation (CTA).
- Rejection and concomitant viral reactivation caused by cytomegalovirus and other herpes family viruses are common after the immediate postoperative period in facial and hand CTA recipients.
- Treatment of cytomegalovirus in CTA recipients has been associated with significant difficulties, including drug-related neutropenia and ganciclovir-resistant infection.
- Fungal infection is an uncommon complication of facial or hand CTA.

INTRODUCTION

Composite tissue allotransplantation (CTA) is a novel surgical procedure in which multiple tissue types, often including skin, skeletal muscle, bone, and peripheral ganglia, are transplanted to improve both the function and esthetic appearance of injured or missing tissue. The field is nascent: the first hand transplant was performed 15 years ago,[1] and the first partial face transplant was performed 7 years ago.[2] Important interrelated goals of this young field include defining optimal immunosuppression, accurately diagnosing and treating rejection, and anticipating and preventing infectious complications.

More than 50 upper extremity transplants, approximately 20 face transplants, and a handful of other composite transplant procedures, including trachea,[3,4] knee,[5] and abdominal wall transplants,[6] have been performed worldwide. Although there have been detailed reports of the immunosuppressive regimens used and the functional outcomes of many face[2,7–16] and hand transplant programs,[17–21] infectious disease

Disclosures: S.P. Hammond has received research grant support from Merck.
Division of Infectious Diseases, Brigham and Women's Hospital, Harvard Medical School, 75 Francis Street, PBB-A4, Boston, MA 02115, USA
E-mail address: shammond2@partners.org

Infect Dis Clin N Am 27 (2013) 379–393
http://dx.doi.org/10.1016/j.idc.2013.02.007
0891-5520/13/$ – see front matter © 2013 Elsevier Inc. All rights reserved.

id.theclinics.com

complications and antimicrobial prophylactic practices (with a few exceptions)[22-25] have been reported infrequently and with limited detail. Based on the available literature, it is clear that CTA generally requires significant immunosuppression, and thus, the theoretic risk for opportunistic infections in this patient population is high. Furthermore, acute rejection is common after CTA and can be difficult to distinguish from other conditions like rosacea, thereby potentially leading to increased treatment of rejection with increased concomitant risk for opportunistic infection.[13]

The purpose of this article is to review the documented infectious complications associated with CTA and prophylactic practices. Despite the limitations both in the small number of transplants performed to date as well as the variability in reporting of infectious complications, certain common infectious complications have emerged that will allow for a rational approach to infection prevention in this population in the future.

BACKGROUND/BASIC PRINCIPLES

As solid organ transplantation has become more common over the last 3 decades, treating and preventing transplant-associated infections has become increasingly important. The infectious risk in recipients of solid organ transplant depends on 2 factors: the epidemiologic exposures and the net state of immunosuppression of the recipient.[26,27] Furthermore, as articulated by Fishman and Rubin in 1998,[27] the types of infections seen after solid organ transplant vary based on the time lag between the transplant and the presentation with infection and whether the recipient has been treated for rejection recently. Infections that develop early after transplantation are typically related to the surgical procedure itself (surgical site infection), the initial hospital stay after transplantation (nosocomial infection), or rarely the donor (donor-derived infection). Infections that develop after the immediate postoperative period but within the first 6 months after transplant or in recipients who were recently treated for rejection are typically caused by opportunists. Infections that develop 6 months or more after transplant in patients without recent rejection are typically caused by community-acquired pathogens. Although these principles describe recipients of solid organ transplant, they also apply to CTA recipients.

The infection risk in CTA recipients in particular is also affected by the significant amount of induction and maintenance immunosuppression required for graft survival in the first few years. Typically, hand and facial CTA recipients are treated with induction immunosuppression, including antithymocyte globulin or alemtuzumab, pulse-dose steroids, and mycophenolate mofetil. The typical maintenance immunosuppressive regimen after induction with antithymocyte globulin includes prednisone, tacrolimus, and mycophenolate mofetil, whereas the maintenance regimen after induction with alemtuzumab typically includes tacrolimus and mycophenolate mofetil only. Other types of immunosuppression have been used, including adjunctive extracorporeal photopheresis.[11] Despite the routine use of significant induction immunosuppression, rejection is common during the first year after composite transplantation.

The complex anatomy of many CTAs also affects the infection risk specific to CTA recipients. For example, most face transplants involve transplantation of skin, bone, nerve, skeletal muscle, and mucosal surfaces. The mucosal surfaces are typically colonized with donor flora that can result in local infection. Furthermore, transplanted donor lymph node and salivary gland tissue can become a source for inflammatory and infectious complications.[14,24] Thus, although the general infectious risks for composite transplantation are predictable, the specific anatomic details of each case, particularly with cases of face transplantation, are crucial to try to prevent both immediate and long-term postoperative complications.

FACE TRANSPLANTATION

Because both partial and full facial CTA are so novel, the number of cases on which to base a review of infectious complications is limited. There are detailed reports describing the procedural aspects of transplantation and subsequent course of 15 face CTA recipients.[2,7–16,28] Infectious complications have been reported in 11 of these recipients and are summarized in **Table 1**.

Each partial and full face transplant involves unique anatomic details,[31] such as the presence of mucosal tissue of the mouth or sinuses and transplantation of donor lymph tissue, which specifically affect the infectious risk. Organ donors are often hospitalized for some time before organ donation. Although direct transmission of nosocomial pathogens from facial CTA donor to recipient has not been reported, hospitalization of the donor before transplantation may increase the risk for colonization of mucosal surfaces with resistant hospital-acquired pathogens that could later cause serious infection in the recipient. In addition, acute rejection requiring augmented immunosuppression is common after facial CTA, which probably also increases the risk for infectious complications with this procedure.[32,33]

Early Postoperative Infection

In the immediate posttransplant period, bacterial infections including pneumonia, surgical site infection, and bacteremia are the most commonly reported infectious complications (see **Table 1**). In particular, bacterial pneumonia developed early after transplantation in affected recipients. Three of the 11 recipients with infectious complications developed gram-negative bacterial pneumonia within 48 hours of transplantation. One recipient had infection caused by a community pathogen, *Haemophilus influenzae*, and apparently had a mild clinical course.[24] In contrast, the other 2 recipients with early postoperative pneumonia had hospital-associated pathogens, including *Pseudomonas aeruginosa* in 1 case[11] and *Pseudomonas aeruginosa*, *Serratia marcesans*, and *Proteus mirabilis* in the other.[24] These 2 patients had severe clinical manifestations, including acute respiratory distress syndrome in 1 and septic shock in the other, although both recovered with antibiotic therapy. The recipient with polymicrobial pneumonia had undergone simultaneous face and bilateral hand transplantation and subsequently lost both hand allografts as a consequence of hypotension caused by the infection.

Knoll and colleagues[24] have suggested that the 2 pneumonias reported in their cohort resulted from aspiration of upper respiratory or gastric secretions during the prolonged transplant procedure itself. In order to prevent this early infection, their center plans to include elevation of the head of the operating table as well as the use of a cuffed endotracheal tube with suction capabilities for future potential face transplantation procedures.

Surgical site infection was also a common and serious infectious complication early after facial CTA. Among the 11 facial CTA recipients in whom infectious complications have been reported, 3 developed gram-negative surgical site infection. Reported pathogens include *Pseudomonas aeruginosa*, *Acinetobacter baumannii*, and 1 polymicrobial infection caused by *Pseudomonas aeruginosa* and *Candida albicans*.

Details regarding the exact timing and severity of infection are lacking in the case of the *Acinetobacter* infection, although the patient reportedly required prolonged intensive care but recovered.[30] In the other 2 cases, infection developed during the second

Table 1
Infectious complications after facial composite tissue allotransplantation

	Early (0–2 mo)	Intermediate and/or after Rejection (2–9 mo)	Late (>9 mo)
Bacterial	Pneumonia (day 1–2)	—	Pneumonia
	• Pseudomonas[11]		• Presumed bacterial (5 y)[28]
	• Haemophilus[14,24]		
	• Pseudomonas/Serratia/Proteus[14,24]		
	Surgical site infection (day 8–47)	—	—
	• Pseudomonas[11]		
	• Acinetobacter[30]		
	• Pseudomonas/Candida[14,24]		
	Bacteremia (day 1–47)	Bacteremia	—
	• Enterobacter[30]	• Enterobacter, streptococci, coagulase-negative staphylococci (day 110)[14,24]	
		• Pseudomonas, coagulase-negative staphylococci (exact timing not indicated)[23]	
	—	Clostridium difficile-associated diarrhea	Clostridium difficile-associated diarrhea
		• Day 100[14,24]	• With concomitant Aeromonas (13 mo)[23]
	Other bacterial infections (day 26–47)	Other bacterial infections	Other bacterial infections
	• Superinfected sialocele[24]	• Parotitis (day 96)[14,24]	• Bacterial conjunctivitis (11 mo)[24]
	• Zygomatic fluid collection[24]		• Recurrent parotitis (2 and 3 y)[24]
	• Tracheobronchitis[30]		
Viral	Early CMV reactivation	CMV reactivation	CMV reactivation
	• CMV viremia[a] (weeks 3 and 7)[30]	• GCV-resistant viremia (day 65)[11,12]	• Syndrome (15 mo)[24]
		• Gastritis (7 mo)[24]	
		• Recurrent viremia (8 mo)[23]	
	HSV reactivation	HSV reactivation	HSV reactivation
	• Lips (day 5)[11]	• Lips (day 185)[9]	• Chin (14 mo)[24]
	Other viral reactivation/infection	Other viral reactivation/infection	Other viral reactivation/infection
	• HCV (day 10)[24]	• Moluscum contagiosum (7 mo)[9]	• Viral gastroenteritis (9 mo)[24]
Fungal	Fungal infection	Fungal infection	—
	• Candida/Pseudomonas surgical site infection as above[14,24]	• Majocchi granuloma (6 mo)[24]	

Abbreviations: CMV, cytomegalovirus; GCV, ganciclovir; HCV, hepatitis C virus; HSV, herpes simplex virus.
a CMV viremia has been reported during this period in only 1 face transplant recipient who was treated preemptively for CMV reactivation.

and third weeks after transplantation. In the case of the monomicrobial *Pseudomonas* infection, the site involved both facial allograft and a hand allograft transplanted at the same time; the facial CTA infection reportedly required repeated debridement and led to partial facial graft necrosis and death.[11] In the case of the polymicrobial infection with *Pseudomonas* and *Candida*, the infection site was associated with a submandibular fluid collection, which was drained. The patient recovered from the infection on a prolonged course of antibiotics.[24]

A handful of viral reactivations have been reported in the immediate posttransplant period, including recurrent hepatitis C virus (HCV) viremia, herpes simplex virus (HSV) infection of the lips, and cytomegalovirus (CMV) viremia. Recurrent HCV was reported at day 10 after transplant in a recipient who had previously been diagnosed with HCV and treated with a full course of interferon and ribavirin, with virologic response, before undergoing transplantation.[24] CMV viremia was reported at week 3 and again at week 7 in a face transplant recipient at risk for CMV who did not receive antiviral prophylaxis and was instead monitored preemptively for reactivation.[30]

Intermediately Timed Posttransplant Infections

Viral infections in general, and those caused by CMV in particular, are the most commonly reported infectious complication in facial CTA recipients who are beyond the immediate posttransplant period but still within 2 to 9 months of transplantation. Other reported viral infections during this period include molluscum contagiosum involving the allograft and reactivation of HSV.

CMV reactivation is common in facial CTA recipients (**Table 2**). Of the 12 facial CTA recipients in whom CMV serostatus has been reported, 11 were at risk for CMV reactivation from either donor or recipient pretransplant CMV seropositivity (the twelfth was CMV donor and recipient seronegative before transplantation [D–/R–]). Of these 11, 8 were in the highest-risk category for CMV reactivation: donor CMV seropositive and recipient seronegative (D+/R–).

Three D+/R– facial CTA recipients (and none of the other recipients at risk for CMV) developed reactivation between 2 and 9 months after transplantation. All 3 had relatively complicated courses. One recipient developed CMV viremia on day 65 after transplant, concurrent with an episode of acute rejection.[11,12] Viremia developed despite valganciclovir prophylaxis and the patient subsequently required an 8-week course of intravenous foscarnet for ganciclovir-resistant CMV. Another recipient developed refractory leukopenia as a result of valganciclovir prophylaxis, which was stopped after 5 months.[23,34] CMV viremia then developed at 8 months in this recipient and was treated with an investigational antiviral agent because of valganciclovir-associated leukopenia. The third facial CTA recipient who developed CMV reactivation during this period presented with CMV gastritis and viremia 7 months after transplantation and 1 month after CMV prophylaxis had finished.[24] His course was uncomplicated after valganciclovir treatment was initiated.

Bacterial infections during the intermediate period were less common than early after transplant. Two bacterial infections reported in this period were late nosocomial infections that occurred 3 to 4 months after transplant. These infections included *Clostridium difficile*-associated diarrhea and polymicrobial bacteremia potentially related to an indwelling venous catheter (vs a decayed tooth).[14,24] Both were treated with antibiotics without event. Another bacterial infection reported during this period was unilateral bacterial parotitis, which may have been related to parotid duct narrowing.[24] Parotitis recurred in this facial CTA recipient 2 and 3 years after transplant but did not recur after parotid duct dilation.

Table 2
CMV in facial composite tissue allotransplant recipients

CTA Recipient	CMV Status	Prophylaxis, Duration	CMV Reactivation	CMV-Related Complications
29-yo man[11]	D+/R–	Valganciclovir, 6 mo	Viremia, 9 wk	Ganciclovir-resistant infection; treated with foscarnet
37-yo man[11]	D+/R–	Valganciclovir, 6 mo	—	—
33-yo man[11]	D+/R–	Valganciclovir, 6 mo	—	—
30-yo man[7]	D+/R–	Valganciclovir, at least 4 mo	—	—
45-yo woman[23]	D+/R–	Ganciclovir/valganciclovir 5 mo	Viremia, 8 mo	Refractory ganciclovir-associated neutropenia requiring alternative antiviral agent
35-yo man[30]	D+/R–	Preemptive monitoring	Viremia, 3 and 7 wk	—
59-yo man[24]	D+/R–	Valganciclovir, 13 mo	Syndrome, 15 mo	—
25-yo man[24]	D+/R+	Valganciclovir, 6 mo	Gastritis, 7 mo	—
30-yo man[24]	D+/R–	Valganciclovir, 6 mo	—	—
57-yo woman[24]	D+/R+	Valganciclovir, 4 mo	—	—
37-yo man[8]	D–/R+	Valganciclovir, duration unknown[a]	—	—

Abbreviations: D+, donor seropositive; D–, donor seronegative; R+, recipient seropositive; R–, recipient seronegative; yo, year old.
[a] Limited follow-up available for this case.

Invasive fungal infection has been reported in only a single patient during this period. Majocchi granuloma, an invasive dermatophyte infection, caused by *Trichophyton rubrum*, was observed 6 months after transplantation.[24] The infection was successfully treated with a 3-month course of terbinafine. This is the only non-*Candida* fungal infection that has been reported in a facial CTA recipient.

Late Posttransplant Infections

Most of the infectious complications more than 9 months after transplantation are caused by late viral reactivation episodes, community-acquired infections, and infections specifically related to the anatomy of the transplanted tissue. Both HSV and CMV reactivation have been reported during this period in the context of recent completion of antiviral prophylaxis.[24] The reported community-acquired infections include presumed viral gastroenteritis in the context of a local outbreak and bacterial pneumonia responsive to antibiotics.[24,28] The late infections related to the anatomy of transplanted tissue include recurrent bacterial parotitis caused by a stenotic parotid duct, as discussed earlier, and allograft palpebral conjunctivitis around an ocular prosthesis, which was successfully treated with topical antibiotics.[24]

HAND TRANSPLANTATION

Although more hand CTA procedures have been performed worldwide than facial CTA, infectious complications in hand transplant recipients have mostly been reported in limited detail in case series from individual centers and in a few large compila-tions.[3,32,35] Only a few publications have systematically reviewed or described infec-tious complications in this population.[22,25] Missing details (such as pretransplant CMV donor and recipient serologic status in some recipients) make it challenging to draw definitive conclusions about how best to manage and prevent infections after hand CTA.

Although the anatomy of hand transplantation does not involve the mucosal sur-faces believed to contribute to the risk of infection in facial CTA, rejection requiring augmentation of systemic immunosuppression is common and likely increases the risk for infectious complications specifically in hand CTA recipients. In 2 recent reviews of 8 bilateral hand transplant recipients at 2 different centers, all recipients experienced at least 1 episode of rejection during the first year after transplant.[18,21] Similarly, a recent report that compiled international hand transplant experience from 1998 to 2010 reported that 85% of recipients in this group developed acute rejection within the first year of transplantation.[32]

Table 3 summarizes the infectious complications reported in hand CTA recipients. Viral infections in general, and specifically viruses in the herpes virus family, caused the largest number of infectious complications reported after hand CTA.

Early Postoperative Infection

Although facial CTA recipients have been reported to develop bacterial infections with some frequency immediately after transplantation, this is an uncommon compli-cation in hand CTA. The only 2 early postoperative bacterial infections reported in hand CTA recipients (bacterial pneumonia and surgical site infection) both occurred in recipients who also received concomitant facial and hand allografts (see **Table 3**).[11,24]

Early viral reactivation is the most commonly reported postoperative infectious complication during the first 2 months after hand CTA. HSV reactivation involving the face developed 8 weeks after transplant in a single recipient.[3,21] Early CMV reactivation has been reported in 4 hand transplant recipients, including 2 with CMV disease and 2 with viremia.[25,37]

Schneeberger and colleagues[25] reported CMV viremia in 3 hand CTA recipients during the second month after transplant, 1 of whom later developed CMV syndrome characterized by fevers and malaise in the setting of recurrent CMV viremia. All were at risk for CMV based on donor or recipient seropositivity for CMV and thus all were on prophylactic oral ganciclovir before reactivation developed. Oral ganciclovir (the only oral option for CMV prophylaxis at the time that these patients were transplanted) does not achieve serum levels comparable to intravenous therapy or oral valganciclo-vir. Thus, the development of early CMV viremia after transplant in the context of oral ganciclovir prophylaxis was not entirely unexpected and raised concern for ganciclovir-resistant infection. However, no genotypic resistance was found in the single case that was tested.

Two of the patients in this report developed rejection shortly after CMV reactivation developed, and a third was treated for acute rejection 2 weeks before the develop-ment of CMV viremia. The development of CMV soon before or after rejection was diagnosed in these patients mimics the complicated relationship between CMV reac-tivation and rejection seen in solid organ transplant recipients.[26,27] All 3 had difficult treatment courses, with relapsing viremia in the setting of antiviral intolerance and repeated treatment of rejection.

Chlemonski and colleagues[37] reported CMV gastritis in a D–/R– hand CTA recip-ient not on prophylaxis 1 month after transplantation. The patient was treated with

Table 3
Infectious complications after hand composite tissue allotransplantation

	Early (0–2 mo)	Intermediate or After Rejection (2–9 mo)	Late (>9 mo)	Timing Not Reported
Bacterial	Surgical site/graft infection • Pseudomonas (day 15)[a,11] Other bacterial infections • Polymicrobial Pneumonia (day 2)[a,24]	Surgical site/graft infection • Osteomyelitis, Staphylococcus aureus (5 mo)[21,32,43] Other bacterial infections • Mucositis (3 mo)[21]	—	Other bacterial infections • Clostridium difficile-associated diarrhea[22,36]
Viral	Early CMV reactivation • CMV disease (gastritis, day 28)[b,19,37] • CMV viremia (day 34–53)[25] Other viral reactivation • HSV reactivation (8 wk)[3,21]	CMV Reactivation • CMV disease (colitis, 2–4 mo)[3,29,38,42] • CMV viremia (6 mo)[25] Other viral reactivation • Recurrent VZV (6, 7, 9 mo)[39,44] Other viral infections • HPV of graft (8 mo)[22,40]	Other viral reactivation • VZV (1.5 y)[6,7] • EBV infection (1.5 y)[15]	CMV Reactivation • CMV viremia[36] Other viral reactivation • HSV reactivation[17] Other viral infections • Severe presumed viral URI[22]
Fungal	Cutaneous infection • Tinea (7 wk)[3]	—	Invasive infection • Alternaria alternata (2 y)[22,41]	Cutaneous infection • Tinea (recurrent in some)[3,17,29,42]

Abbreviations: CMV, cytomegalovirus; EBV, Epstein-Barr virus; HPV, human papilloma virus; HSV, herpes simplex virus; URI, upper respiratory tract infection; VZV, varicella zoster virus.

a Combined face and hand transplant recipient.

b Occurred in a single patient reportedly CMV D–/R– on no prophylaxis; CMV viremia occurred in 3 recipients who were all receiving oral ganciclovir prophylaxis.

intravenous ganciclovir and reduction in immunosuppression, with improvement, but subsequently developed acute rejection. The timing of the infection after transplantation is suggestive of reactivation as opposed to new infection. Because there was a delay of several months between the time that recipient CMV serologies were checked and transplantation, the investigators suggested that primary infection may have occurred before transplantation.

A single early postoperative superficial fungal infection caused by tinea has been reported.[3] The infection developed 7 weeks after transplantation and responded to topical antifungal treatment.

Intermediately Timed Posttransplant Infections

Viral infections were also common in hand CTA recipients beyond the immediate posttransplant period but still within 2 to 9 months of transplantation. Reported viral infections include varicella zoster virus (VZV) reactivation, common warts involving the allograft, and CMV viremia and disease.

Recurrent dermatomal VZV involving the leg developed in 1 hand CTA recipient.[17,39] Episodes of VZV developed at 6, 7, 9, and 18 months after transplantation, beginning around the time that valganciclovir prophylaxis (given for 6 months) ended.

Extensive warts caused by human papilloma virus involving the allograft developed in a bilateral forearm CTA recipient 8 months after transplantation.[22,40] The patient had been treated for rejection twice with antithymocyte globulin, then later with alemtuzumab, before developing veruccae. Topical cidofovir gel applied to the warts led to regression, although they reportedly intermittently flared thereafter with changes in immunosuppression.[40]

CMV reactivation was common during the intermediate period after transplantation and was specifically seen in patients who had recently finished a relatively short course of prophylaxis or had to stop valganciclovir-based prophylaxis before the planned duration because of drug-induced neutropenia. CMV colitis developed in 2 hand CTA recipients 2.5 and 3.5 months after transplantation. A CMV D+/R− recipient developed CMV colitis 3.5 months after transplantation, approximately 2 weeks after completing a 3-month course of oral ganciclovir prophylaxis.[20,38,42] The other patient developed CMV colitis concurrent with acute rejection approximately 2 weeks after valganciclovir and mycophenolate were stopped because of neutropenia.[20,42] Both patients cleared their CMV infection with antiviral therapy. CMV viremia developed in a CMV D+/R+ hand CTA recipient 6 months after transplantation, 1 month after valganciclovir prophylaxis was truncated early because of drug-induced neutropenia refractory to granulocyte colony-stimulating factor.[25]

Bacterial infections during the intermediate period after hand CTA were uncommon. A single episode of osteomyelitis of the ulna caused by *Staphylococcus aureus* has been reported.[21,32,43] The infection reportedly resolved with removal of hardware and prolonged systemic antibiotic therapy. Oral mucositis in the context of neutropenia has also been reported.[21]

Late Posttransplant Infections

Only a few infectious complications have been reported late after transplant. These complications include 2 viral infections: recurrent VZV 18 months after transplant (as described earlier)[17,39] and Epstein-Barr virus infection (not further characterized) in a different recipient, also 18 months after transplant.[21]

One invasive fungal infection has been reported in this population as a result of an injury sustained in the community. A hand CTA recipient developed a local swelling on the thigh after penetrating trauma from organic material. The lesion was excised surgically and a diagnosis of *Alternaria alternata* was made. The patient was treated with liposomal amphotericin B subsequently followed by oral itraconazole with complete resolution.[22,41]

Other Infections

A handful of other infections have been reported in hand CTA recipients, without details regarding the timing of the infection. At least 2 hand CTA recipients have developed *Clostridium difficile*-associated diarrhea after transplantation, which was treated without reported complications.[22,36]

Several additional viral infections, including 1 other episode of HSV reactivation[17] and 1 episode of severe presumed viral upper respiratory tract infection, have been reported.[22] In addition, 3 other CTA recipients have developed CMV reactivation after transplantation but the details of the timing of reactivation, the severity of the illness (viremia vs end-organ disease), the response to treatment, and the pretransplant donor and recipient CMV serostatus were not reported.[36] Including these 3 cases, 10 hand CTA recipients developed CMV reactivation after transplantation.

In addition, tinea, or noninvasive cutaneous fungal infection, has been reported in several hand CTA recipients.[3,17,29,42] The location of these infections (including whether any involved an allograft) and when infection developed has not been described. All reports indicate that treatment with topical antifungal agents led to resolution.

CHRONIC PRETRANSPLANT INFECTIONS

The outcomes in solid organ transplant recipients with chronic viral hepatitis and human immunodeficiency virus (HIV) infection are the subject of extensive study. The international experience with CTA in individuals with hepatitis B virus, HCV, and HIV infections is limited. Some centers performing CTA procedures have treated HIV infection or chronic viral hepatitis as exclusion criteria for transplantation.[17,42] Only 2 CTA recipients with chronic viral infections have been reported.

Knoll and colleagues[24] reported that a 59-year-old man with recently treated chronic HCV underwent partial facial CTA. Although he had finished a full course of pegylated interferon α and ribavirin therapy with virologic response (HCV virus load was undetectable before transplantation), he developed HCV reactivation 10 days after transplantation. His HCV has remained untreated since.

Cavadas and colleagues[44] reported that a 42-year-old man with HIV infection underwent lower facial CTA. The patient had a CD4 count more than 400 and an undetectable virus load on highly active antiretroviral therapy before transplant. At 16 months after transplant, HIV replication reportedly remained fully suppressed.

PREVENTION OF INFECTION

There are no published guidelines to direct the prophylactic use of antimicrobial agents in CTA recipients in the short-term or long-term after transplantation. Determining the optimal prophylaxis for a particular center or recipient is challenging for several reasons. First, the available data are difficult to interpret. Case series describing CTA recipients sometimes include exact details on prophylactic agents used and the durations, whereas other reports leave this information out. Of the centers that do include details, there is significant heterogeneity in prophylaxis practices.[24] Furthermore, as shown in **Tables 1** and **3**, the infectious complications in facial and hand CTA recipients vary significantly. Rejection requiring augmentation of systemic immunosuppression is common in both facial and hand transplantation and potentially increases and prolongs the risk for infection in this population.

Bacterial Infections

Most centers performing facial CTA and some performing hand CTA procedures have described antibacterial prophylaxis practices.[11,23,24] However, practices are varied in terms of both the antibiotic choice and duration.[24] As shown in **Table 1**, the early infectious complications reported after facial transplantation are predominately bacterial, including early pneumonia and surgical site infection. On a theoretic basis, the pathogens of concern are those that colonize the skin and mucosal surfaces of the donor and recipient such as streptococci. Thus early postoperative antibacterial prophylaxis with agents active against typical colonizers of the mouth is indicated. Gordon and colleagues[23] stressed the importance of tailoring the antimicrobial regimen based on donor or recipient colonization with resistant pathogens. Knoll and colleagues[24] described adding an antipseudomonal agent to their perioperative antibiotic regimen based on commonly noted donor or recipient colonization with resistant gram-negative pathogens. Among the centers that have published details, broad-spectrum antibiotics with a third-generation or fourth-generation cephalosporin or a β-lactam/β-lactamase combination drug with or without vancomycin are typically used.

The appropriate duration of prophylaxis for face transplant recipients is not clear. Some centers only use prophylaxis for 48 hours,[11] whereas others use prophylaxis for more than a week.[23] Gordon and colleagues[23] suggest continuation of the initial perioperative antibiotics until sutures heal.

In contrast, bacterial infections are uncommon early after transplant in hand CTA recipients who did not concurrently undergo facial CTA. Therefore it is not clear that prolonged or broad-spectrum antibiotics are indicated.

Viral Infections

For both facial and hand CTA recipients CMV is the most common and problematic viral infection, despite the use of prophylaxis at most centers. Overall, CMV reactivation is most common during the intermediate period after CTA. Many CMV reactivation episodes were reported early after transplant (in 1 facial CTA recipient and several hand CTA recipients, as shown in **Tables 1** and **3**), but in all cases, the affected recipients were either on no prophylaxis or were on suboptimal prophylaxis with oral ganciclovir, which is no longer used as a first-line agent, because of poor oral absorption. Given the substantial risk of CMV reactivation in CTA recipients and the reported complications with CMV infection (including drug-induced neutropenia, ganciclovir-resistant CMV infection, and possibly increased risk of rejection), most centers use prophylaxis with valganciclovir. One center recently reported early CMV reactivation with a favorable outcome in a facial CTA recipient who was monitored preemptively for CMV reactivation without systemic prophylaxis.[30]

For centers choosing prophylaxis, the optimal duration is unclear. One facial CTA recipient developed CMV viremia more than a year after transplant shortly after finishing a 13-month course of valganciclovir prophylaxis.[24] Most centers give prophylaxis for at least 3 to 6 months.

As with solid organ transplant recipients, CMV risk likely depends on CMV donor and recipient serologic status, with CMV D+/R− recipients at highest risk. Because CTA is not a life-sustaining procedure, to mitigate the risk of CMV infection in CMV-seronegative recipients, some centers choose not to offer transplantation with a CMV-seropositive donor to these candidates.[23,25] Other centers choose to offer transplantation to seronegative recipients with seropositive donors with the use of prophylaxis, as is given to CMV-seropositive recipients.

Other herpes virus infections are also problematic after CTA, as shown in **Tables 1** and **3**. Specifically, HSV reactivation was common in facial CTA recipients and was also seen in a few hand CTA recipients. Recurrent dermatomal VZV reactivation was also reported in a hand transplant recipient.[17,39] Both HSV and VZV should be effectively prevented with valganciclovir prophylaxis. For CMV D–/R– recipients not receiving valganciclovir and all patients at centers that use preemptive monitoring for CMV, acyclovir or valacyclovir prophylaxis should be considered.

Fungal Infections

In general, fungal infections are uncommon after CTA. The risk for invasive fungal infection early after transplant is significant in facial CTA recipients, whereas hand CTA recipients seem to have negligible risk for invasive infection during this period. For facial CTA recipients, sinus and oral mucosal colonization with *Candida* in addition to bacteria, as described earlier, is of concern. Knoll and colleagues[24] reported *Candida* surgical site infection in the 1 facial CTA recipient in their cohort who did not receive initial postoperative antifungal prophylaxis. Based on the theoretic and proven risk, fungal prophylaxis should be considered for facial CTA recipients in the immediate postoperative period.

Several hand transplant recipients have reportedly developed superficial tinea infection. In all reported cases, the infection responded to topical treatment without complication, and thus prophylaxis is not clearly indicated.

Other Pathogens of Concern

Neither *Pneumocystis jirovecii* pneumonia (PCP) nor toxoplasmosis has been reported in CTA recipients after transplant. However, both are preventable infectious complications of concern in this population.

The risk of PCP in solid organ transplant recipients and other patients with depressed CD4 T-lymphocyte counts or chronic steroid use is well known.[27,45] Predictably, CTA recipients are also likely at significant risk. Most CTA centers that have described their prophylactic practices have included trimethoprim-sulfamethoxazole prophylaxis for at least 6 months.[11,22,24,42]

Toxoplasma gondii is a parasitic infection that is particularly prevalent in certain geographic areas, including Europe. Primary infection results in parasite encystation in muscle and occasionally visceral organs of the host. With the large amount of striated muscle present in composite grafts (hand allografts in particular), there is potential for donor-to-recipient transmission of toxoplasma, as has occurred with seronegative heart transplant recipients with a seropositive donor.[46] In addition, seropositive recipients may be at some lesser risk for reactivation after CTA, as shown with other solid organ transplants. The risk for development of active toxoplasmosis is likely highest in the first 3 months after transplantation.[46] Prophylaxis with trimethoprim-sulfamethoxazole is the most effective regimen, and thus the PCP prophylaxis practices at most CTA centers also provide toxoplasma prophylaxis.

SUMMARY

Composite transplantation is a nascent field in which the surgical technique, typical immunosuppressive regimen, and treatment of rejection are evolving. All of these aspects of CTA affect the risk for posttransplant infectious complications. Based on the detailed reports describing these early facial and hand CTA procedures, certain patterns of infectious complications have emerged.

Although the immediate postoperative risk for serious bacterial or candidal infection is high in facial transplant recipients, it is less in hand CTA recipients. Both groups are at significant risk for rejection and viral infections after the immediate postoperative period during the first year after transplant. CMV in particular has caused significant infection-related morbidity after both facial and hand CTA and has been associated with significant treatment-related toxicities, such as neutropenia. Despite the significant immunosuppression required to maintain a composite transplant, invasive fungal infection is an uncommon complication in this population, with the only serious infections occurring in 1 recipient early after facial CTA in the absence of antifungal prophylaxis and in a hand CTA recipient late after transplant as the result of a traumatic injury with organic matter. Based on these observations and the known infectious risks for pathogens like *Pneumocystis* and *Toxoplasma* in other solid organ transplant recipients, a rational approach to antimicrobial prophylaxis and infection treatment is possible.

REFERENCES

1. Dubernard JM, Owen E, Herzberg G, et al. Human hand allograft: report on first 6 months. Lancet 1999;353:1315.
2. Devauchelle B, Badet L, Lengele B, et al. First human face allograft: early report. Lancet 2006;368:203.
3. Barker JH, Francois CG, Frank JM, et al. Composite tissue allotransplantation. Transplantation 2002;73:832.
4. Knott PD, Hicks D, Braun W, et al. A 12-year perspective on the world's first total laryngeal transplant. Transplantation 2011;91:804.
5. Diefenbeck M, Wagner F, Kirschner MH, et al. Outcome of allogeneic vascularized knee transplants. Transpl Int 2007;20:410.
6. Agarwal S, Dorafshar AH, Harland RC, et al. Liver and vascularized posterior rectus sheath fascia composite tissue allotransplantation. Am J Transplant 2010;10:2712.
7. Barret JP, Gavalda J, Bueno J, et al. Full face transplant: the first case report. Ann Surg 2011;254:252.
8. Dorafshar AH, Bojovic B, Christy MR, et al. Total face, double jaw, and tongue transplantation: an evolutionary concept. Plast Reconstr Surg 2013;131(2): 241–51.
9. Dubernard JM, Lengele B, Morelon E, et al. Outcomes 18 months after the first human partial face transplantation. N Engl J Med 2007;357:2451.
10. Guo S, Han Y, Zhang X, et al. Human facial allotransplantation: a 2-year follow-up study. Lancet 2008;372:631.
11. Lantieri L, Hivelin M, Audard V, et al. Feasibility, reproducibility, risks and benefits of face transplantation: a prospective study of outcomes. Am J Transplant 2011; 11:367.
12. Lantieri L, Meningaud JP, Grimbert P, et al. Repair of the lower and middle parts of the face by composite tissue allotransplantation in a patient with massive plexiform neurofibroma: a 1-year follow-up study. Lancet 2008; 372:639.
13. Pomahac B, Pribaz J, Eriksson E, et al. Restoration of facial form and function after severe disfigurement from burn injury by a composite facial allograft. Am J Transplant 2011;11:386.
14. Pomahac B, Pribaz J, Eriksson E, et al. Three patients with full facial transplantation. N Engl J Med 2012;366:715.

15. Sicilia-Castro D, Gomez-Cia T, Infante-Cossio P, et al. Reconstruction of a severe facial defect by allotransplantation in neurofibromatosis type 1: a case report. Transplant Proc 2011;43:2831.
16. Siemionow M, Papay F, Alam D, et al. Near-total human face transplantation for a severely disfigured patient in the USA. Lancet 2009;374:203.
17. Cavadas PC, Landin L, Thione A, et al. The Spanish experience with hand, forearm, and arm transplantation. Hand Clin 2011;27:443.
18. Hautz T, Engelhardt TO, Weissenbacher A, et al. World experience after more than a decade of clinical hand transplantation: update on the Innsbruck program. Hand Clin 2011;27:423.
19. Jablecki J. World experience after more than a decade of clinical hand transplantation: update on the Polish program. Hand Clin 2011;27:433.
20. Kaufman CL, Breidenbach W. World experience after more than a decade of clinical hand transplantation: update from the Louisville hand transplant program. Hand Clin 2011;27:417.
21. Petruzzo P, Dubernard JM. World experience after more than a decade of clinical hand transplantation: update on the French program. Hand Clin 2011;27:411.
22. Bonatti H, Brandacher G, Margreiter R, et al. Infectious complications in three double hand recipients: experience from a single center. Transplant Proc 2009; 41:517.
23. Gordon CR, Avery RK, Abouhassan W, et al. Cytomegalovirus and other infectious issues related to face transplantation: specific considerations, lessons learned, and future recommendations. Plast Reconstr Surg 2011;127:1515.
24. Knoll B, Hammond SP, Koo S, et al. Infections following facial composite tissue allotransplantation– single center experience and review of the literature. Am J Transplant 2013;13(3):770–9.
25. Schneeberger S, Lucchina S, Lanzetta M, et al. Cytomegalovirus-related complications in human hand transplantation. Transplantation 2005;80:441.
26. Fishman JA. Infection in solid-organ transplant recipients. N Engl J Med 2007; 357:2601.
27. Fishman JA, Rubin RH. Infection in organ-transplant recipients. N Engl J Med 1998;338:1741.
28. Petruzzo P, Testelin S, Kanitakis J, et al. First human face transplantation: 5 years outcomes. Transplantation 2012;93:236.
29. Breidenbach WC, Gonzales NR, Kaufman CL, et al. Outcomes of the first 2 American hand transplants at 8 and 6 years posttransplant. J Hand Surg Am 2008;33:1039.
30. BenMarzouk-Hidalgo OJ, Cordero E, Gomez-Cia T, et al. First face composite-tissue transplant recipient successfully treated for cytomegalovirus infection with preemptive valganciclovir treatment. Antimicrobial Agents Chemother 2011;55:5949.
31. Siemionow M, Ozturk C. An update on facial transplantation cases performed between 2005 and 2010. Plast Reconstr Surg 2011;128:707e.
32. Petruzzo P, Lanzetta M, Dubernard JM, et al. The international registry on hand and composite tissue transplantation. Transplantation 2010;90:1590.
33. Yi C, Guo S. Facial transplantation: lessons so far. Lancet 2009;374:177.
34. Gordon CR, Abouhassan W, Avery RK. What is the true significance of donor-related cytomegalovirus transmission in the setting of facial composite tissue allotransplantation? Transplant Proc 2011;43:3516.

35. Lanzetta M, Petruzzo P, Dubernard JM, et al. Second report (1998-2006) of the international registry of hand and composite tissue transplantation. Transpl Immunol 2007;18(1):1–6.
36. Lanzetta M, Petruzzo P, Vitale G, et al. Human hand transplantation: what have we learned? Transplant Proc 2004;36:664.
37. Chelmonski A, Jablecki J, Szajerka T. Insidious course of cytomegalovirus infection in hand transplant recipient: case report, diagnostics, and treatment. Transplant Proc 2011;43:2827.
38. Jones JW, Gruber SA, Barker JH, et al. Successful hand transplantation. One-year follow-up. Louisville Hand Transplant Team. N Engl J Med 2000;343:468.
39. Cavadas PC, Landin L, Ibanez J. Bilateral hand transplantation: result at 20 months. J Hand Surg Eur Vol 2009;34:434.
40. Bonatti H, Aigner F, De Clercq E, et al. Local administration of cidofovir for human papilloma virus associated skin lesions in transplant recipients. Transpl Int 2007; 20:238.
41. Bonatti H, Lass-Florl C, Zelger B, et al. Alternaria alternata soft tissue infection in a forearm transplant recipient. Surg Infect (Larchmt) 2007;8:539.
42. Ravindra KV, Buell JF, Kaufman CL, et al. Hand transplantation in the United States: experience with 3 patients. Surgery 2008;144:638.
43. Petruzzo P, Badet L, Gazarian A, et al. Bilateral hand transplantation: six years after the first case. Am J Transplant 2006;6:1718.
44. Cavadas PC, Ibanez J, Thione A. Surgical aspects of a lower face, mandible, and tongue allotransplantation. J Reconstr Microsurg 2012;28:43.
45. Yale SH, Limper AH. Pneumocystis carinii pneumonia in patients without acquired immunodeficiency syndrome: associated illness and prior corticosteroid therapy. Mayo Clin Proc 1996;71:5.
46. Derouin F, Pelloux H. Prevention of toxoplasmosis in transplant patients. Clin Microbiol Infect 2008;14:1089.

Parasitic Infections in Solid Organ Transplant Recipients

Laura O'Bryan Coster, MD

KEYWORDS

- Toxoplasmosis • Chagas disease • *Leishmania* • *Acanthamoeba* • *Strongyloides*
- Parasitic infection • Malaria • Transplantation

KEY POINTS

- The 4 modes of parasitic transmission in solid organ transplant (SOT) recipients are donor-derived disease, reactivation disease, blood-transfusion transmission, and de novo infection.
- The risks for parasitic SOT infections differ by transplanted organ and degree or type of immunosuppressive therapy.
- Trimethoprim-sulfamethoxazole (TMP-SMX) prophylaxis of D+/R− *Toxoplasma* cardiac transplant recipients has dramatically reduced the incidence of life-threatening toxoplasmosis.
- The optimal length and dosing of TMP-SMX toxoplasmosis prophylaxis for high-risk SOT recipients (cardiac-seronegative recipients or SOT recipients on high-dose immunosuppressive therapy) is unclear.
- The occurrence of donor-derived and reactivated Chagas disease has brought attention to the need for targeted donor and recipient screening of *Trypanosoma cruzi* in the United States.
- When the SOT donor or recipient is seropositive for *T cruzi*, microbiological and *T cruzi* polymerase chain reaction (PCR) monitoring of the blood assists in early diagnosis and preemptive therapy.
- The diagnosis of visceral leishmaniasis requires a high degree of suspicion and can be made by parasitologic evaluation of the bone marrow or spleen, in combination with ancillary testing such as PCR, serology, and culture.
- Preevaluation testing and treatment of *Strongyloides*-seropositive patients can prevent high-morbidity hyperinfection and disseminated disease after transplantation.

The author has no financial conflicts to disclose.
Department of Infectious Diseases, Georgetown University Hospital, 3800 Reservoir Road, Washington, DC 20007, USA
E-mail address: laura.o.coster@gunet.georgetown.edu

Infect Dis Clin N Am 27 (2013) 395–427
http://dx.doi.org/10.1016/j.idc.2013.02.008
0891-5520/13/$ – see front matter © 2013 Elsevier Inc. All rights reserved.

INTRODUCTION

Parasitic infections are a relatively uncommon complication in solid organ transplant (SOT) recipients in the United States. In addition, parasitic infections are also rare in the general population and are often acquired as a result of travel to other endemic areas throughout the world. The phenomena of globalization will likely contribute to increased rates of parasitic infections in SOT patients.

The majority of serious posttransplant parasitic infections are protozoal infections. Specifically of concern are protozoa, for example, *Trypanosoma cruzi*, which establish lifelong latency in the recipient or donor and have the ability to transform into lethal opportunistic infections during posttransplant immunosuppression. Given the complex management issues, most of this review is devoted to the opportunistic protozoa *Toxoplasma gondii* and *T cruzi*.

Many helminthic diseases, such as *Ascaris* infection and schistosomiasis, are not opportunistic infections after transplantation, and do not differ significantly from infection in an immunocompetent individual.[1] A notable exception after a transplant is *Strongyloides*, a long-lived, often innocuous infection, which portends a mortality rate of greater than 50% when hyperinfection syndrome occurs as a result of massive larval proliferation and autoinfection after SOT immunosuppression.[2–4]

Modes of Transmission

Appropriate suspicion of a parasitic infection in SOT requires insight into clinical manifestations (**Table 1**) as well as knowledge of the 4 modes of transmission of parasitic diseases in SOT: (1) reactivation of a dormant parasitic infection in the recipient; (2) donor-derived parasitic infection; (3) blood-transfusion transmission of the parasitemic phase of the parasite; and (4) de novo transmission (**Table 2**).

In the pretransplant screening period the ethnic, travel, and geographic history of the transplant recipient and of the donor (especially in the case of a living donor) must be closely investigated. This aspect is of particular importance for Hispanic patients, who represent nearly 20% of renal transplant candidates in the United States and have an increased risk not only for reactivation of posttransplant latent tuberculosis but also for *Strongyloides stercoralis*, leishmanias (visceral and cutaneous), and *T cruzi*.[5–7] Targeted pretransplant screening of recipients and donors for tropical parasitic infections allows for: institution of appropriate measures to eradicate the parasite before transplant (eg, treatment of *Strongyloides*); posttransplant prophylaxis of SOT patients at high risk of reactivation (eg, *Toxoplasma* D+/R−); and posttransplant infection surveillance for those at risk for donor-derived or reactivated disease (eg, *T cruzi* polymerase chain reaction [PCR]). Where appropriate, pretransplant diagnostic testing may include blood smears (eg, where malaria is a concern), serologies (eg, *Toxoplasma*), and stool assays (especially in a patient with diarrhea or eosinophilia) (**Table 3**).

In the immunocompromised, acute Chagas disease has been accidently transmitted by organs or blood transfusions from infected donors in the United States. The list of donor-derived parasitic infections has grown to include: *T cruzi*, *S stercoralis*, malaria, filariasis, visceral leishmaniasis (VL), and *Balamuthia mandrillaris*. Often, failure to recognize symptoms and risk factors can delay diagnosis and increase mortality. Life-threatening transfusion-associated *Babesia* and malaria have been reported in SOT patients, and should be suspected with posttransfusion fevers.[8,9]

Type of Organ Transplant and Risk

Not surprisingly, kidney transplantation, the most commonly transplanted organ, accounts for the majority of parasitic infections reported. However, because of more

Table 1
Clinical manifestation and treatment of important parasitic diseases in SOT

	Clinical Syndromes	When Disease Occurs Post Transplant	Treatment
Toxoplasma gondii	Myocarditis Encephalitis Pneumonitis Chorioretinitis	First 3 mo: Donor-related (D+/R−) disease More than 3–6 mo: Reactivation disease De novo disease Rejection immunosuppressive therapy	1. Pyrimethamine and sulfadiazine 2. Pyrimethamine and clindamycin (sulfa-allergic) 3. Intravenous pyrimethamine + trimethoprim-sulfamethoxazole
Trypanosoma cruzi	Myocarditis Encephalitis Panniculitis	First 3 mo: Donor-derived disease Reactivation disease with induction therapy More than 3–6 mo: Reactivation disease with rejection therapy	1. Benznidazole 2. Nifurtimox
Visceral *Leishmania*	Hepatomegaly Splenomegaly Pancytopenia Wasting Fever of unknown origin	First 6 mo: Liver transplantation Reactivation disease with induction therapy More than 18 mo: Renal transplantation De novo infection	1. Liposomal amphotericin
Strongyloides	Purpuric rash Abdominal pain Pneumonitis Gram-negative Meningitis Sepsis	First 6 mo: Most cases	1. Ivermectin 2. Ivermectin + albendazole for disseminated disease

intensive immunosuppressive regimens, parasitic infections have the potential to be more invasive in heart, lung, intestinal, and liver transplant patients. Cardiac transplantation poses a special risk in the case of donor-derived Chagas disease or toxoplasmosis infection, where myocarditis of the allograft can be lethal. In cardiac transplantation for end-stage chagasic cardiomyopathy, reactivation is anticipated and treated expectantly. Small bowel transplantation (SBT) presents unique risks for parasitic infection because of lengthy and intensive immunosuppressive regimens and the fact that the intestinal transplant itself can harbor a massive amount of microorganisms. Intestinal protozoa infections reported in SBT include microsporidia, *Isospora* (*Cystoisospora*) *belli*, and *Cryptosporidium*.[9–11] In human immunodeficiency virus (HIV) transplantation patients, parasitic opportunistic infections such as *Cryptosporidium* have been reported.[12] Protozoa accounted for 1% of the infections diagnosed in a series of HIV-infected liver transplant patients in the United States.[13]

Immunosuppressive Agents and the Risk of Parasitic Infection

The type of immunotherapy used in transplant affects the severity of parasitic infection (**Table 4**). The major treatment strategies for acute T-cell–mediated rejection, including

Table 2
Modes of parasite transmission in SOT

	Reactivation of Latent Infection Post Transplant	Donor Transmission	Transmission Through Blood Transfusion Post Transplant	De Novo Infection Post Transplant
Toxoplasma gondii	Rare	Especially with D+/R− heart transplants	No	Yes, especially in hyperendemic countries
Trypanosoma cruzi	Yes	Yes	Rare	Yes
Visceral *Leishmania*	Yes	Rare	Possible	Yes
Free-living amoeba	Unknown	*Balamuthia mandrillaris*	No	*Acanthamoeba castellani*
Alimentary protozoa	Unknown but possible	Unknown but possible in small bowel transplant	No	Yes
Babesia	Unknown	Yes (hematopoietic stem cell transplant)	Yes	Yes
Malaria	Rare (*Plasmodium malariae*)	Yes	Yes	Yes
Strongyloides	Yes	Rare	No	Possible

corticosteroids, antithymocyte globulin, and OKT-3, all increase the risk of opportunistic parasitic infections after transplantation. Antithymocyte globulin (ATG), which is used in induction and rejection therapy, increases the risk of severe posttransplant toxoplasmosis,[14–16] Chagas disease,[17] and malaria.[18] OKT-3, a monoclonal antibody against the CD3 T-cell receptor, has also been implicated as a risk for disseminated toxoplasmosis.[14,19] High-dose steroids used in rejection increase the risk of posttransplant active toxoplasmosis,[14,16,20] *T cruzi*,[21] and *Strongyloides*[22] infections.

Mycophenolic acid, an antimetabolite used in immunosuppressive maintenance therapy, greatly increases reactivation of *T cruzi*,[21,23–25] but conversely may exert an antimicrobial effect against *Pneumocystis jiroveci* pneumonia (PJP). Cyclosporine, a calcineurin inhibitor, presents a similar paradox: high levels increase the risk of *T cruzi* reactivation,[23,26] yet there is compelling evidence that cyclosporine is actually protective against *Strongyloides*.[2] The calcineurin inhibitor tacrolimus, by contrast, has no parasiticidal activity against *Strongyloides*.[2]

The induction monoclonal antibodies, alemtuzumab and basiliximab, may also increase the risk of parasitic infections in SOT. In one case of *Toxoplasma* encephalitis, the renal transplant recipient had received both basiliximab and ATG immunotherapy.[16] In a descriptive study, 10% of patients on alemtuzumab induction or rejection therapy developed opportunistic infections after SOT. The one parasitic opportunistic infection attributable to alemtuzumab therapy in this series was *Toxoplasma* pneumonitis in a lung transplant patient.[27]

TOXOPLASMOSIS
Epidemiology

Toxoplasmosis is a rare but potentially lethal infection in SOT recipients. This protozoan is common worldwide, with acquisition based on: the local customs of consuming raw

Table 3
SOT pretransplant screening of parasites

	Recipient	Donor
Toxoplasma gondii	Serologic testing for cardiac transplant recipients	Serologic testing of donors not mandatory but recommended for cardiac transplant
Trypanosoma cruzi	Targeted screening of those from endemic areas or who have received blood transfusions in Latin America. Two different FDA-approved serologic assays recommended	EIA screening tests recommended for Hispanic donors. CDC consultation for confirmatory tests if the screening test is positive
Leishmania	No data. Consider serologic testing for recipients from areas endemic for VL and veterans who served in Middle East endemic areas	Not recommended
Alimentary parasites	If eosinophilia or from endemic area: check stool O and P and *Strongyloides* serology. Urine O and P for renal transplant	If risk factors consider screening for SBT donors and live SOT donors by stool O and P and *Strongyloides* serology
Malaria	Consider blood smear if appropriate risks	No approved screening tests Consideration of IFA testing, blood smear, and PCR testing if donor from endemic area
Strongyloides	With risk factors, *Strongyloides* serology and stool O and P	If risk factors, consider for SBT donors and live donors by stool O and P and *Strongyloides* serology

Abbreviations: CDC, Centers for Disease Control and Prevention; EIA, enzyme immunoassay; FDA, Food and Drug Administration; IFA, indirect fluorescent antibody; O and P, ova and parasites; PCR, polymerase chain reaction; SBT, small bowel transplant; VL, visceral leishmaniasis.

meat of animals; accidental ingestion of cat excreta through contaminated food or environmental exposure; and transplacental transmission. Cats are the definitive hosts of this parasite. The protozoan establishes lifelong dormancy in the tissue cysts as a bradyzoite in the muscle, myocardium, brain, and eyes. In the United States, 10% to 40% of people have latent infection with *T gondii* determined by serologic testing. Worldwide, the prevalence of toxoplasmosis is greater than 50%.[28,29] Of note, antitoxoplasma immunoglobulin (Ig)G antibodies are found in more than 80% of the general population in Chile and France.[30]

Donor-Derived Transmission

Before the institution of trimethoprim-sulfamethoxazole (TMP-SMX) prophylaxis in SOT, cardiac transplantation recipients D+/R− for toxoplasmosis had a 50% to 75% risk of life-threatening disseminated toxoplasmosis.[31–35] Given the persistence of encysted *Toxoplasma* in the myocardium, cardiac transplant patients are at a substantially greater risk for donor-transmitted toxoplasmosis in comparison with liver, lung, or kidney transplant patients.[36–38] During posttransplantation immunosuppression, the encysted bradyzoites (from the donor) transform into proliferating tachyzoites, which can destroy infected cells and cause necrotizing inflammation. In the

Table 4
Risks for parasitic disease in SOT based on type of immunosuppression

	Increased Risks	Decreased Risks
Toxoplasma gondii	ATG, OKT-3, high-dose steroids for rejection Alemtuzumab ? Basiliximab D+/R− *T gondii* serostatus	TMP-SMX prophylaxis R+ *T gondii* serostatus
Trypanosoma cruzi	ATG, high-dose steroids for rejection Mycophenolic Acid Cyclosporine (high dose)	Nonmycophenolic acid regimen
Plasmodium falciparum	? ATG	
Strongyloides	High-dose steroids for rejection ?ATG	Cyclosporine

Abbreviations: ATG, antithymocyte globulin; TMP-SMX, trimethoprim-sulfamethoxazole.

case of the seronegative patient who lacks toxoplasmosis-specific immunity, the infection can become disseminated and lethal.[39] Donor-derived toxoplasmosis most commonly occurs within the first 3 months after transplant during induction immunosuppressive therapy.[31–33]

Reactivation and De Novo Transmission

For cardiac transplant recipients who are toxoplasmosis-seropositive before transplant, reactivation of latent infection is rare. Typically reactivation infections are less severe than donor-derived infections, depending on the degree of immunosuppression. Distinct from donor-transmitted toxoplasmosis disease whereby cardiac transplant cases predominate, reactivation can occur in the toxoplasmosis-seropositive recipient independent of the type of transplant.[38] The risk of reactivation of toxoplasmosis is associated with lymphocyte-depleting therapy, as well as residency in a country with high seroprevalence.[38,40] Transplant patients can also develop de novo infection, especially in highly endemic countries such as Spain.[36] Blood-transfusion transmission of toxoplasmosis is a theoretical risk after transplantation; however, because of its short parasitemic phase it is likely infrequent.[41]

Noncardiac Solid Organ Transplant

There are rare worldwide reports of toxoplasmosis disease in noncardiac transplant patients. The rarity of toxoplasmosis may be explained by the near universal use of TMP-SMX prophylaxis for *P jiroveci* in all SOT patients since 1988. Another factor explaining the infrequency of donor-related infection in noncardiac patients is that unlike the heart, cysts do not typically persist in the liver, kidney, pancreas, and intestines.[30,36] In a review of 52 noncardiac cases of toxoplasmosis in SOT recipients reported in the international literature, 42% were donor related, 21% were secondary to reactivation, and 37% were of unknown cause. Organ-transmitted disease had a much higher rate of dissemination and mortality than reactivation disease in this review.[14] In this same series, 65% of noncardiac SOT patients survived with timely anti-toxoplasmosis treatment.[14] Lethal toxoplasmosis disease after renal transplantation is generally reported in the first 90 days posttransplant when immunosuppression is the highest.[42] Toxoplasmosis has been reported after liver,[36,43,44] kidney,[36,39,45] multiorgan (liver-pancreas, liver-kidney-pancreas),[46] and intestinal transplantation.[14]

Risk Factors for Toxoplasmosis in a Matched Case-Control Study

In an extensive retrospective Spanish study of 15,800 SOT patients, only 22 recipients developed toxoplasmosis. Predictably, cardiac transplantation patients had a significantly higher rate of toxoplasmosis than kidney or liver transplant patients (occurring in 0.61% of heart transplantations vs 0.08% of liver and kidney transplantations). The risk for toxoplasmosis infection in this matched case-control study included: negative serostatus before transplant, diagnosis of cytomegalovirus (CMV) infection, and high-dose prednisone. Although all of the patients of this series had received either TMP-SMX or pyrimethamine prophylaxis, they had completed therapy by the time active infection developed. Eighty-one percent of toxoplasmosis infections were primary infections occurring within the first 6 months after transplant. The donor status information was incomplete in this study, but 40% of the cases had a known D+/R− status.[36] Of toxoplasmosis-infected patients, 22.7% (5 of 22) had disseminated disease and 13.6% (3 of 22) died. The investigators concluded that for patients who are seronegative before transplant, prophylaxis should be continued for at least 6 months (longer if on intensified immunosuppression) with close follow-up, especially in high-prevalence areas.[36]

Clinical

The severity of toxoplasmosis disease depends on the degree of immunosuppression of the host and the timing of appropriate antitoxoplasmosis therapy. Initial symptoms of toxoplasmosis can be nonspecific, with pyrexia, and respiratory and neurologic symptoms. Severe manifestations include chorioretinitis, myocarditis, encephalitis, pneumonitis, and multiorgan failure.[36] The mortality rate of disseminated disease is estimated at as high as 80%.[47]

In reports of cardiac transplantation of D+/R− patients, by the time toxoplasmosis myocarditis of the allograft has been recognized, the disease is life-threatening with dissemination to other organs, especially the lungs and brain.[19,30,33,48] In an illustrative case of presumed donor-derived disease in a cardiac transplant patient who did not receive prophylaxis, intracellular T gondii was not detected until the fourth weekly endomyocardial biopsy, when the patient was already symptomatic with fever and pneumonitis.[48] Despite initiation of therapy the patient died, with the autopsy revealing ventricular dilation and wall thickening with abundant protozoa in the cardiomyocytes, as well as dissemination to the brain and lungs.[48] Toxoplasmosis myocarditis can be misdiagnosed as rejection, with lethal sequelae if immunosuppression is intensified.[19]

Patients with Toxoplasma pneumonitis can present with a productive cough and dyspnea.[47] Often the pneumonitis is associated with disseminated disease and multiorgan failure.[30] On imaging, Toxoplasma pneumonia is characterized by diffuse pulmonary infiltrates and opacities, similar to PJP.[1,43,47]

Central nervous system (CNS) manifestations occur in 10% to 25% of transplant recipients with toxoplasmosis.[49–53] Toxoplasmosis encephalitis (TE) in SOT is marked by headache, altered mental status, seizures, focal neurologic deficits, hemiparesis, and ataxia.[16,32,46] ATG induction therapy and lack of toxoplasmosis prophylaxis were risk factors shared in 2 cases of cerebral toxoplasmosis after multiorgan transplant (liver-pancreas and liver-pancreas-kidney).[46] Basiliximab induction and ATG rejection therapy may have contributed to the development of CNS toxoplasmosis in a renal transplant patient who presented 7 months after TMP-SMX prophylaxis was discontinued.[16]

In the majority of cases, donor-related toxoplasmosis disease occurs within the first 3 months after transplant,[14,32] whereas reactivation and reinfection or de novo infection occur later after transplant.[14,32] Late-onset disease (>3 months after transplant) has been noted when immunosuppression is extended or augmented, as in the case of organ rejection or antilymphocyte therapies, and after discontinuation of toxoplasmosis prophylaxis.[14,16,19]

Diagnosis

Definitive diagnosis of toxoplasmosis requires the identification of parasites in biopsy samples. When myocarditis presents in cardiac transplant patients, endomyocardial biopsy is crucial in differentiating infection from rejection. In *Toxoplasma* myocarditis, tachyzoites and cysts can be found in the myocardium.[32,54,55] PCR and immunochemistry can further confirm the histologic diagnosis in myocarditis.[46] Lung biopsy can also reveal bradyzoites.[47]

Toxoplasma trophozoites can also be detected in the blood, cerebrospinal fluid (CSF), bone marrow, peritoneal fluid, and bronchoalveolar lavage (BAL), and may provide a rapid diagnosis.[39,43,44,48,54] In cases of pneumonitis where it is difficult to differentiate toxoplasmosis from *P jiroveci* on BAL, immunohistochemical staining for *Toxoplasma* can be instrumental in confirming the diagnosis.[47]

Seroconversion of serum anti-*T gondii* IgG/IgM antibodies by enzyme-linked immunosorbent assay (ELISA) can assist in the diagnosis during reactivation or new infection. However, seroconversion may not occur in severely immunocompromised patients in early infection.[44] Seroconversion after transplant in seronegative recipients should lead to a high level of disease surveillance, but should not be interpreted as active disease. Only 1 of 8 patients who seroconverted after cardiac transplant in a cohort study where patients were treated with thrice-weekly TMP-SMX developed active toxoplasmosis.[19] In reactivated toxoplasmosis an increase in antibody levels may occur, but does not do so reliably.[15]

Serum *Toxoplasma* PCR testing assists in the diagnosis and monitoring of disease.[40] A positive toxoplasmosis PCR of the BAL[43] or CSF[36] helps to establish disease and is valuable in making an early diagnosis. A positive PCR of a blood sample, especially with evidence of organ involvement, should alert for disseminated disease.[44] However, a positive PCR of the blood without evidence of organ involvement does not confirm a diagnosis of acute disease.[39] In the case of disseminated *Toxoplasma* infection, PCR of BAL, CSF or blood can assist in determining the length of therapy and management of immunosuppression.[40,56]

TE can be diagnosed by the presence of tachyzoites and cysts on brain biopsy, with confirmation by immunohistochemistry. The presence of tachyzoites in the CSF or positive PCR of the CSF can also make the diagnosis of TE. Although the toxoplasmosis PCR assay of CSF is highly specific, it varies in sensitivity and should not be used to exclude the diagnosis of CNS toxoplasmosis.[32,38,39,57,58] Likewise, tachyzoites are only occasionally seen on CSF analysis of TE, and their absence should not rule out CNS disease. In transplant patients with toxoplasmosis encephalitis, focal necrosis with ring-enhancing lesions on magnetic resonance imaging (MRI) is the most common radiologic finding.[16] However, radiologic manifestations in TE after SOT may be atypical and diffuse.[39,46]

Treatment

The preferred regimen for toxoplasmosis in transplantation is combination treatment with pyrimethamine and sulfadiazine, which synergistically act against the tachyzoites during active infection or reactivation.[36] This first-choice regimen is available only in oral form.[54] Alternative agents include pyrimethamine and clindamycin (especially in sulfa-allergic patients). Intravenous TMP-SMX is another option, depending on availability. In a patient with post–liver transplant toxoplasmosis who had ileus, intravenous clindamycin and intravenous TMP-SMP were curative.[43] Atovaquone and sulfadiazine or pyrimethamine are alternatives; however, there are few data on the effectiveness of the regimen, especially in the treatment of SOT patients.[30] Of note, treatment with pyrimethamine, a folic acid antagonist, is always accompanied with leucovorin "rescue."

Prophylaxis

Prophylactic treatment with TMP-SMX for 6 months in heart and liver transplant recipients reduces the risk of infection by *T gondii*, as well as infection by *Listeria monocytogenes*, *Nocardia asteroides*, and *P jeroveci*.[37] In fact, lack of toxoplasmosis prophylaxis is characteristic of approximately75% of toxoplasmosis cases reported in SOT.[39] Current American Society of Transplantation (AST) recommendations are that PJP prophylaxis is administered for at least 6 to 12 months after transplantation in centers having a prevalence of 3% to 5%.[59] With the relatively decreased immunosuppression compared with other transplantations, many renal transplant centers administer prophylaxis with TMP-SMX for a period of 3 to 6 months.[37]

TMP-SMX double-strength thrice weekly is sufficient for suppression of toxoplasmosis in the majority of cardiac transplant patients. In a United States study of 417 cardiac transplant patients who received prophylaxis of thrice-weekly TMP-SMX (160 mg/800 mg), only 1 case of acute toxoplasmosis occurred in a D+/R– patient.[19] Of note, this patient was treated for acute rejection with OKT-3. Given these data, with increasing immunosuppression for rejection, daily double-strength TMP-SMX or addition of pyramethamine should be considered for prophylaxis.[19]

Patients who have received antilymphocyte therapies or who have undergone treatment for acute rejection episodes are at higher risk of developing opportunistic infections, including PJP and toxoplasmosis, and these patients should receive a longer course of TMP-SMX.[16] In fact, extending prophylaxis beyond a 6- to 12-month period, and even lifelong prophylaxis, is recommended at many centers that perform heart, liver, lung, or SBT.[59] Longer duration or lifelong prophylaxis has also been proposed for patients with a history of chronic CMV or prior PJP.[59]

For sulfa-allergic patients pyrimethamine prophylaxis can be used, but this is less effective than TMP-SMX.[39] The combination of dapsone or atovaquone with pyrimethamine and folinic acid has been used as effective alternative toxoplasmosis prophylaxis in HIV patients, but these regimens are not well studied in SOT.[54] For posttransplant toxoplasmosis secondary prophylaxis is recommended, as there is no agent to eradicate the bradyzoite cyst stage; however, the length of prophylaxis is not well defined. Maintenance therapy should be given when T-cell–depleting regimens are continued.[40,43,54] To avoid new infection, SOT recipients are advised to avoid cat boxes and to avoid undercooked meat.

Screening for Toxoplasmosis

Toxoplasmosis antibody screening of recipients is typically performed before cardiac transplantation, but is not routinely tested for other organs in the United States. Serologic screening of the donor for toxoplasmosis is not mandatory in the United States.[30] In cardiac transplantation, the screening is important to determine recipients who are toxoplasmosis seronegative, as this becomes particularly relevant if high-level immunosuppression is needed for rejection, or if toxoplasmosis prophylaxis is not tolerated. In one cautionary case, a patient who developed toxoplasmosis after heart transplant had a false-positive toxoplasmosis antibody test in the setting of intravenous IgG therapy, and did not receive appropriate prophylaxis.[47]

In the United States, noncardiac SOT patients are not screened for toxoplasmosis, given the low risk. A retrospective Canadian study of 1006 noncardiac transplant recipients revealed a relatively low toxoplasmosis seropositivity rate of 13% for donors and 18% for recipients. In this study only 39% of patients received TMP-SMX therapy (the 14-year study spanned a time period before the advent of TMP-SMX prophylaxis), yet there were only 4 cases of seroconversion and no active disease.[60] In France, where prevalence of toxoplasmosis is high, serologic screening is obligatory for the donor, and is commonly performed for the recipient before all organ transplantations.[39]

CHAGAS DISEASE
Epidemiology

In the United States, T cruzi is rare in autochthonous form, and is primarily imported through Hispanic immigration. It is estimated that 300,000 people in the United States are infected with T cruzi.[61] This high number of asymptomatic T cruzi–infected individuals poses a serious health concern given the potential of the disease to progress to severe cardiac and gastrointestinal chronic disease, or transform into an aggressive opportunistic infection with immunosuppression.

T cruzi is estimated to infect 8 to 10 million people in Latin America, with a geographic range from Mexico to Argentina.[23,61–63] Approximately 80% of the endemic South American cases are acquired through the bite of a tritomine "assassin bug" in the setting of substandard housing in a forested area. In South America, because of urbanization blood-transfusion transmission now accounts for nearly 5% to 20% of cases.[25] The incidence of congenital infection in Latin America is estimated at 15,000 cases per year.[64–66] Concerningly, outbreaks of oral chagasic disease with severe clinical manifestations have been reported throughout South America.[67]

Congenital, transfusion-transmitted, and transplant-transmitted Chagas disease have all been documented in the United States.[68–71] In the 5 years after T cruzi enzyme immunoassay (EIA) blood-bank screening was initiated in 2007, 1600 T cruzi–seropositive donors have been confirmed in the United States, with the highest seropositivity rates reported in Florida and California.[62,72,73]

Clinical Disease in Immunocompetent Persons

There are 3 different stages of Chagas disease. Acute infection is typically self-limited and relatively asymptomatic, or may be marked by a chagoma, fever, lymphadenitis, and hepatosplenomegaly. More rarely, acute Chagas disease can manifest as a potentially lethal meningoencephalitis or myocarditis.[74–76] In the acute stage, the transmitted trypomastigotes enters the host cells as amastigotes, the intracellular replicating form. After immune resolution, the chronic indeterminate stage lasts 10 to 30 years: it is during this asymptomatic stage that transfusion-related infections occur. With ongoing inflammation and fibrosis with chronic disease, 20% to 30% of infected patients go on to develop cardiomyopathy and/or gastrointestinal disease (megaesophagus or megacolon).[62,74]

Chagas Cardiomyopathy and Transplantation

For patients with end-stage chagasic cardiomyopathy heart disease (CCHD), cardiac transplant is a proven and accepted therapy. In Brazil it currently is the third most common etiologic determinant of cardiac transplant.[74] In a large Brazilian cohort, the survival rate for chagasic cardiac transplantation exceeded that of other cardiac transplantations, with a 12-year survival rate of 46% for CCHD versus 22% for ischemic cardiomyopathy.[77] The successful outcome of chagasic cardiac transplant contrasts strikingly with the low 9% life expectancy at 10 years for CCHD patients.[78] In the United States, chagasic heart transplant has been performed in more than 25 patients.[79] In the one article describing cardiac transplant for CCHD in 2 patients in the United States, both patients were clinically well without reactivation of Chagas disease after long-term follow-up.[80]

Reactivation of acute Chagas disease after transplantation for CCHD occurs in 27% to 43% of recipients.[21,81] Over the decades, however, cardiac transplantation for CCHD has evolved, with an immunosuppression regimen that optimizes the balance between reactivation and acute rejection. In a retrospective analysis by Bocchi and Firelli[77] of CCHD cardiac transplant patients from 1983 to 1999, 2 patients died of acute *T cruzi*, 1 with acute chagasic myocarditis of the transplanted heart. Throughout the 1990s, reduction of cyclosporine levels in cardiac transplants improved survival and lowered rates of reactivation of Chagas disease.[23,26] In an early series of Chagas cardiac transplant patients, there was an increased risk of malignant neoplasm reported (4.3% in one large series), possibly related to high doses of cyclosporine.[23,77]

Steroid therapy and multiple rejection episodes are also related to an increased risk of *T cruzi* reactivation.[21] A 6-fold higher rate of *T cruzi* reactivation is associated with mycophenolate mofetil (MMF) in comparison with azathioprine. Avoidance of MMF is controversial, however, as there is some evidence that MMF is associated with lower rejection and decreased mortality.[21,25,63,81] Because of severe immunosuppression and the increased risk for reactivation, authors of a recent Spanish review recommend avoidance of both antithymocyte globulin and MMF in chagasic cardiac transplantation.[17]

Management of reactivation in Chagas heart disease transplantation has improved with the advancement of diagnostic tests, which allow for early and preemptive therapy and improved survival. Current posttransplant monitoring for *T cruzi* reactivation uses weekly serum Chagas PCR testing, as well as microscopic evaluation for presence of trypomastigotes in fresh blood or the buffy coat during the first 2 months after transplant.[74,82] Endomyocardial biopsy (EMB) is repeated routinely after transplant to rule out rejection or infection, with microscopic evaluation for the presence of amastigotes and *T cruzi* PCR testing of biopsy material. With early recognition of reactivation, a standard course of benznidazole or nifurtimox leads to excellent clinical outcomes.[74,78,83–86]

Reactivation disease in cardiac transplantation typically manifests as asymptomatic parasitemia or fever. Chagasic subcutaneous nodules are often an early manifestation of reactivation disease.[21] When myocarditis occurs after cardiac transplant, EMB is necessary to confirm the etiology. Chagasic myocarditis manifested as atrioventricular block in a case report of myocarditis after cardiac transplant.[87] CNS Chagas disease is rare after cardiac transplantation, but has presented as a large brain mass in the setting of high-dose MMF for rejection.[24]

Reactivation-Related Infection in Noncardiac SOT

There is evidence that patients with asymptomatic chronic Chagas disease can safely receive noncardiac transplantation with close surveillance for reactivation. The risk of reactivation in Chagas disease differs according to the organ transplanted, with a predictably higher rate of reactivation in cardiac transplantation. Reactivation risk also increases with intensive immunosuppressive therapy. In an Argentinean renal transplant study, 21.7% (5 of the 23) of patients with chronic Chagas disease had early reactivation of Chagas disease. Two of the cases were diagnosed by surveillance of blood parasitemia. Three of these patients presented with chagasic panniculitis, which was diagnosed by the presence of *T cruzi* amastigotes in the skin biopsies. All 5 patients were treated with benznidazole, with resolution of parasitemia.[88,89] A relatively low rate of 19% reactivation was also found for liver transplant patients with chronic Chagas disease.[25] *T cruzi* reactivation has also occurred in lung transplant patients.[82,88] Chagasic reactivation in noncardiac SOT transplant patients presents during heightened immunotherapy, either early after transplant or later with rejection immunotherapy.[25,82]

In a small series of renal transplant patients with chronic Chagas disease, reactivation occurred in patients on a mycophenolic acid maintenance regimen, but in none of the patients who were not treated with mycophenolic acid.[25] Reactivated Chagas disease in renal transplant patients on mycophenolic acid therapy has been associated with severe disease, including graft failure with amastigotes present on renal biopsy,[90] encephalitis,[25] and lethal myocarditis.[91] Reactivation disease was determined as the mode of transmission in a Swiss renal transplant patient with lethal myocarditis based on *T cruzi* seropositive testing of pretransplant archived sera and extensive South American travel history.[91]

Similar to CCHD management, patients seropositive for *T cruzi* in noncardiac SOT can be managed with PCR surveillance, with treatment initiated early for asymptomatic parasitemia or chagasic skin involvement.[88] Proposed contraindications to transplantation of noncardiac organs in patients with chronic Chagas disease include grade 2 or greater myocardiopathy, or gastrointestinal disease (megaesophagus or megacolon).[82]

Donor-Derived Chagas Disease

Alarmingly, in 2001 Chagas disease was transmitted from a cadaveric donor from Central America to 3 SOT recipients in the United States. Fortuitously, the diagnosis was made when trypanomastigotes were found on a blood smear of a febrile pancreatic kidney transplant patient 1 month after transplant. Subsequently, a liver and a kidney recipient from the same donor were found to be culture positive for *T cruzi*. Although all patients received nifurtimox, 2 of the 3 transplant patients died. The multiorgan transplant patient, who received the most intensive immunosuppressive therapy, relapsed after completion of 4 months of nifurtimox treatment and died of chagasic myocarditis 2 weeks into the second course of nifurtimox therapy. Although not directly linked to Chagas disease, the liver recipient died of hepatic and renal failure. It was the kidney transplant patient who survived, possibly in relation to a less immunosuppressive regimen or early treatment.[69]

The first reports of *T cruzi* donor transmission by cardiac transplantation surprisingly occurred in 2 cardiac recipients from the Los Angeles area in 2005 and 2006. On retrospective testing, both cadaveric donors were seropositive for *T cruzi*. One donor was an American born to a Mexican mother, who had traveled to an area endemic for Chagas disease for whom vector or congenital transmission both were possibilities. The other donor was from Central America, with unknown risk.[62,70] Both cardiac transplant patients presented in the second month after transplant with a febrile illness; one of the patients had an abdominal rash, possibly a panniculitis, which cleared with treatment. Diagnosis was confirmed by presence of *T cruzi* by peripheral smear, and by positive blood culture and serum Chagas PCR. Both had negative serologies. Only 1 of the 2 cardiac transplant patients had amastigotes on endomyocardial biopsy. With antitrypanosomal therapy both patients cleared their parasitemia; however, both died of unrelated causes.[62,70]

The cardiac transplant recipient who had biopsy-proven donor-derived chagasic myocarditis had symptoms before diagnosis. His initial immunosuppression regimen included mycophenolic acid. During the 6 weeks after transplant his ejection fraction decreased with diffuse hypokinesis and elevated troponin levels, findings which prompted increased steroid treatment for presumed rejection. At 8 weeks after transplant he was admitted for fever, failure to thrive, and anorexia. Diagnosis of Chagas disease was made swiftly by presence of blood smear trypomastigotes and intracellular amastigotes on cardiac biopsy. On nifurtimox therapy, his parasitemia cleared after 1 week; repeat cardiac biopsies were negative for amastigotes at weeks 2 and 6 of therapy; and troponin levels returned to normal. His immunotherapy was decreased. The patient died 4 months after transplant with evidence of acute cellular rejection, without evidence of *T cruzi* on autopsy cardiac biopsy.[62,70] The patient received mycophenolate and high-dose steroids, both known risk factors for reactivation of chagasic disease, although reduction in his immunotherapy may have ultimately contributed to his death.

Of interest, 6 other patients had received liver or kidney transplantations from the aforementioned 2 infected organ donors; however, none of these patients showed evidence of *T cruzi* infection and remained negative by repeat serology, smear, culture, and PCR surveillance.[62,70] By 2010, in the United States an additional 14 transplant recipients had received organs from 7 donors.

T cruzi–positive donors included heart-kidney, pancreatic, liver, and kidney transplant donors.[92,93] From United States transplantation data available from the Centers for Disease Control and Prevention (CDC), the percentage of recipients who developed donor-transmitted Chagas disease from seropositive donors varied according to transplanted organ, specifically 67% (2 of 3) for heart, 18% (2 of 11) for kidney, and 29% (2 of 7) for liver.[62,69,70,92] There were 3 cases of Chagas disease transmission in the United States (2 heart recipients and 1 liver recipient) whereby the donor was identified as seropositive early after transplant; and with prospective monitoring, early diagnosis, and treatment, all patients survived.[74,92]

Use of Seropositive Donors for Transplant

To address high donor shortages in Latin America, donors seropositive for *T cruzi* have been used in renal and liver transplantation. These transplants can be performed safely with close posttransplant surveillance for disease. In a 1999 study of renal transplant recipients who received transplants from a known *T cruzi*–seropositive donor, only 18.7% (3 of 16) of the recipients developed acute Chagas disease as diagnosed by blood parasitemia. The complications in this early study included fever, bone marrow suppression, and relapse; however, all recovered with therapy.[88] Liver transplantation performed in Argentina using *T cruzi*–infected donors had a good outcome; with close monitoring for infection using the Strout method, 22% (2 of 9) were found to have asymptomatic parasitemia and were treated successfully with benznidazole.[94–96] One case of liver transplantation with a known seropositive donor was performed as an emergency transplantation. The patient was treated preemptively with benznidazole once parasitemia developed, and did well clinically.[97] Heart transplants from *T cruzi*–seropositive donors are an obvious contraindication.[62] There are few data concerning the safety of using *T cruzi*–seropositive donors for transplantations that involve high-level immunosuppression, such as lung, pancreas, and intestinal. Chagasic gastrointestinal disease in a donor would be a contraindication for SBT.

De Novo Infection

There is minimal literature on de novo infection of vector-transmitted Chagas disease after transplantation. De novo infection was suspected in the case of 2 renal transplant patients in South America (D−/R− *T cruzi*–seronegative pretransplant) who had asymptomatic *T cruzi* seroconversion late after transplant on return to Chagas disease hyperendemic areas.[88] Given the therapeutic benefits of benznidazole for recently infected individuals, de novo infected SOT patients should be treated.[61,88]

Blood Transfusion

Blood-transfusion transmission was suspected in a case of a Chilean renal transplant patient who died of acute Chagas disease after transplant.[98] Chagas disease has also been transmitted through bone marrow transplantation.[99] Blood-transfusion transmission is a possible cause of acute infection after SOT, particularly with platelet transfusions, which have the highest risk of all blood products for transmitting Chagas disease.[68,100]

Diagnosis/Monitoring

When the donor or recipient is seropositive for T cruzi, recipients are monitored closely with PCR testing of the serum, and direct parasitologic tests (eg, Strout method).[25,97,101,102] PCR and direct parasitic evaluation require parasitemia and are typically insensitive for diagnosing chronic infection. Likewise, serology used to diagnose chronic infection is inadequate for the diagnosis of acute disease in the immunocompromised, although it is helpful if seroconversion occurs.

PCR is more sensitive than microscopy and is increasingly used for the diagnosis of acute Chagas disease and monitoring for reactivation, relapse, and cure.[82,103] T cruzi PCR has been used in endomyocardial biopsy for monitoring reactivation in cardiac transplant patients. PCR is also used for the diagnosis of chagasic skin nodules.[86] The CDC reference laboratory simultaneously uses 3 PCR assays that correspond to different regions of the T cruzi genome to maximize sensitivity and specificity. It has been recommended that at least 2 PCR assays should be used to increase accuracy. PCR extraction from the buffy coat further increases sensitivity.[103]

Direct detection of T cruzi parasites can be made by evaluation of the blood, CSF, or tissue biopsy. Careful parasitologic examination of biopsy materials is necessary when the diagnosis of Chagas disease is unclear. In a case of chagasic encephalitis where the CSF was negative for trypomastigotes, amastigotes on brain biopsy established the diagnosis. In this case, the MRI findings of a mass lesion with micronodular enhancement were indistinguishable from Toxoplasma encephalitis.[24] A misdiagnosis of rejection by repeated endomyocardial biopsies led to lethal myocarditis in a CCHD transplant patient; amastigotes were found retrospectively on an early endomyocardial biopsy.[87]

Treatment

Benznidazole and nifurtimox are effective in eradicating trypomastigote and amastigote forms, leading to a 70% cure in patients with acute disease.[61,62] Both drugs are available through the CDC under an investigational protocol. Benznidazole is considered the treatment of choice for acute Chagas disease, given a comparatively more favorable side-effect profile. Frequent side effects of benznidazole include allergic dermatitis, paresthesias, and anorexia. Rarely, bone marrow depression and liver toxicity occur. Nifurtimox is the second-line drug, as side effects of nausea, vomiting, weight loss, irritability, and insomnia make the drug difficult to tolerate. Neuropathy is a late but serious side effect.[61] Posaconazole was shown to be curative in a patient with acute Chagas disease secondary to Lupus.[17]

Prophylaxis

Given the risks of toxicity from trypanocidal treatment and lack of evidence of an obvious benefit, prophylactic therapy is not recommended for patients who are seropositive for T cruzi or have received transplants from seropositive donors.[21,26,78]

Prophylactic antitrypanosomal therapy has been used after cardiac transplant for CCHD[78,80] and in renal transplantation with known seropositive donors.[101] There are no prospective studies to support pretransplant treatment or posttransplant prophylaxis in the case of *T cruzi*–seropositive recipients. In the case of living donors who are *T cruzi* antibody positive, predonation treatment of the donor has been performed for bone marrow transplant donors, but it is unclear whether this prevents transmission.[99] There is no known role for secondary prophylaxis after resolution of acute Chagas disease in the SOT patient.[74]

Screening Recipients

There are no guidelines for screening recipients of organ transplant for *T cruzi* in the United States. Targeted testing of transplant recipients who have lived in an endemic area or who have received a blood transfusion in Latin America is strongly advised. At least 2 different Food and Drug Administration (FDA)-approved *T cruzi* serologic assays with different antigens or techniques (eg, EIA and indirect fluorescent antibody [IFA] or radioimmune precipitation assay [RIPA] test) should be used simultaneously to increase sensitivity and specificity.

Transplant Donor Screening

In Latin America, organ donor and recipient screening for *T cruzi* by serologic testing is standard. By contrast, organ donor screening has been inconsistently performed in the United States. In 2008, less than 20% of United States organ procurement organizations (OPOs) screened for *T cruzi* in organ donors. Of the 993 organ donors screened for Chagas disease in 2008, 0.6% were seropositive for *T cruzi*, which led to elimination of 5 donors and 17 organs.[104,105]

Recent United States guidelines by the multidisciplinary Chagas in Transplant Working Group (CTWG) propose that all OPOs screen donors for *T cruzi* who are from Mexico, Central America, or South America.[92] Either of the two FDA-approved EIA screening tests (Ortho EIA and Abbot Prism) for blood or organ donor screening are recommended for initial screening. To increase the specificity of blood donor screening in the United States, a secondary confirmatory test, such as a RIPA test, is used. If a screening test is positive for a transplant donor, the CTWG recommends consultation with the CDC and a local transplant infectious disease specialist for additional confirmatory testing. In the case of a cadaveric transplant, timely confirmation testing and ability to make decisions about the organ's usability are essential.[92]

Autochthonous Transmission

Autochthonous Chagas disease in the United States is rare but has been reported in Texas, California, Louisiana, and Mississippi. Sixteen cases of autochthonous chronic *T cruzi* infection have been identified in the United States through blood-bank surveillance.[106,107] Although a low probability, clinicians need to consider de novo or reactivation of autochthonous posttransplant Chagas disease from the southern United States with appropriate clinical signs.

LEISHMANIASIS
Epidemiology

Leishmaniasis is an intracellular protozoan parasite that infects macrophages and is spread by the bite of a sandfly. Dogs serve as a major domestic animal reservoir. Its wide domain spans nearly 100 countries worldwide.[108] The approximately 20 different species of *Leishmania* are classified clinically as: cutaneous leishmaniasis

(CL), which occurs in the Old World (Northern Africa, Middle East) and New World (Latin America) forms; mucocutaneous leishmaniasis (ML), primarily a South American disease; and visceral leishmaniasis (VL), 90% of which is found in India, Bangladesh, Nepal, Sudan, and Brazil.[108] VL is usually caused by *Leishmania donovani* and *Leishmania infantum* (also called *Leishmania chagasi*). With the AIDS epidemic, a dramatic increase of VL occurred in intravenous drug users in southwestern Europe.[109] A worldwide estimate of the prevalence of *Leishmania* is approximately 12 million cases, although this is likely an underestimation.

Clinical Manifestations

VL, although potentially deadly, is subclinical in most cases and establishes lifelong latency. Acute VL has an insidious onset manifested by fever, hepatosplenomegaly, bone marrow suppression, and hepatic dysfunction, and ultimately is lethal without treatment. In the setting of T-cell defects, such as HIV or immunosuppressive therapy for organ transplant or autoimmune disease, VL can reactivate with severe disease and can be complicated by relapsing episodes.[110] Rare cases of transfusion-mediated and congenital VL have been reported.[110,111]

Visceral Leishmaniasis in SOT

In SOT recipients VL is rare, with fewer than 100 cases reported in the literature, primarily in renal transplant patients.[112–115] Transplant centers in Southern Europe account for two-thirds of the cases reported, with Italy having the highest prevalence.[116–118] The majority of posttransplant VL is linked to reactivation or primary infection in an endemic area. Donor-transmitted *Leishmania* has been reported twice; one case of fatal VL was transmitted from a "purchased" kidney from an Indian donor.[116]

Of the cases reported in the literature, VL after SOT occurs most commonly in renal transplantation and accounts for more than 75% of the reported cases. VL occurs less commonly in liver, lung, and heart transplantation.[112,119–122] There are rare case reports of VL in pancreatic and combined kidney-pancreas transplant patients.[112,123,124] Recrudescence of dormant infection has been the most often cited cause of infection after SOT, based on evidence of seropositive serology before transplant.[113,114,119–121]

VL presents after transplant at a median of 18 months for renal transplant as compared with 6 months for liver transplant.[112] In endemic countries, posttransplant incubation periods of greater than 18 months, when immunosuppression is lower, may represent de novo VL infection.[115] Shorter incubations, such as in one case series of 5 kidney transplant patients who presented early in the first month of surgery (range 7–32 days), may indicate reactivation disease when immunosuppression is at the greatest level.[115] In the case of relapse in an endemic area, it is impossible to distinguish between reactivation of the same strain and de novo infection without evaluation by restriction fragment length polymorphism or PCR sequencing.[125] When symptoms of VL occur in a patient from a nonendemic area, previous travel has to be evaluated, as in one case in the Netherlands where the patient had traveled to an endemic area of Greece before transplant.[123] Even in endemic countries, the diagnosis may remain elusive, with a median delay between symptoms and diagnosis of 1 month.[112]

Clinical

In SOT, VL presents in a manner same as for immunocompetent patients: as a pyrexial illness associated with hepatosplenomegaly, wasting, hypoalbuminemia, and pancytopenia.[124,126] Like Chagas disease, the severity depends on when the diagnosis is made and how quickly treatment is initiated.[112]

Fatal disseminated leishmaniasis involves infection of the spleen, liver, and bone marrow. With delayed treatment, multiorgan failure and death result.[119,121] Unusual manifestations of VL include ophthalmitis, kala-azar dermal leishmanias, and laryngeal and tongue involvement.[125,127–130] In a Brazilian report, L chagasi caused colonic leishmaniasis in a liver transplant patient.[131] Acute renal graft dysfunction with evidence of amastigotes on renal biopsy has been reported.[115,125] VL has also been complicated with coexistent infections, such as tuberculosis.[113,121]

Cutaneous Leishmaniasis

There are few cases of CL after SOT. Recurrence of cutaneous leishmaniasis has been described in HIV[132] as well as in organ transplant recipients.[130,133] A Brazilian case of Leishmania (Viannia) braziliensis, typically a cause of CL, caused fatal disseminated disease after renal transplantation, with parasites discovered in skin, bone marrow, bone, and eyes (aqueous humor and vitreous body).[127]

Diagnosis

Typically the diagnosis of VL is made by direct examination of amastigotes on bone marrow and spleen aspiration, with a 98% specificity.[112] Splenic aspiration is a higher-yielding, yet riskier, procedure, with sensitivities of greater than 95%.[112] Antibody detection and PCR may have a higher sensitivity in detection of VL in early disease when compared with bone marrow biopsy, and should be used as an adjunct to diagnosis.[112,115] The CDC can be contacted for diagnostic assistance including Leishmania PCR, serology, and microscopic evaluation of culture and biopsy, as many of these tests are not commercially available.[79]

Limitations of VL antibody detection include false negatives in early disease or in immunocompromised patients (especially in AIDS), cross-reactivity with T cruzi, and low sensitivity in cutaneous disease.[134] Serologic testing can also be negative in patients with asymptomatic Leishmania infection.[110]

The recombinant kinesin antigen (rK39) antibody ELISA has a high sensitivity and specificity of (>95% and 98%, respectively) for VL in immunocompetent patients.[135] In SOT patients with active VL, the rK39 ELISA demonstrated a sensitivity of 94%.[112] In a prospective Italian transplant study, rK-39 antigen testing was used as a screening test in posttransplant patients given a high incidence of VL. The rK39 antigen test revealed early disease in 5 (1.2%) of the 396 kidney recipients.[115] In this study, 1.2% (5 of 396) of patients had rising rK39 antigen titers with concomitant fever and cytopenias (only 2 of 5 had bone marrow evaluation and both were negative), and all were treated with Liposomal amphotericin B (L-AmB) with clinical resolution.[115]

Leishmania PCR (to either the kinetoplast DNA or ribosomal RNA genes) is a very sensitive test for diagnosis and follow-up of transplant patients.[112] The PCR has an estimated sensitivity of 91% for diagnosing VL in SOT, a much higher sensitivity than parasitic smear evaluation or culture.[112] It can be used on peripheral blood; however, sensitivity is greatest when used on splenic or bone marrow aspirates.[112]

Treatment

L-AmB is a well-tolerated FDA-approved treatment for VL, with cure rates as high as 95%.[108] In VL of SOT patients, cure rates of 84% have been reported.[124] Pentavalent antimony was the historical treatment for all forms of Leishmania; however, its multiple side effects including pancreatitis, myalgias, and electrocardiogram abnormalities make it undesirable for use in VL.

Miltefosine is the only oral agent available for VL, and leads to cure rates of greater than 90% of patients with VL.[108] It is not FDA-approved but can be obtained through an Investigational New Drug (IND) application from the CDC.

Treatment and Reactivation

Relapse of VL is a difficult management issue after transplant in SOT recipients. In a review by Simon and colleagues,[125] there were 19 published cases of relapsing VL in renal transplant patients. The mean number of recurrences was 1.7 (range 1–5), at a mean of 13 months apart. Combination therapy with miltefosine and L-AmB was used successfully in 2 cases of relapse.[108,125,128] Secondary prophylaxis with either L-AmB or miltefosine has been effective in VL relapses, and such prophylaxis should be considered with relapses related to high-level immunosuppressive therapy after transplant.[125,136,137] Leishmania PCR may be helpful in monitoring relapse.[125]

Recipient Screening

There is no consensus on screening at-risk organ recipients for Leishmania. Transplant candidates from VL endemic countries as well as United States veterans who have served in VL-endemic areas of the Middle East should be considered for screening before transplant. In a screening study of Hispanic transplant candidates in the United States, 10.4% (5/38) had low positive Leishmania titers by a commercially available IFA assay; however, given the diversity of Leishmania species it was unclear if the patients were at risk for reactivation disease. Larger prospective studies, especially in VL-endemic countries, are necessary to clarify the role of pretransplant testing.[5] Because of the rarity of donor-related disease, donor screening is not recommended.[98]

Blood Transfusion

Cases of transfusion-associated VL have been rarely reported in the international literature, although there are no reported cases of transfusion-transmitted Leishmania in posttransplant patients.[138] Because of the cases of atypical CL with visceral involvement that occurred in US military personnel in the Middle East, the US Armed Services Blood Program prohibits blood donation for 1 year after leaving an endemic area.[111]

FREE-LIVING AMOEBAS

The 3 species of free-living amoebas, Acanthamoeba castellani, Naegleria fowleri, and B mandrillaris, are rare but life-threatening illnesses. Acanthamoeba and B mandrillaris cause granulomatous amoebic encephalitis (GAE), whereas Naegleria presents as a lethal meningoencephalitis.

In SOT, Acanthamoeba carries a risk of disseminated disease in patients who develop cutaneous ulcers after exposure to water. To date it has been reported in liver, lung, and renal transplant patients.[139–141] The initiating symptom is typically a cutaneous lesion, and if diagnosis is made early, patients can recover. The finding of Acanthamoeba in a cutaneous biopsy of a lung transplant patient led to early and curative treatment with L-AmB and voriconazole therapy.[141] Acanthamoeba rhinosinusitis in a lung transplant patient was cured with debridement and amphotericin, voriconazole, and caspofungin therapy.[139] Fatal disseminated Acanthamoeba has been reported to involve the skin, sinuses, lung, brain, and bones.[142,143] Transplant patients who survive disseminated disease have received complex pentamidine-based or amphotericin-based regimens.[140] The first case of nonfatal Acanthamoeba cerebral CNS abscess in SOT was successfully managed with surgical excision and TMP-SMX and rifampin.[140] The diagnosis of acanthamebiasis is made by visualization of the trophozoites and cysts on tissue biopsy. Immunofluorescent staining and culture can assist in diagnosis.[141,142] PCR can also be used for *Acanthamoeba* genotyping.[141] An amphotericin-based regimen in combination with other agents, such as azoles, is the most commonly used treatment strategy for this rare disease.[141]

A multivisceral transplant recipient died of *B mandrillaris* meningitis 2 days after alemtuzumab rejection therapy. Alemtuzumab was not a primary factor of this lethal infection, as the patient was symptomatic before therapy; however, it may have accelerated the disease.[27]

From 2009 to 2010 in the United States there were 2 unusual groupings of donor-transmitted *B mandrillaris* from 2 different donors who died of a CNS process. One donor died of encephalitis. The other donor was a Hispanic landscaper who died of a stroke-like syndrome, and had a large skin lesion on his back of 6 months' duration.[144,145] Of note, Hispanic ethnicity is a proposed risk factor for *B mandrillaris* infection.[145] In each "outbreak," 2 transplant recipients from each donor developed GAE. GAE was diagnosed by the presence of amoebas on brain biopsy or CSF evaluation. *B mandrillaris* was confirmed by both PCR and culture. Two other recipients from each donor were not infected. Of the 4 recipients who developed granulomatous amoebic encephalitis, only 1 survived. Treatment of this rare infection is unclear; however, the survivor of GAE, a renal transplant recipient, received miltefosine, pentamidine, sulfadiazine, flucytosine, fluconazole, and azithromycin therapy.[144,145]

In contrast to *B mandrillaris*, multiple organs were safely transplanted from a donor who died of *N fowleri* meningoencephalitis.[146]

ALIMENTARY PROTOZOA

Intestinal amebiasis, balantidiasis, and giardiasis are examples of protozoal infections that may cause an occasional diarrheal illness after transplant, but are otherwise not especially pathogenic in the transplant patient. By contrast, *Cryptosporidium* and microsporidia can be life-threatening in the immunocompromised.

Isospora (*Cystoisospora*) *belli* is a rarely reported cause of transplant diarrhea in patients from Turkey and South America. An intestinal transplant patient with *C belli* who presented with increased ostomy output, dehydration, and abdominal pain was successfully treated with TMP-SMX and immunosuppression reduction.[10] TMP-SMX prophylaxis incidentally covers the intestinal protozoa *C belli* and *Cyclospora cayetanensis*.

Cryptosporidium is an intracellular protozoan known to cause outbreaks in immunocompetent hosts exposed to communal contaminated water sources.[147] It has a worldwide distribution, with a notably higher prevalence in developing countries.[148] In AIDS and transplant patients it can cause lethal diarrhea with malabsorption and weight loss. It has been reported in liver, intestinal, pancreatic, and kidney transplant patients and in posttransplant HIV patients.[9,12,149–154] It is especially problematic in pediatric transplant patients. Sclerosing cholangitis in liver transplant patients causes significant morbidity, necessitating surgical intervention and even retransplantation.[150] *Cryptosporidium* enteritis in SOT is complicated by increases in tacrolimus levels, presumably secondary to poor absorption.[147] The diagnosis of *Cryptosporidium* is made primarily by modified acid-fast staining of stool cysts. The stool *Cryptosporidium* antigen ELISA assists in the diagnosis, and has a sensitivity of 98.7%.[149] There is no optimal therapy for *Cryptosporidium*, and eradication is a challenge. Successful treatment of a pediatric renal transplant patient was achieved with spiramycin, nitazoxanide, and paromomycin therapy, and close monitoring of the tacrolimus levels.[149]

Reduction of immunosuppressive therapy may be necessary to control severe infection.[9] Because of persistent and relapsing disease, it is important to guide treatment by follow-up stool studies.

Microsporidia are intracellular spore-forming protozoa that cause disease in the immunocompromised host. In SOT, microsporidiosis has been reported in kidney transplants in the majority of cases, but also has been described in heart, lung, liver, intestinal, and pancreas-kidney transplants.[11,148,155,156] Diarrhea is the major clinical manifestation in SOT. *Enterocytozoon bieneusi*, which is resistant to treatment, is the most commonly encountered species in SOT.[11] Disseminated disease presents with protean manifestations of fever, keratoconjunctivitis, CNS involvement, cholangitis, cough, and thoracic/abdominal pain,[9,11,155] and is associated with a high mortality rate of 33%.[148] Leakage from a duodenal-vesicular anastomosis site was a proposed route of dissemination in a pancreas-kidney transplant patient.[155] The diagnosis of microsporidiosis is made by modified trichrome staining of spores in stool or urine (in the case of kidney transplant patients).[9] *Encephalitozoon* species-specific PCR testing is only available in research laboratories. In invasive disease microsporidia have been discovered in urine samples, stool, sputum, conjunctival scrapings, and brain and kidney biopsies.[11] Immunofluorescent staining of biopsy material is used for species identification. There is no fully eradicating therapy; however, albendazole (which only works against non–*E bieneusi* infections), metronidazole, and decreasing immunosuppression have all been used for therapy in *E bieneusi* infection in SOT.[11,155,156]

BABESIOSIS

Babesia, endemic to the United States and Europe, has been reported in 6 transplant patients by transfusion transmission (5 cases) or tick bite (1 case).[9] Transfusion-related *Babesia* typically occurs from August through December, reflecting the seasonality. Babesia is hardy and can survive blood-bank processing of freezing and glycerol treatment.[157]

Infection with *Babesia* can become quickly lethal in asplenic SOT patients.[157] In SOT, hemolytic anemia and fever in a patient who has received a blood transfusion should prompt examination of peripheral blood smears to rule out *Babesia*. Babesiosis attributed to blood transfusion has been reported in renal[9,158] and cardiac[159] transplant recipients. Unusual manifestations in renal transplant patients include impaired graft function[158] and hemophagocytic syndrome in an asplenic transplant patient.[9,160] Severe disease can present with high parasitemia, disseminated intravascular coagulation, congestive heart failure, respiratory distress, splenic infarction, and renal failure.[9] De novo babesiosis was lethal in an asplenic patient who lived in Northern Indiana 2 years after liver transplant.[161] In severe cases of *Babesia* with overwhelming parasitemia, SOT patients have been treated with intravenous clindamycin and quinine sulfate, and exchange transfusion.[9,161] In patients who can tolerate oral therapy, atovaquone and azithromycin is an equally effective regimen.[162] Reduction in immunosuppression is also used in severe disease.[158,162] It is important to educate SOT patients, especially those with asplenia, about risk and avoidance of tick bites in *Babesia*-endemic areas.

MALARIA

Malaria is a rarely reported and unexpected cause of posttransplant infection in non-endemic countries. Because of the high mortality of *Plasmodium falciparum* infection, a heightened index of suspicion must be present with unexplained fever after transplantation, especially in cases where an organ or blood donor has had exposure to an endemic area. Posttransplant malaria has occurred mainly through donor-related infection, and less frequently through blood transfusions and de novo infection. Reactivation malaria after transplant is rare but has been described with *Plasmodium malariae*.[1] As would be expected, posttransplant malaria is more common in transplant centers in malaria-endemic countries such as in India. Of note, all 4 major *Plasmodium* species have been reported following transplants.[18,163]

Donor-transmitted malaria has occurred in heart, liver, and renal transplant recipients. In general, kidney transplant patients fare well and present later than other infected transplant recipients; this is likely related to less intense immunosuppressive regimens. Theoretically the washing of organs should remove parasitized red blood cells, but by virtue of being the most commonly transplanted organ, the majority of donor-reported cases are reported in kidney transplant recipients.[8,18] Donor-transmitted malaria is especially fatal in liver transplantation. In donor-derived disease of liver transplant patients, the allograft harbors parasitized hepatocytes, contributing to early-onset and high-level parasitemia. Malaria is further complicated in liver transplantation, as antimalarial therapy can be hepatotoxic and can contribute to graft failure.[18,164]

Unexpected donor-transmitted *P falciparum* led to significant morbidity and mortality in 2 French SOT recipients. The cadaveric donor had a history of travel to Togo but was not screened for malaria. The liver allograft recipient was incidentally diagnosed with *P falciparum* by blood smear while asymptomatic; fortunately, treatment was initiated early and despite a comatose period the patient survived. The heart transplant recipient was symptomatic with fever and neurologic symptoms by the time treatment was started, and died of multiorgan failure. The investigators proposed that the antilymphocyte globulin therapy contributed to the severity of disease in the heart transplant patient. The 2 kidney transplant patients who received organs from the same donor were empirically treated before the development of any symptoms of malaria, and did well.[18]

In general, *Plasmodium vivax* is a more benign infection and presents later than *P falciparum*. *P vivax* was transmitted from a donor from Zaire (whose predonor screening for malaria by smear was negative) to 2 Swiss kidney transplant recipients. Although both patients had parasitemia, they recovered quickly with treatment.[165] A case of donor-derived *P vivax* in a liver transplant patient was complicated by hepatotoxicity from chloroquine and primaquine therapy. Although the patient's parasitemia resolved with antimalarial therapy, he died months later from graft failure. Hepatotoxicity from the antimalarial therapy was a proposed contributory factor.[163]

In 2009, the CDC received 2 reports of transfusion-related malaria and 1 case transmitted by stem cell transplant. Of note, the stem cell transplant donor was a relative from West Africa.[10] Blood-transfusion–transmitted malaria was responsible for 7.5% of the cases of malaria in SOT recipients in one international series.[9] In the United States, *Plasmodium ovale* was transmitted to a liver transplant patient via platelet transfusion from a donor who had traveled to an endemic area. With chloroquine therapy, the patient recovered without incident.[166–168]

Severe *P falciparum* malaria is treated by intravenous artesunate (available by IND) or quinidine (which requires telemetry monitoring). In uncomplicated *P falciparum*, artemisinin combinations or atovaquone-proguanil are the treatments of choice for SOT patients. The other treatment options for uncomplicated *P falciparum*, quinine or mefloquine, significantly interact with calcineurin inhibitors. *P vivax*, *P ovale*, and *P malariae* can all be treated with chloroquine.

Donor Screening

In the United States there are no approved tests to screen donated blood, stem cells, or organs for malaria. Screening of donor organs from endemic areas by thick and thin smear and PCR or antibody testing is recommended. The IFA can be used as a screen to determine if a donor has ever been infected with *Plasmodium*.[9] In investigations of transfusion-transmitted and transplantation-transmitted cases, infected donors are most often identified by antibody tests, as parasitemia by blood smear evaluation and even PCR can be insensitive. Prevention of transfusion and transplant-related malaria requires careful assessment of the donor's travel history.[169,170]

STRONGYLOIDES
Epidemiology

Strongyloides is an intestinal nematode that infects more than 10 million persons worldwide, mainly in tropical and semitropical areas. The infection is transmitted by cutaneous contact with soil contaminated with human waste. In the United States it exists in the temperate areas of the southeastern United States, including the Appalachian region, and is associated with low socioeconomic status, institutionalization, mining, and alcoholism.[22] This nematode has the rare ability to persist by autoinoculation with low-level replication and minimal symptoms. In the immunocompromised, the autoinoculation syndrome can be accelerated to a level of life-threatening hyperinfection (50% mortality rate) and disseminated strongyloidiasis (80% mortality rate).[2,22]

Clinical Manifestations in SOT

Strongyloides hyperinfection most commonly results from reactivation of dormant disease. It has been reported with renal, liver, heart, and lung transplantation.[2,171–176] T-cell–depleting therapies, such as corticosteroids and antithymocyte globulin, increase susceptibility to hyperinfection.[22] Although uncommon, donor-related Strongyloides transmission has occurred through intestinal, renal, renal-pancreas, and heart allografts.[177–182] In the case of an intestinal transplant patient, *Strongyloides* was presumed to be transmitted through the allograft of a Honduran donor. However, the other organ recipients who received transplants from this recipient were not affected.[182] By contrast, a single donor transmitted *Strongyloides* infection to both recipients: a liver recipient who developed hyperinfection syndrome and a pancreas-kidney transplant recipient who had gastrointestinal symptoms.[181]

Of interest is that cyclosporine is strongly parasiticidal against *Strongyloides*. Since the introduction of cyclosporine into renal transplantation in the 1990s, hyperinfection rates have been greatly reduced.[22] In fact, the majority of cases reported occur in patients who are treated with cyclosporine-sparing regimens. One case of *Strongyloides* hyperinfection occurred in a renal transplant patient on cyclosporine who was suspected to have donor-derived infection.[180]

In SOT, strongyloidiasis can present early with vague gastrointestinal symptoms. With accelerated autoinfection, hyperinfection symptoms correlate with larval migration, causing pyrexia, gastrointestinal pain, bloody diarrhea, ileus, and pneumonitis with bilateral infiltrates.[182] Intestinal and pulmonary obstruction are rare complications. A purpuric rash can occur in the area of larva currens. With dissemination, sepsis or meningitis with gram-negative bacteria results from seeding from the gastrointestinal tract or lungs. Eosinophilia may be a clue to infection, although it is often absent with steroid therapy.[22,31,182] Most cases of *Strongyloides* in SOT occur in the first 6 months after transplant.[9]

Diagnosis

Diagnosis of *Strongyloides* is made by direct identification of larvae in stool or duodenal aspiration.[176] Repeat testing is recommended because of the low sensitivity of stool testing. The agar plate culture technique can increase larval detection to a sensitivity of 78% to 96%.[31] Skin biopsy findings of larvae in a purpuric or petechial rash can lead to an early and life-saving diagnosis.[177] In disseminated infection, larvae have also been identified in bronchial aspirates, sputum, serum, CSF, urine, stool, skin lesions, and peritoneal fluid.[182] Serology is not sensitive or specific in diagnosing new infection. Other limitations of serology are inability to distinguish between past or present infection, cross-reactivity with other helminthic infections, and false-negative results in disseminated infection.[173]

Treatment

Treatment of hyperinfection syndrome and dissemination includes ivermectin and albendazole therapy. Broad-spectrum antibiotics are initiated if bacteremia, meningitis, or pneumonitis is suspected. Moreover, a reduction in immunosuppression is necessary; it is important that steroids be tapered rapidly.[2] In patients with ileus, administration of the medications can be done via nasogastric tube. Ivermectin is available in intravenous, subcutaneous, or enema formulations.[179,182] Treatment should continue for at least 2 weeks after parasitologic cure is achieved, and longer if high-level immunosuppression is necessary.[179]

Screening

Recipients and donors from worldwide endemic areas should be screened for *Strongyloides* by serology. United States recipients from rural southeastern states, particularly with risk factors, should also receive pretransplant screening. The screening ELISA detects IgG to the filariform larvae and has a sensitivity of approximately 85%. In the case of an immunosuppressed transplant candidate with unexplained eosinophilia or abdominal symptoms, multiple stool specimens with agar plate cultures should be used to increase the yield.[31,182] With evidence or suspicion of *Strongyloides*, pretransplant candidates and live donors should be treated with ivermectin before transplant. Human T-lymphocytic virus type 1 is associated with hyperinfection; however, it is no longer a requirement for SOT donor screening.[183]

SUMMARY

Cumulative experiences in parasitic diseases in SOT over the past decades have had an impact on changes in transplant practices with respect to infectious disease. Based on early studies of life-threatening toxoplasmosis infection in *Toxoplasma* D+/R− cardiac recipients, pretransplant serotesting and TMP-SMX prophylaxis are now routine in cardiac transplantation. The pioneering of heart transplantation for chagasic cardiac disease in South America has provided a model for early and sensitive diagnostic surveillance and preemptive treatment of *T cruzi*. In the European and Brazilian literature, cases of VL in SOT patients have quadrupled over the past 3 decades,[112] and have led to the development of valuable strategies for the diagnosis and treatment of VL reactivation. With awareness of the risk factors and lethality of the hyperinfection syndrome in *Strongyloides*, infection is now prevented by targeted pretransplant screening and treatment of infected recipients.

There are management issues in parasitic infections of SOT recipients that remain unresolved. More study is needed to define those transplant recipients at risk of toxoplasmosis who require higher doses or longer duration of toxoplasmosis prophylaxis. Now that donor-derived Chagas disease has been documented in the United States and the possibility of reactivation *T cruzi* of SOT recipients in the United States exists, targeted and standardized screening of donors and recipients is a priority. Adequate screening testing for recipients at risk for reactivated VL is currently lacking. More effective treatment strategies for severe infection with *Cryptosporidium*, microsporidiosis, *Acanthamoeba*, and *B mandrillaris* in SOT also need to be developed. With the increases in international travel and transplantation abroad, our understanding of parasitic disease in SOT will continue to evolve.

REFERENCES

1. Barsoum RS. Parasitic infections in organ transplantation. Exp Clin Transplant 2004;2:258–67.
2. Roxby A, Gottlieb G, Liaye A. Strongyloidiasis in transplant patients. Clin Infect Dis 2009;49(9):1411–23.
3. Schaeffer MW, Buell JF, Gupta M, et al. Strongyloides hyperinfection syndrome after heart transplantation: case report and review of the literature. J Heart Lung Transplant 2004;23:905–11.
4. Schad GA. Cyclosporine may eliminate the threat of overwhelming strongyloidiasis in immunosuppressed patients. J Infect Dis 1986;153:178.
5. Fitzpatrick MA, Caicedo JC, Stosor V, et al. Expanded infectious diseases screening program for Hispanic transplant candidates. Transpl Infect Dis 2010;12:336–41.
6. Franco-Paredes C, Jacob J, Hildron A, et al. Transplantation and tropical infectious diseases. Int J Infect Dis 2010;14:e189–96.
7. Gill J, Madhira BR, Gjertson D, et al. Transplant tourism in the United States: a single-center experience. Clin J Am Soc Nephrol 2008;3:1820–8.
8. Machado CM, Levi JE. Transplant-associated and blood transfusion-associated tropical and parasitic infections. Infect Dis Clin North Am 2010;26(2):225–41.
9. Muñoz P, Valerio M, Puga D, et al. Parasitic infections in solid organ transplant recipients. Infect Dis Clin North Am 2010;24(2):461–95.
10. Gruz F, Fuxman C, Errea A, et al. *Isospora belli* infection after isolated intestinal transplant. Transpl Infect Dis 2010;12(1):69–72.
11. Galván AL, Sánchez AM, Valentín MA, et al. First cases of microsporidiosis in transplant recipients in Spain and review of the literature. J Clin Microbiol 2011;49(4):1301–6.
12. Beatty G, et al. HIV-related predictors and outcomes in 275 liver and/or kidney transplant recipients, 2011. 6th IAS Conference of HIV Pathogenesis, Treatment and Prevention, Rome, Italy. July 2, 2011. p. 17–20. Abstract # MOAB0105.
13. Miro J, Blanes M, Norman F, et al. Infections in solid organ transplantation in special situations: HIV-infection and immigration. Enferm Infecc Microbiol Clin 2012;30(2):76–85.
14. Campbell A, Goldberg C, Madid M, et al. First case of toxoplasmosis following small bowel transplantation and systematic review of tissue-invasive toxoplasmosis following noncardiac solid organ transplantations. Transplantation 2006; 81(3):408–17.
15. Gallino A, Maggiorini M, Kiowski W, et al. Toxoplasmosis in heart transplant recipients. Eur J Clin Microbiol Infect Dis 1996;15(5):389–93.
16. Malhotra P, Rai SD, Hirschwerk D. Duration of prophylaxis with trimethoprim-sulfamethoxazole in patients undergoing solid organ transplantation. Infection 2012;40:473–5.
17. Pinazo MJ, Espinosa G, Gallego M, et al. Successful treatment of a patient with chronic Chagas diseases and systemic lupus erythematosus. Am J Trop Med Hyg 2010;82:583–7.

18. Chiche L, Lesage A, Duhamel C, et al. Posttransplant malaria: first case of transmission of *Plasmodium falciparum* from a white multiorgan donor to four recipients. Transplantation 2003;75:166–8.
19. Baden LR, Katz JT, Franck L, et al. Successful toxoplasmosis prophylaxis after orthotopic cardiac transplantation with Trimethoprim-sulfamethoxazole. Transplantation 2003;75:339–43.
20. Fishman JA. Prevention of infection caused by *Pneumocystis carinii* in transplant recipients. Clin Infect Dis 2001;33:1397–405.
21. Campos SV, Stabelli TM, Amato Neto V, et al. Risk factors for Chagas disease reactivation after heart transplant. J Heart Lung Transplant 2008;27:597–602.
22. Keiser P, Nutman T. *Strongyloides stercoralis* in the immunocompromised population. Clin Microbiol Rev 2004;17(4):208–17.
23. Bacal F, Silva CP, Pires PV, et al. Transplantation for Chagas' disease: an overview of immunosuppression and reactivation in the last two decades. Clin Transplant 2010;24(2):E29–34.
24. Bestetti RB, Rubio F, Ferraz Filho JR, et al. *Trypanosoma cruzi* infection reactivation manifested by encephalitis in a Chagas heart transplant recipient. Int J Cardiol 2013;163(1):e7–8.
25. Chagas Disease Argentine Collaborative Transplant Consortium, Casadei D. Chagas' disease and solid organ transplantation. Transplant Proc 2010;42:3354–9.
26. Bocchi EA, Giovanni E, Mocelin AO, et al. Heart transplantation for chronic Chagas' disease. Ann Thorac Surg 1996;61:1727–33.
27. Peleg A, Husain S, Kwak E, et al. Opportunistic infections in 547 organ transplant recipients receiving alemtuzumab, a humanized monoclonal CD-52 antibody. Clin Infect Dis 2007;44:204–12.
28. Israelski DM. Prevalence of Toxoplasma infection in a cohort of homosexual men at risk of AIDS and toxoplasmic encephalitis. J Acquir Immune Defic Syndr 1993;6:414.
29. Roghmann MC, et al. Decreased seroprevalence for *Toxoplasma gondii* in Seventh Day Adventists in Maryland. Am J Trop Med Hyg 1999;60:790–2.
30. Derouin F, Pelloux H, ESCMID Study Group on Clinical Parasitology. Prevention of toxoplasmosis in transplant patients. Clin Microbiol Infect 2008;14:1089–101.
31. Kotton CN, Lattes R, AST Infectious Diseases Community of Practice. Parasitic infections in solid organ transplant recipients. Am J Transplant 2009;9:S234–51.
32. Luft B, Naot Y, Araujo F, et al. Primary and reactivated toxoplasma infection in patients with cardiac transplants: clinical spectrum and problems in diagnosis in a defined population. Ann Intern Med 1983;99:27–31.
33. Montoya J, Giraldo L, Efron B, et al. Infectious complications among 620 consecutive heart transplant patients at Stanford University Medical Center. Clin Infect Dis 2001;33:629–40.
34. Nissapatorn V, Leong TH, Lee R. Seroepidemiology of toxoplasmosis in renal patients. Southeast Asian J Trop Med Public Health 2011;42(2):237–47.
35. Orr K, Gould F, Short G, et al. Outcome of *Toxoplasma gondii* mismatches in heart transplant recipients over a period of 8 years. J Infect 1994;29:249–53.
36. Fernandez-Sabe N, Cervera C, Farinas C, et al. Risk factors, clinical features, and outcomes of toxoplasmosis in solid-organ transplant recipients: a matched case-control study. Clin Infect Dis 2012;54(3):355–61.
37. Fishman JA. Infection in solid-organ transplant recipients. N Engl J Med 2007;357:2601–14.

38. Robert-Gangneux F, Dardé ML. Epidemiology of and diagnostic strategies for toxoplasmosis. Clin Microbiol Rev 2012;25(2):264–96.
39. Contreras M. Seroepidemiology of human toxoplasmosis in Chile. Rev Inst Med Trop Sao Paulo 1996;38:431–5.
40. Patrat-Delon S, Gangneux JP, Lavoue S. Correlation of parasite load determined by quantitative PCR to clinical outcome in a heart transplant patient with disseminated toxoplasmosis. J Clin Microbiol 2010;48(7):2541–5.
41. Dodd RY. Transmission of parasites by blood transfusion. Vox Sang 1998; 74(Suppl 2):161–3.
42. Martina MN, Cervera C, Esforzado N, et al. Toxoplasma gondii primary infection in renal transplant recipients. Two case reports and literature review. Transpl Int 2011;24:e6–12.
43. Barcan LA, Dallurzo ML, Clara LO, et al. Toxoplasma gondii pneumonia in liver transplantation: survival after a severe case of reactivation. Transpl Infect Dis 2002;4:93–6.
44. Botterel F, et al. Disseminated toxoplasmosis, resulting from infection of allograft, after orthotopic liver transplantation: usefulness of quantitative PCR. J Clin Microbiol 2002;40:1648–50.
45. Sukthana Y, Chintana T, Damrongkitchaiporn S, et al. Serological study of Toxoplasma gondii in kidney recipients. J Med Assoc Thai 2001;84:1137–41.
46. Hommann M, Schotte U, Voigt R, et al. Cerebral toxoplasmosis after combined liver-pancreas-kidney and liver-pancreas transplantation. Transplant Proc 2002; 34:2294–5.
47. Monaco S, Monaghan S, Stamm J. Toxoplasmosis in a post-transplant bronchoalveolar lavage. Diagn Cytopathol 2011;40(7):629–33.
48. Hermanns B, Brunn A, Schwarz E, et al. Fulminant toxoplasmosis in a heart transplant recipient. Pathol Res Pract 2001;197:211–5.
49. Muñoz P, Valerio M, Palomo J, et al. Infectious and non-infectious neurologic complications in heart transplant recipients. Medicine (Baltimore) 2010;89:166–75.
50. Ritter ML, Pirofski L. Mycophenolate mofetil: effects on cellular immune subsets, infectious complications and antimicrobial activity. Transpl Infect Dis 2009;11(4): 290–7.
51. Sever MS. Outcome of living unrelated (commercial) renal transplantation. Kidney Int 2001;60(4):1477–83.
52. Walker M, Kublin J, Zunt JJ. Parasitic central nervous system infections in immunocompromised hosts. Clin Infect Dis 2006;42:115–25.
53. Aubert D, Foudrinier I, Villena J, et al. PCR for diagnosis and follow-up of two cases of disseminated toxoplasmosis after kidney grafting. J Clin Microbiol 1996;34:1347.
54. Sanchez Mejia A, Debrunner M, Cox E, et al. Acquired toxoplasmosis after orthotopic heart transplantation in a sulfonamide-allergic patient. Pediatr Cardiol 2011;32(1):91–3.
55. Singh N. Toxoplasma gondii pneumonitis in a liver transplant recipient: implications for diagnosis. Liver Transpl Surg 1996;2:299–300.
56. Porter S, Sande MA. Toxoplasmosis of the central nervous system in the acquired immunodeficiency syndrome. N Engl J Med 1992;327:1643–8.
57. Joseph P. Optimization and evaluation of a PCR assay for detecting toxoplasmic encephalitis in patients with AIDS. J Clin Microbiol 2002;40:4499–503.
58. Karras A, Thervet E, Legendre C, Groupe Cooperatif de transplantation d'Ile de France. Hemophagocytic syndrome in renal transplant recipients: report of 17 cases and review of literature. Transplantation 2004;77:238–43.

59. Martin SI, Fishman JA, AST Infectious Diseases Community of Practice. Pneumocystis pneumonia in solid organ transplant recipients. Am J Transplant 2009;9:S227–33.
60. Gourishankar S, Doucette K, Fenton J. The use of donor and recipient screening for toxoplasma in the era of universal trimethoprim sulfamethoxazole prophylaxis. Transplantation 2008;85(7):980–5.
61. Bern C. Antitrypanosomal therapy for chronic Chagas' disease. N Engl J Med 2011;364:2527–34.
62. Kun H, Moore A, Mascola L, et al. Transmission of *Trypanosoma cruzi* by heart transplantation. Clin Infect Dis 2009;48(11):1534–40.
63. Machado F, Jelicks L, Kirchhoff L, et al. Chagas' heart disease: report on recent developments. Cardiol Rev 2012;20(2):53–65.
64. Buekens P, Almendares O, Carlier Y, et al. Mother-to-child transmission of Chagas disease in North America: why don't we do more? Matern Child Health J 2008;12:283–6.
65. Pan American Health Organization. Estimación cuantitativa de la enfermedad de Chagas en las Americas. [Quantitative estimation of Chagas disease in the Americas]. OPS/HDM/CD/425–06. Washington, DC: Pan American Health Organization; 2006.
66. Perez-Mazliah DE, Alvarez MG, Cooley G, et al. Sequential combined treatment with allopurinol and benznidazole in the chronic phase of *Trypanosoma cruzi* infection: a pilot study. J Antimicrob Chemother 2013;68(2):424–37.
67. Bechimol Barbosa PR. The oral transmission of Chagas' disease; an acute form of infection responsible for regional outbreaks. Int J Cardiol 2006;112(1):132–3.
68. CDC. Blood donor screening for Chagas Disease-United States, 2006-2007. MMWR Morb Mortal Wkly Rep 2007;56(7):141–3.
69. CDC. Chagas disease after organ transplantation—United States, 2001. MMWR Morb Mortal Wkly Rep 2002;51:210–2.
70. CDC. Chagas disease after organ transplantation—Los Angeles, California, 2006. MMWR Morb Mortal Wkly Rep 2006;55:798–800.
71. CDC. Congenital transmission of Chagas disease—Virginia, 2010. MMWR Morb Mortal Wkly Rep 2012;61(26):477–9.
72. Stramer SL, Foster G, Townsend R, et al. *Trypanosoma cruzi* antibody screening in US blood donors: one year experience at the American Red Cross. Transfusion 2008;48(Suppl):2A.
73. Vazquez MC. Chagas disease and transplantation. Transplant Proc 1996;28:3301–3.
74. Bern C. Chagas' disease in immunosuppressed host. Curr Opin Infect Dis 2012;25(4):450–7.
75. Bern C, Montgomery S. An estimate of the burden of Chagas' disease in the United States. Clin Infect Dis 2009;49:e52–4.
76. Bern C, Montgomery S, Herwaldt B, et al. Evaluation of Chagas disease in the United States: a systematic review. JAMA 2007;298(18):2171–81.
77. Bocchi EA, Fiorelli A. The paradox of survival results after heart transplantation for cardiomyopathy caused by *Trypanosoma cruzi*. First Guidelines Group for Heart Transplantation of the Brazilian Society of Cardiology. Ann Thorac Surg 2001;71:1833–8.
78. de Carvalho VB, Sousa EF, Vila JH, et al. Heart transplantation in Chagas' disease. 10 years after the initial experience. Circulation 1996;94:1815–7.
79. Tanowitz HB, Machado FS, Jelicks LA, et al. Perspectives on *Trypanosoma cruzi*-induced heart disease (Chagas disease). Prog Cardiovasc Dis 2009;51(6):524–39.

80. Blanche C, Aleksic I, Johanna J, et al. Heart transplantation for Chagas' cardio-myopathy. Ann Thorac Surg 1995;60:1406–9.
81. Bestetti RB, Theodoropoulos TA. A systematic review of studies on heart transplantation for patients with end-stage Chagas' heart disease. J Card Fail 2009; 15:249–55.
82. Pinazo MJ, Miranda B, Rodríguez-Villar C, et al. Recommendations for management of Chagas disease in organ and hematopoietic tissue transplantation programs in nonendemic areas. Transplant Rev (Orlando) 2011;25(3):91–101.
83. Diez M, Favaloro L, Bertolotti A, et al. Usefulness of PCR strategies for early diagnosis of Chagas disease reactivation and treatment in heart transplantation. Am J Transplant 2007;7:1633–40.
84. Gascon J, Bern C, Pinazo MJ, et al. Chagas disease in Spain, the United States and other non-endemic countries. Acta Trop 2010;115(1–2):22–7.
85. Godoy H, Guerra C, Viegas R, et al. Infections in heart transplant recipients in Brazil: the challenge of Chagas' disease. J Heart Lung Transplant 2010;29: 286–90.
86. Maldonado C, et al. Using polymerase chain reaction in early diagnosis of re-activated *Trypanosoma cruzi* infection after heart transplantation. J Heart Lung Transplant 2004;23(12):1345–8.
87. Bestetti RB, Cury PM, Theodoropoulos TA, et al. *Trypanosoma cruzi* myocardial infection reactivation presenting as complete atrioventricular block in a Chagas' heart transplant recipient. Cardiovasc Pathol 2004;13:323–6.
88. Riarte A, Luna C, Sabatiello R, et al. Chagas' disease in patients with kidney transplants: 7 years of experience 1989-1996. Clin Infect Dis 1999;29:561–7.
89. Rodrigues Coura J, de Castro SL. A critical review on Chagas disease chemotherapy. Mem Inst Oswaldo Cruz 2002;97:3–24.
90. Arias LF, Duque E, Ocampo C, et al. Detection of amastigotes of *Trypanosoma cruzi* in a kidney graft with acute dysfunction. Transplant Proc 2006;38(3):885–7.
91. Kocher C, Segerer S, Schleich A, et al. Skin lesions, malaise, and heart failure in a renal transplant recipient. Transpl Infect Dis 2012;14(4):391–7.
92. Chin-Hong PV, Schwartz BS, Bern C, et al. Screening and treatment of Chagas Disease in organ transplant recipients in the United States: recommendations from the Chagas in Transplant Working Group. Am J Transplant 2011;11: 672–80.
93. Chocair PR, Sabbaga E, Amato Neto V, et al. Kidney transplantation: a new way of transmitting Chagas disease. Rev Inst Med Trop Sao Paulo 1981;23:280–2.
94. McCormack L, Quinonez E, Goldaracena N, et al. Liver transplantation using Chagas-infected donors in uninfected recipients: a single- center experience without prophylactic therapy. Am J Transplant 2012;12:2832–7.
95. Moore K, Mascola L, Steurer F, et al. Transmission of Trypanosoma by heart transplantation. Clin Infect Dis 2009;48(11):1534–40.
96. Moreira OC, Ramirez JD, Velazquez E. Towards the establishment of a consensus real-time qPCR to monitor *Trypanosoma cruzi* parasitemia in patients with chronic Chagas disease cardiomyopathy: a substudy from the BENEFIT trial. Acta Trop 2013;125(1):23–31.
97. Barcan L, Luna C, Clara L, et al. Transmission of *T. cruzi* infection via liver transplantation to a nonreactive recipient for Chagas' disease. Liver Transpl 2005; 11(9):1112–6.
98. Martin-Davila P, Fortun J, Loqez-Velez R, et al. Transmission of tropical and geographically restricted infection during solid-organ transplantation. Clin Microbiol Rev 2008;21(1):60–96.

99. Atclas J, Sinagra A, Dictar M, et al. Chagas' disease in bone marrow transplantation: an approach to preemptive therapy. Bone Marrow Transplant 2005;36: 123–9.

100. Kessler D, Shi P, Avecilla ST, et al. Results of lookback for Chagas' disease since the inception of donor screening at New York Blood Center. Transfusion 2012. http://dx.doi.org/10.1111/j.1537-2995.2012.03856.x.

101. Sousa A, Lobo MC, Barbosa RA. Chagas seropositive donors in kidney transplantation. Transplant Proc 2004;36:868–9.

102. Souza FF, Castro ES, Marin Neto JA, et al. Acute chagasic myocardiopathy after orthotopic liver transplant with donor and recipient serologically negative for T. cruzi: a case report. Transplant Proc 2008;4:875–8.

103. Qvarnstrom Y, et al. Sensitive and specific detection of Trypanosoma cruzi DNA in clinical specimens using a multi-target real-time PCR approach. PLoS Negl Trop Dis 2012;6(7):e1689.

104. Schwartz B, Paster M, Ison M. Organ donor screening practices for Trypanosoma cruzi infections among US Organ Procurement Organizations. Am J Transplant 2011;11:848–51.

105. Silva N, O'Bryan L, Medeiros E, et al. Trypanosoma cruzi meningoencephalitis In HIV-infected patients. J Acquir Immune Defic Syndr Hum Retrovirol 1999;20(4): 342–9.

106. Cantey P, Stramer S, Townsend R, et al. The United States Trypanosoma cruzi infection study: evidence for vector-borne transmission of the parasite that causes Chagas disease among United States blood donors. Transfusion 2012;52:1922–30.

107. Carvalho MF, de Franco MF, Soares VA. Amastigotes forms of Trypanosoma cruzi detected in a renal allograft. Rev Inst Med Trop Sao Paulo 1997;39:223–6.

108. Murray HW. Review: leishmaniasis in the United States: treatment in 2012. Am J Trop Med Hyg 2012;86:434–40.

109. Fernández-Guerrero ML, et al. Visceral leishmaniasis in immunocompromised patients with and without AIDS: a comparison of clinical features and prognosis. Acta Trop 2004;90(1):11–6.

110. Bogdan C. Leishmaniasis in rheumatology, haematology and oncology: epidemiological, immunological and clinical aspects and caveats. Ann Rheum Dis 2012;71(Supp II):i60–6.

111. Cardo LJ. Leishmania: risk to the blood supply. Transfusion 2006;46(9):1641.

112. Antinori S, Cascio A, Paravicinic C, et al. Leishmania among organ transplant recipients. Lancet Infect Dis 2008;8:191–9.

113. Ersoy A, Gullulu M, Usta M, et al. A renal transplant recipient with pulmonary tuberculosis and visceral leishmaniasis: review of superimposed infections and therapy approaches. Clin Nephrol 2003;60:289–94.

114. Moulin B, Ollier J, Bouchouareb D, et al. Leishmaniasis: a rare cause of unexplained fever in a renal graft recipient. Nephron 1992;60:360–2.

115. Veroux M, Corona D, Giuffrida G, et al. Visceral leishmaniasis in the early post-transplant period after kidney transplantation: clinical features and therapeutic management. Transpl Infect Dis 2010;12:387–91.

116. Badaro R, Benson D, Eulalio MC, et al. rK39: a cloned antigen of Leishmania chagasi that predicts active visceral leishmaniasis. J Infect Dis 1996;173(3): 758.

117. Basset D, Faraut F, Marty P, et al. Visceral leishmaniasis in organ transplant recipients; 11 new cases and a review of the literature. Microbes Infect 2005;7: 1370–5.

118. Berenguer F, Gómez-Campdera F, Padilla B, et al. Visceral leishmaniasis (Kala-azar) in transplant recipients. Transplantation 1998;65:1401–4.
119. Frapier JM, Abraham B, Dereure J, et al. Fatal visceral leishmaniasis in a heart transplant recipient. J Heart Lung Transplant 2001;20:912–3.
120. Horber FF, Lerut JP, Reichen J, et al. Visceral leishmaniasis after orthotopic liver transplantation: impact of persistent splenomegaly. Transpl Int 1993;6:55–7.
121. Morales P, Torres JJ, Salavert M, et al. Visceral leishmaniasis in lung transplantation. Transplant Proc 2003;35:2001–3.
122. Moroni G, Bossi L. Don't forget visceral leishmaniasis in transplant patients. Nephrol Dial Transplant 1995;10:563–4.
123. Aardema H, Sijpkens YW, Visser LG. Pancytopenia in a simultaneous pancreas and kidney transplant: an unexpected cause: a case of visceral leishmaniasis in a transplant recipient. Clin Nephrol 2009;71:460–2.
124. Rodriguez CN, et al. Leishmaniasis visceral en un paciente con diabestes tipo 1 y transplante aislado de pancreas. Endocrinol Nutr 2011;58:375–7 [in Spanish].
125. Simon I, Wissing KM, Del Marmol V, et al. Recurrent leishmaniasis in kidney transplant recipients: report of 2 cases and systematic review of the literature. Transpl Infect Dis 2011;13:397–406.
126. Oliveira CM, Oliveira ML, Andrade SC, et al. Visceral leishmaniasis in renal transplant recipients; clinical aspects, diagnostic problems and response to treatment. Transplant Proc 2008;40:755–60.
127. Gontijo CM, Pacheco RS, Orefice F, et al. Concurrent cutaneous, visceral and ocular leishmaniasis caused by Leishmania (Viannia) braziliensis in a kidney transplant patient. Mem Inst Oswaldo Cruz 2002;97:751–3.
128. Hernández-Pérez JM, Jimenez-Martinez E, et al. Visceral leishmaniasis (kala-azar) in solid organ transplantation: report of five cases and review. Clin Infect Dis 1999;29:918–21.
129. Jha PK, Vankalakunti M, Siddini V, et al. Postrenal transplant laryngeal and visceral leishmaniasis—a case report and review of the literature. Indian J Nephrol 2010;22(4):301–3.
130. Roustan G, Jimenez JA, Gutierrez-Solar B, et al. Post-kala-azar dermal leishmaniasis with mucosal involvement in a kidney transplant recipient: treatment with liposomal amphotericin B. Br J Dermatol 1998;138:526–68.
131. Araujo SA, Queiroz TC, Cabral MM. Colonic leishmaniasis followed by liver transplantation. Am J Trop Med Hyg 2010;83(2):209.
132. Couppie P, Clyti E, Sobesky M, et al. Comparative study of cutaneous leishmaniasis in human immunodeficiency virus (HIV)-infected patients and non-HIV-infected patients in French Guiana. Br J Dermatol 2004;151:1165–71.
133. Fernandes IM, Baptista MA, Barbon TR, et al. Cutaneous leishmaniasis in kidney transplant recipient. Transplant Proc 2002;34:504–5.
134. Sabbatini M, et al. Visceral leishmaniasis in renal transplant recipients: is it still a challenge to the nephrologist? Transplantation 2002;73:299–301.
135. Gatti S, Gramegna M, Klersy C, et al. Diagnosis of visceral leishmaniasis: the sensitivities and specificities of traditional methods and a nested PCR assay. Ann Trop Med Parasitol 2004;98(7):667–76.
136. Marquez N, Sa R, Coelho F, et al. Miltefosine for visceral leishmaniasis relapse treatment and secondary prophylaxis in HIV-infected patients. Scand J Infect Dis 2008;40:523–6.
137. Massimo S, Pisani A, Ragosta A, et al. Visceral leishmaniasis in renal transplant recipients: is it still a challenge to the Nephrologist? Transplantation 2002;73(2):299–301.

138. Otero A, et al. Occurrence of *Leishmania donovani* DNA in donated blood from seroreactive Brazilian blood donors. Am J Trop Med Hyg 2000;622:128–31.
139. Young AL, Leboeuf NR, Tsiouris SJ, et al. Fatal disseminated *Acanthamoeba* infection in a liver transplant recipient immunocompromised by combination therapies for graft-versus-host disease. Transpl Infect Dis 2010;12(6):529–37.
140. Fung KT, Dhillon AP, McLaughlin JE, et al. Cure of *Acanthamoeba* cerebral abscess in a liver transplant patient. Liver Transpl 2008;14(3):308–12.
141. Walia R, Montoya JG, Visvesvera GS, et al. A case of successful treatment of cutaneous *Acanthamoeba* infection in a lung transplant recipient. Transpl Infect Dis 2007;9(1):51–4.
142. Duarte AG, Sattar F, Granwehr B, et al. Disseminated acanthamoebiasis after lung transplantation. J Heart Lung Transplant 2006;25(2):237–40.
143. Steinberg JP, Galindo RL, Kraus ES, et al. Disseminated acanthamoebiasis in a renal transplant recipient with osteomyelitis and cutaneous lesions: case report and literature review. Clin Infect Dis 2002;35:e43–9.
144. CDC. Transplant-transmitted *Balamuthia mandrillaris*—Arizona, 2010. MMWR Morb Mortal Wkly Rep 2010;59:1182.
145. CDC. *Balamuthia mandrillaris* transmitted through organ transplantation—Mississippi, 2009. MMWR Morb Mortal Wkly Rep 2010;59(36):1165–70.
146. Bennett WM, Nespral JF, Rosson MW, et al. Use of organs for transplantation from a donor with primary meningoencephalitis due to *Naegleria fowleri*. Am J Transplant 2008;8(6):1334–5.
147. Bonatt H, Barroso RG II, Swyer CN, et al. *Cryptosporidium enteritis* in solid organ transplant recipients: multicenter retrospective evaluation of 10 cases reveals and association with elevated tacrolimus concentrations. Transpl Infect Dis 2012;14(6):635–48.
148. Muñoz P, Valerio M, Eworo A, et al. Parasitic infections in solid organ transplant recipients. Curr Opin Organ Transplant 2011;16:565–75.
149. Acikgoz Y, Ozkaya O, Bek K, et al. Cryptosporidiosis: a rare and severe infection in a pediatric renal transplant recipient. Pediatr Transplant 2012;16:E115–9.
150. Campos M, Jouzdani E, Sempoux C, et al. Sclerosing cholangitis associated to cryptosporidiosis in liver-transplanted children. Eur J Pediatr 2000;159:113–5.
151. Denkinger CM, Harigopal P, Ruiz P, et al. *Cryptosporidium parvum* associated Sclerosing cholangitis in a liver transplant patient. Transpl Infect Dis 2008;10:133–6.
152. Minz M, Udgiri NK, Heer MK, et al. Cryptosporidiasis in live related renal transplant recipients: a single center experience. Transplantation 2004;77:1916–7.
153. Pozio E, Rivasi F, Caccio SM. Infection with *Cryptosporidium hominis* and reinfection with *Cryptosporidium parvum* in a transplanted ileum. APMIS 2004;112:309–13.
154. Udgiri N, Minz M, Kashyap R, et al. Intestinal cryptosporidiasis in living related renal transplant recipients. Transplant Proc 2004;36(7):2128–9.
155. Carlson JR, Li L, Helton CL, et al. Disseminated microsporidiosis in a pancreas/kidney transplant recipient. Arch Pathol Lab Med 2004;128:e41–3.
156. Mohindra AR, Lee MW, Visvesvara G, et al. Disseminated microsporidiosis in a renal transplant recipient. Transpl Infect Dis 2002;4:102–7.
157. Gubernot DM, Lucey CT, Lee KC, et al. Babesia infection through blood transfusions: reports received by the US Food and Drug Administration, 1997-2007. Clin Infect Dis 2009;48(1):25–30.
158. Perdrizet GA, Olson NH, Krause PJ, et al. Babesiosis in a renal transplant recipient acquired through blood transfusion. Transplantation 2000;70:205–8.

159. Lux JZ, Weiss D, Linden JV, et al. Transfusion-associated babesiosis after heart transplant. Emerg Infect Dis 2003;9:116–9.
160. Slovut DP, Benedetti E, Matas AJ. Babesiosis and hemophagocytic syndrome in an asplenic renal transplant recipient. Transplantation 1996;62:537–53.
161. Berman KH, Blue DE, Smith DS, et al. Fatal case of babesiosis in postliver transplant patient. Transplantation 2009;87(3):452–3.
162. Kotton CN. Transplant tourism and donor-derived parasitic infections. Transplant Proc 2011;43:2448–9.
163. Fischer L, Sterneck M, Claus M, et al. Transmission of malaria tertiana by multi-organ donation. Clin Transplant 1999;13:491.
164. Crafa F, Gugenheim J, Di Marzo L, et al. Possible transmission of malaria by liver transplantation. Transplant Proc 1991;23:2664.
165. Holzer BR, Gluck Z, Zambelli D, et al. Transmission of malaria by renal transplantation. Transplantation 1985;39(3):315–6.
166. Talabiska D, Komar M, Wytock D, et al. Post-transfusion acquired malaria complicating orthotopic liver transplantation. Am J Gastroenterol 1996;91(2):376–9.
167. Turkmen A, Sever MS, Ecder T, et al. Post transplant malaria. Transplantation 1996;62:1521–3.
168. Gupta RK, Jain M. Renal transplantation: potential source of microfilarial transmission. Transplant Proc 1998;30(8):4320–1.
169. Mali S. Malaria surveillance—United States, 2009. MMWR Surveill Summ 2011; 60(3):1–15.
170. Mungai M, Tegtmeier G, Chamberland M, et al. Transfusion-transmitted malaria in the United States from 1963 through 1999. N Engl J Med 2001;344:1973–8.
171. Arango C, Arango C, Seas C. A 29-year-old renal transplant recipient with acute respiratory failure. Am J Trop Med Hyg 2012;86(6):911–2.
172. Balagopal A, Mills L, Shah A, et al. Detection and treatment of *Strongyloides* hyper infection syndrome following lung transplantation. Transpl Infect Dis 2009; 11(2):149–54.
173. Grover I, Davila R, Subramony C, et al. *Strongyloides* infection in a cardiac transplant recipient: making a case for pretransplantation screening and treatment. Gastroenterol Hepatol 2011;7(11):763–6.
174. Sen S, Dawwa M, Nash K, et al. Uncomplicated strongyloidiasis in a liver transplant recipient on steroid-free immunosuppression. Transpl Infect Dis 2010;12:184–5.
175. Simpson WG. Disseminated *Strongyloides stercoralis* infection. South Med J 1993;86:821–5.
176. Lattes R, Linares L, Radisic M. Emerging parasitic infections in transplantation. Curr Infect Dis Rep 2012;14:642–9.
177. Brugemann J, Kampinga G, Riezebos-Brilman A, et al. Two donor-related infections in a heart transplant recipient: one common, the other a tropical surprise. J Heart Lung Transplant 2010;29:1433–7.
178. DeVault GA. Opportunistic infections with *Strongyloides stercoralis* in renal transplantation. Rev Infect Dis 1990;12:653–71.
179. Hamillton K, Abt P, Rosenbach M, et al. Donor-derived *Strongyloides stercoralis* infections in renal transplant recipients. Transplantation 2011;91(9):1019–24.
180. Palau LA, Pankey GA. *Strongyloides* hyperinfection in a renal transplant recipient receiving cyclosporine: possible *Strongyloides stercoralis* transmission by kidney transplant. Am J Trop Med Hyg 1997;57:413–5.
181. Rodriguez-Hernandez MJ, Ruiz-Perez-Pipaon M, Canas E, et al. *Strongyloides stercoralis* hyperinfection transmitted by liver allograft in a transplant recipient. Am J Transplant 2009;9(11):2637–40.

182. Patel G, Arvelakis A, Sauter BV, et al. *Strongyloides* hyperinfection syndrome after intestinal transplantation. Transpl Infect Dis 2008;10(2):137–41.
183. Morris M, Fischer S, Ison M. Infections transmitted by transplantation. Infect Dis Clin North Am 2010;24:497–514.

Travel Medicine and the Solid-Organ Transplant Recipient

Jessica Rosen, MD

KEYWORDS

- Solid-organ transplant • Immunosuppression • Travel • Travel medicine • Vaccine
- Vaccination • Malaria • Traveler's diarrhea

KEY POINTS

- Solid-organ transplant recipients (SOTRs) are traveling, and awareness of this fact before and after transplant can help protect patients.
- A careful risk assessment of the patient and the trip can help guide advice to the patient.
- Some vaccinations may be contraindicated in SOTRs, and those that are not may have decreased efficacy.
- There are no current data to support that vaccination with inactivated vaccines increases the risk of graft rejection.
- Traveler's diarrhea and its complications can be more severe in SOTRs.
- There are many drug interactions between transplant medications and medications for malaria prophylaxis and traveler's diarrhea.

INTRODUCTION

The number of international travelers is steadily increasing worldwide; the total number of international arrivals is expected to reach 1 billion in 2012.[1] Given the increasing commonality and ease of international travel, the likelihood of travel by those with underlying medical issues, including solid-organ transplantation, is presumably increasing also. As solid-organ transplant patients return to their usual routines, travel needs may arise for leisure, visiting friends and relatives, or for business. This review discusses the epidemiology of travel by solid-organ transplant recipients (SOTRs), the current knowledge and gaps in knowledge about the risks of travel in this population, and the best available strategies to reduce risk.

Travel Epidemiology

Most studies on travel patterns of SOTRs have involved single transplant centers ranging from 200 to more than 1100 patients.[2–4] Most of the patients included are renal and liver transplant recipients, and the data may be somewhat difficult to

Medstar Georgetown University Hospital, Division of Infectious Diseases and Travel Medicine, 3800 Reservoir Road NW, Washington, DC 20007, USA
E-mail address: jdr9@gunet.georgetown.edu

Infect Dis Clin N Am 27 (2013) 429–457
http://dx.doi.org/10.1016/j.idc.2013.02.009
0891-5520/13/$ – see front matter © 2013 Elsevier Inc. All rights reserved.

id.theclinics.com

generalize. However, the rates of travel outside North America and/or Western Europe agree fairly well between studies, from 27% to 36%. The percent traveling to tropical areas or areas with increased infection risk was 16% to 48%.

Looking at which SOTRs are more likely to travel, in 1 study, almost two-thirds of SOTRs traveling after transplant were foreign born.[4] Not only are foreign-born SOTRs traveling more but they are more likely to travel to higher risk areas. A study from the Mayo Clinic reported that 29% of foreign-born SOTRs traveled to areas at higher risk of infectious diseases compared with only 6% of patients born in the United States or Canada.[2] In terms of the degree of immunosuppression at the time of travel, 2 studies report only 6% to 8% of SOTR travelers traveled within the first year of transplant.[2,3] The amount of pretravel advice that SOTRs sought out before travel varied greatly from only 4% to 67%. The most common source of medical recommendations on travel was the transplant physician in all of the studies.

Expanding beyond the confines of single transplant center studies, data were recently presented from Global TravEpiNet, a nationwide consortium of US travel clinics, showing that 1.4% of the 25,711 travelers were identified as immunocompromised. Of the immunocompromised patients, 14% were SOTRs. Eighty percent of the immunocompromised travelers were visiting low or low-middle income countries, and there was no difference in rates of travel to highest risk regions between immunocompromised and nonimmunocompromised travelers. India was the most frequent destination. Immunocompromised travelers were more likely to stay in the home of a relative than nonimmunocompromised travelers, a situation that is associated with increased risk of infection.[5]

Assessing Risk

Knowing that SOTRs are traveling to areas associated with increased risk of infection, the provider needs to know how best to assess the individual's risk based on the traveler and the itinerary. Determining actions to take based on risk may be subjective, as there are different levels of comfort with risk. One traveler, provider, or even governmental agency such as the Centers for Disease Control and Prevention (CDC), may hear that the risk of illness is 1 in 1 million and believe that that represents a negligible risk, whereas another may focus on the fact that it is not an impossibility. The safest environment for any individual, including an SOTR, is living in a bubble. We allow ourselves and our patients to live outside a bubble and it is impossible to draw a line in the sand about when the risk based on health status and the environment outweighs the benefit. The best we can do is help our patients weigh those risks, and then offer them advice and any prophylaxis available to minimize that risk as much as possible.

It is estimated overall that 20% to 70% of travelers who spend 1 month in a developing country will develop illness of some sort. Eight percent of travelers will be ill enough to seek medical care, and about 4% of these will be serious enough to require hospitalization.[6] In a study comparing 345 travelers with underlying conditions with healthy travelers, the incidence of self-reported travel-related illness was about twice as high in those with underlying medical conditions. Gastrointestinal symptoms, fever, and respiratory problems were the most frequently reported. Of patients on immunosuppressants, 33% reported travel-related disease.[7] This differed from the results of a prospective study at 2 Dutch travel clinics comparing travelers on immunosuppressants and their nonimmunocompromised travel companions. In this study, only skin infections were more frequent than in controls, but there were no differences with regard to fever, diarrhea, respiratory illness, or the need for medical attention.[8]

In 4 studies of SOTR travelers reporting rates of illness, 8% to 29% of patients had complications during or immediately after travel.[2–4,9] Fevers, diarrheal illnesses, and respiratory infections were the most commonly reported illnesses. Hospitalization rates for ill travelers ranged from 0% to 50%. Among the 4 studies (totaling more than 500 SOTR travelers), there were only 2 reported episodes of graft rejection, which may not differ significantly from the expected rate. However, acute rejection during travel, especially in settings where medical care may be suboptimal even for healthy individuals, could be associated with poor outcome. One study reported that 43% of ill patients sought medical care locally while on their trip.[2] In 1 small study, there was no significant difference in observed complications based on the immunosuppressive regimen[9] and data were not presented in the remaining studies.

Assessment of risk in the individual SOTR

The first step in advising SOTRs who plan to travel is to assess their net immunosuppression, taking into account the time since their transplant, immunosuppressive regimen, any recent episodes of rejection, any immunomodulating infections such as cytomegalovirus (CMV), and comorbidities. Some antirejection strategies, such as lymphocyte-depleting therapies can produce prolonged T-cell and B-cell deficits and increase infection risk long after the therapy is completed.[10] Although most authorities, including the CDC's Health Information for the International Travel, recommend postponing travel to high-risk destinations until beyond a year after solid-organ transplants,[11] there are few data currently available about the risks of travel early after transplant, with no increased risk seen in a few small series.[2,3,9] Risks may be mitigated by routine prophylaxis such as trimethoprim/sulfamethoxazole (TMP/SMX), which in addition to decreasing the risk of pneumocystis, also likely decreases the risk of travel-related toxoplasmosis, *Isospora*, *Cyclospora*, *Listeria*, and some other gastrointestinal, urinary, and respiratory pathogens. TMP/SMX prophylaxis may also decrease the risk of malaria, as seen in studies of human immunodeficiency virus (HIV)-infected hosts in Africa,[12] although it should not be used alone for malaria prophylaxis because of resistance. Previous vaccinations (especially those done before immunosuppression) may also somewhat mitigate risk, but presumably the efficacy is less than it would be in an immunocompetent traveler.

Travel itinerary assessment and initial considerations

Assessing the precise risk of a traveler for illness in a given location is impossible. For some infections, but certainly not all, there are good data for disease incidence in the local population. However, this may overestimate the disease risk to travelers, who likely have different exposures than the locals, but may also underestimate the travelers' risk because of the immunity of the local population due to past infection or routine vaccination. When collecting data specifically on illness in travelers, it may be difficult to determine where the disease was acquired if the itinerary included several locations. In addition, focusing on travelers presenting acutely during or after travel underestimates the risk of travel-related illnesses that have prolonged incubation periods. In 1 study 10% of travel-related illnesses presented more than 6 months after travel,[13] making them more difficult to link to travel specifics. It is then difficult to establish the total number of travelers to a given location to get the denominator to calculate an incidence rate. Therefore, much of the current data regarding the incidence of travel-related illness are based on extrapolations of the limited data available. Disease risks are not stable over time because new infections continue to emerge and established infections continue to shift, yet for many illnesses, data regarding the incidence of infection in travelers are based on figures collected more than 20 years ago.[14]

Therefore, specific travel plans need to be carefully assessed, looking not only at the destination country but also the specific areas of travel within the country, what activities are planned, the type of accommodation, and the season and duration of the trip. In many countries, infection risk for malaria and yellow fever is not holoendemic; only certain areas have known risk of transmission. A commonly used and authoritative source for up-to-date information about infection risk in a given area can be found on the CDC's Travelers' Health Web site at http://wwwnc.cdc.gov/travel/default.aspx. Longer trips are associated with increased risk of illness, including exposure to malaria and tuberculosis.[15] Weather conditions may also greatly influence risk; for example, there is increased chance of insect-transmitted infections during warm rainy seasons, but increased risk of meningococcus during dry seasons. There are also large differences in risk for travelers who are going on a business trips versus adventure tours versus other reasons for travel. As noted earlier, foreign-born SOTRs are more likely to travel, so it is important to know the increased risks of visiting friends and relatives (VFR). In the United States, VFRs account for more than 50% of cases of malaria.[11] Typhoid is 7 times more likely in VFRs, representing 66% of total cases. Intestinal parasites are 4 times more likely and sexually transmitted infections are also more common.[16] VFRs are twice as likely as other travelers to receive a diagnosis of a vaccine-preventable cause of fever, and are less likely than other travelers to have sought pretravel medical advice.[17]

SOTRs should be advised to speak to their provider before booking trips, so that modifications can be made to the itinerary if necessary. However, a pretravel consultation even the day before travel is better than none at all. An ideal time to speak about potential travel, especially in foreign-born patients, is actually before transplant. This allow some live vaccines that are contraindicated after solid-organ transplant, such as yellow fever vaccine, to be given. There is also a greater likelihood of response to vaccinations before transplant.

Every travel-related medical visit should include assessment of travel risk, advice on minimizing the risk of illness and injury, and provision of appropriate vaccines and prescriptions. For the SOTR, it is essential to ensure that the graft is functioning well, medication levels are achieving their goal, and the patient is overall fit for travel. Medication adherence should be stressed before travel; issues including time changes, carrying medications on their person, and bringing extra medication to avoid the risk of losing pills or unexpectedly having to prolong the trip, must be stressed. It also can be helpful to have a letter from their physician attesting to the medication that they are taking to decrease the risk of confiscation of a large number of pills by customs.

SOTRs should bring a summary of their medical history, including recent laboratory results and a list of current medications, on their trip. They need to consider obtaining medical evacuation insurance, although it may be somewhat cost prohibitive because of their underlying medical issues. Before travel, they should investigate the closest transplant center and experienced specialists available. They need to figure out access to the most state-of-the-art facility possible, and if not possible, they should have an evacuation plan in place. **Box 1** reviews the important components of a travel visit for the SOTR.

Vaccine-Preventable Diseases

In a study of ill returning travelers, more than 50% of patients with vaccine-preventable diseases required hospitalization.[18] Given the serious nature of these infections, vaccines are part of the mainstay of protecting travelers, including SOTRs. However, their efficacy in SOTRs may not match that of a healthy host, and some are contraindicated in immunocompromised patients. Although there has been theoretic concern about rejection from immune stimulation with vaccination, there is no evidence linking

---

Box 1
Practical Tips for the Travel Visit

Assess the health of the traveler

Time since transplant, last episode of rejection, status of graft, additional medical conditions, immunosuppressive regimen and other medications, allergies, immunization history

Assess the risk of the itinerary

Specific destinations, season of travel, duration, travel style, accommodation, activities

Preventive advice

Vaccine-preventable illness (indications, safety, and tolerability and decreased efficacy of vaccines, vaccination of travel companions)

Food and water safety, symptomatic and antibiotic self-treatment of traveler's diarrhea

Malaria prevention (benefits of a particular regimen vs potential adverse reactions)

Insect protection (use of protective clothing, repellents, bed nets, and insecticides)

Exposure risks from locals and other travelers, including sexual health

Environmental hazards

Animal avoidance

Travel medical kits (including extra medication)

Medication adherence

Travel health and medical evacuation insurance

Access to medical care overseas, with investigation of closest transplant facilities

Vaccinations (routine and travel related)

Prescriptions for self-treatment of traveler's diarrhea, antimalarials if indicated, acute mountain sickness prophylaxis if indicated

Letter of yellow fever waiver if needed, attestations to medications, medical summary/latest laboratory results

---

vaccines with graft rejection.[19] The degree of immunosuppression at the time of vaccine administration affects efficacy. It is standard to wait 6 months after transplant, at a time when immunosuppression is generally decreased, to give routine vaccinations so that there is increased chance of attaining a protective antibody response.[19]

In general, efficacy is evaluated in terms of the serologic response to vaccination, as a much larger population than is feasible would be needed to see differences in the development of disease, especially with the less common infections. Although they may not be as accurate a measure after transplant, currently serologies are used to predict disease protection after vaccination, with evaluation of antibody titers before and 4 weeks after vaccination. Unfortunately testing is not always commercially available, and there is little guidance on the steps to take when there is less than the 4-fold increase standardly used as evidence of seroconversion in healthy hosts.[20] There are a reasonable amount of data on a few routine vaccinations used in SOTRs; however, for most vaccines, and particularly for travel-related vaccines, there are few data to evaluate. A systematic review of the literature from 1985 to 2010 was performed to identify prospective controlled studies reporting titers before and after vaccination against influenza, pneumococcal, meningococcal, hepatitis A and B, tetanus, pertussis, varicella, and zoster among patients on immunosuppressive therapies. Of the 972 studies identified, only 15 met the inclusion criteria, and no appropriate studies were found for meningococcal, hepatitis A, hepatitis B, tetanus, pertussis, varicella, or zoster vaccination.[21] Therefore, most advice on travel vaccination in SOTR comes from extrapolation of data from the general population or occasionally from data derived from other immunocompromised hosts. **Table 1** reviews the general

Table 1
Vaccinations for the SOTR Traveler

Vaccine	Indications	Schedule	Comments
Hepatitis A	Recommended for all, especially for areas with intermediate or high risk, and all liver transplant recipients	0 and 6–12 mo, check titers	Immunoglobulin if nonimmune after vaccine or if travel in less than 2 weeks
Hepatitis B	Recommended for all, especially for areas with intermediate or high risk	3- or 4-shot series, check titers	
Influenza	Recommended for all	Annually	Avoid nasal live attenuated vaccine
Japanese encephalitis	Recommended for prolonged or intense exposure in endemic areas during transmission season	0 and 28 d, booster after 1 y if continued/recurrent risk	
Meningococcus	Required for Hajj and Umrah, recommended for travel to meningitis belt or asplenia	Single vaccine, booster every 5 y if continued/recurrent risk	
MMR	Avoid in SOTR	NA	Appropriate for contacts if indicated
Pneumococcus	Recommended for all	One PCV13, PPSV23 >8 wk later, PPSV23 5 y later	
Polio	Recommended for travel to areas where polio cases are still occurring	One-time adult booster in normal host, consider checking titers	Live oral vaccine contraindicated
Rabies	Recommended for travel with high risk of animal exposure	0, 7, 28 d, check titers	May still need human rabies immunoglobulin after exposure
Tetanus/Tdap	Recommended for all	One-time Tdap, then Td every 10 y in normal hosts	Consider checking diphtheria titers
Typhoid	Recommended for travel to areas where there is an increased risk	Every 2 y in normal hosts	Avoid live oral vaccine
Varicella/Zoster	Avoid in SOTR	NA	Appropriate for contacts if indicated
Yellow fever	Avoid in SOTR, document exemption when required	NA	Appropriate for contacts if indicated

indications, contraindications, and schedule of vaccines that may be recommended for the SOTR traveler.

Travel-Related Vaccines

Hepatitis A

In ill travelers presenting to GeoSentinel clinics, hepatitis A was the second most common vaccine-preventable illness.[18] The risk of hepatitis A in nonimmune travelers in developing regions is estimated to be 1 in 1000 per week for the usual tourist routes, and 1 in 200 for more remote travel.[22] In 2007, 85% of travel-related cases in the United States came from Central and South America. Although the risk is higher with travel off the beaten path, cases of travel-related hepatitis A can also occur in developing countries even when travelers stick to the usual tourist activities, accommodation, and restaurants.[11] There are no specific data on hepatitis A infection in SOTRs, but it has been shown to be associated with more fulminant hepatic failure in chronic hepatitis C infections[23] and may also be associated with increased risk in liver transplant recipients.

In healthy adults less than 40 years of age, hepatitis A vaccination, even given just before travel, is sufficient to offer protection. After completing the standard 2 dose series, seroprotective levels in this group persist for at least 5 to 12 years and likely for more than 20 years based on mathematical modeling.[24] However, most studies of hepatitis A vaccine in SOTRs show decreased efficacy compared with healthy adults. Studies of hepatitis A seronegative SOTRs given hepatitis A vaccine using the standard 2-dose series showed 8% to 41% seroconversion 1 month after the first shot and 26% to 97% at 1 month after the second shot.[25,26] SOTRs also have been shown to have more rapid decline of hepatitis A antibody than healthy hosts. In 1 study of SOTRs who initially had shown seroconversion after standard vaccine, the rate of protection after 2 years was 59% in liver transplant recipients and 26% in renal transplant recipients.[27] There are currently no data on what to do for those who have received standard vaccine and no longer have protective hepatitis A antibody levels, or upfront strategies to increase the durability of protection.

An additional strategy for hepatitis A protection is intramuscular gamma globulin, which is 85% to 90% effective at protecting against hepatitis A infection, although this effect is short lived. For less than 3 months of protection, a dose of 0.02 mL/kg is recommended; for 3 to 5 months of protection, a dose of 0.06 mL/kg is recommended.[11] For immunocompromised travelers, including SOTRs, traveling within 2 weeks, the initial dose of hepatitis A vaccine should be given along with immunoglobulin (0.02 mL/kg) at a separate anatomic site.[11] For those who have sufficient time before departure, it would be optimal to check the hepatitis A titer 4 weeks after vaccination, and provide immunoglobulin if they have not reached seroprotective levels.

Meningococcus

Neisseria meningitidis is found worldwide, but the highest incidence of meningococcal disease occurs in the "meningitis belt" that stretches across part of sub-Saharan Africa. In this region, there are periodic epidemics during the dry season (December to June), at which times the rate can be as high as 1000 cases per 100,000. Proof of receipt of meningococcal vaccination is required for people traveling to Mecca during the annual Hajj and Umrah pilgrimages because of past outbreaks.[11]

The meningococcal vaccine has not been studied in adult SOTRs, but in a small study (10 patients) of pediatric SOTRs, the vaccine was shown to be safe and relatively effective. In increase in serum bactericidal antibody titers was seen in all patients. However, 40% had a delayed immune response, which may be relevant to the timing of vaccination before a trip to an endemic region. There was a significant decrease in titers after 6 months, which is important because the standard recommendations for revaccination of those at continued risk is after 5 years.[28] It may be reasonable to check titers and give an earlier booster if protective levels are no longer present. All SOTRs who had splenectomy as part of an intestinal or multivisceral transplant, or for other underlying disease, should get meningococcal vaccination every 5 years, regardless of their travel destination (and a one-time vaccination against *Haemophilus influenza*).

Polio

There are few remaining countries with ongoing cases of wild-type polio, but there is also some risk of transmission from exposure to those shedding vaccine-associated virus. Given the rarity of polio nowadays, there are no data about polio disease in SOTRs, but there are limited data about seroprotection with vaccine.

In a study of 164 adult renal transplant recipients, only 3% showed protective antibody levels against all 3 poliovirus types before an adult booster dose, significantly less than in healthy controls. The difference between rates of seroprotection in SOTRs versus controls was most pronounced for poliovirus type 2. This is particularly relevant to SOTRs traveling to areas where the oral polio vaccine is still used and there may be circulating vaccine-derived polioviruses, because the type 2 oral polio vaccine (OPV) strain seems to spread most readily.[29] Fortunately, the seroprotection rates after an inactivated polio vaccine (IPV) booster were 86% to 92% for each poliovirus type, and there was no significant difference compared with healthy controls.[29]

The current recommendation for travelers to polio endemic regions is for a one-time adult booster dose of IPV if they received standard childhood polio vaccination.[11] There are no separate recommendations in immunocompromised hosts, but antibody levels should likely be checked for SOTRs traveling additional times to endemic areas, and additional booster doses given if antibody levels are below protective levels.

Typhoid

In travelers presenting to GeoSentinel clinics, typhoid fever was the most common vaccine-preventable illness.[18] The risk of *Salmonella typhi* and *paratyphi* is highest in south Asia, but it is also endemic in east and southeast Asia, Africa, the Caribbean, and Central and South America. Travelers visiting friends and relatives are at particularly increased risk. Although typhoid fever is more common during prolonged travel, it has been seen after short trips to endemic areas.[11] *Salmonella* infections can lead to severe complications in SOTRs,[20] but there are less data on *S typhi* and *paratyphi* specifically. Renal transplant patients may be at increased risk of *S typhi* infection of the genitourinary system and be at increased risk of becoming chronic typhoid carriers.[30]

Typhoid vaccine response even in the healthy traveler is believed to be only 50% to 80%,[11] and although it has not been directly studied in SOTRs, it can be presumed that adequate protection is even less likely. In addition, the inactivated vaccine has no protection against *S paratyphi*, whereas the contraindicated oral vaccine offers about 50% protection.[31] Although the live oral typhoid vaccine has not been shown to cause disseminated disease, it is contraindicated in SOTRs because of theoretic risks, in part because of an effective inactivated alternative. There are no commercially available tests to assess for vaccine efficacy.

Yellow fever

The estimated risk of acquiring yellow fever in an unvaccinated traveler during a 2-week stay in an endemic region is approximately 50 per 100,000 in West Africa and 5 per 100,000 in South America.[11] Yellow fever vaccine is a live attenuated virus, and there have been cases of fatal encephalitis following vaccination in immunocompromised hosts.[32] There have been episodes of inadvertent yellow fever vaccination in SOTRs, and a questionnaire from Brazil found 19 physician-reported cases of administration of yellow fever vaccine. In this small series there were no side effects reported voluntarily, but there may have been reporting bias and it is unclear if some of these patients had some baseline immunity from previous vaccination.[33]

It is best to vaccinate potential travelers to areas endemic for yellow fever before transplant if possible, and transplant candidates born in yellow fever endemic areas particularly should be questioned about potential future travel. However, there are no data on how well a pretransplant yellow fever vaccine protects the individual after transplant. In patients immunocompromised from HIV, yellow fever vaccine response was not as robust and immunity waned more rapidly than in immunocompetent controls[34]; similar outcomes can be assumed for SOTRs. Yellow fever serology testing is not commercially available but can be obtained through the CDC in certain circumstances.

At this time, yellow fever vaccination is absolutely contraindicated in all SOTRs, and it is best to alter a traveler's itinerary to avoid endemic areas. If travel to an endemic region is unavoidable, the SOTR should try to avoid the peak season (ie, January to May in South America, and July to October in rural West Africa).[11] When traveling to a yellow fever endemic area without vaccination, strict adherence to insect protection measures is crucial, particularly during dawn and dusk, the *Aedes* mosquito's maximum biting times.[35]

If traveling to a country that requires documentation of yellow fever vaccination in the International Certificate of Vaccination or Prophylaxis, the Medical Contraindication to Vaccination section should be filled out and stamped in an official yellow fever vaccination center. In addition, the traveler should be given a letter of medical exemption on the physician's letterheaded stationary, which should again carry the official stamp. The letter of medical exemption will likely be accepted by some, but not all, governments, and it is possible that the traveler may be denied entrance, quarantined, or be offered immediate vaccination under questionable circumstances to avoid being sent back.[35] To improve the likelihood that the waiver will be accepted by local authorities in the destination country, the CDC suggests that the traveler carry documentation of requirements for waivers obtained from the country's embassy or consulate.[11]

Japanese encephalitis virus

Japanese encephalitis virus (JEV) is the most common vaccine-preventable cause of encephalitis in Asia, although the overall incidence among travelers to Asia is estimated to be less than 1 per 1 million travelers. It is recommended for travelers who will spend at least a month in endemic areas during the JEV transmission season, shorter travel time with more intense exposure risks, travel to areas with an outbreak of JEV, or those unsure of their travel plans.[11] There are no data on JEV in SOTRs or on the efficacy of the vaccine in SOTRs, and there is no commercially available testing for antibody levels. However, Ixiaro, the only vaccine currently available in the United States, is not a live vaccine and presumably has no additional safety concerns for SOTRs.

Rabies

Rabies exists essentially worldwide, but in certain areas, canine rabies remains highly enzootic, including parts of Africa, Asia, and Central and South America. The rate of possible rabies exposure in travelers is roughly 16 to 200 per 100,000 travelers.[11] Even in healthy hosts, once there are signs of disease, rabies causes progressive encephalopathy and death with rare exception. Although there are no specific cases of rabies infection after animal exposure in SOTRs in the literature, several donor-derived cases have been documented.[36,37]

The data on rabies vaccination of SOTRs comes mainly from cases of postexposure prophylaxis (PEP). In a systematic literature review of 16 immunocompromised patients potentially exposed to rabies, 7 did not show the acceptable World Health Organization (WHO) cut-off virus-neutralizing antibody (VNA) titer level at any of the reported measurement points during and after administration of the initial PEP regimen.[38] One of these cases was a renal transplant recipient bitten by a rabid dog, who did not show adequate titers after standard PEP, but did after reduction of his immunosuppression and a second 5-shot series.[39] However, in 8 pediatric SOTRs with bat exposure, all showed adequate seroprotection during standard PEP, though 1 patient showed a delayed response.[40] The CDC recommends that immunosuppressed patients avoid activities for which rabies preexposure prophylaxis is indicated (such as travel to hyperendemic areas), and if preexposure vaccination is given, to have antibody titers checked after vaccination.[11] Because many immuno-compromised hosts, including SOTRs, may not mount adequate antibody responses to preexposure vaccination, some recommend administration of human rabies immu-noglobulin after potential rabies exposure regardless of rabies vaccine status.[41]

Tick-borne encephalitis virus

Tick-borne encephalitis (TBE) virus is endemic in forested areas of Central and Eastern Europe, Russia, and China. The overall risk of acquiring TBE for an unvaccinated visitor to a highly endemic area during the spring to fall transmission season for TBE virus has been estimated at 1 case per 10,000 person-months of exposure.[11] There are no data on TBE in SOTRs, but the vaccine has been studied in a small group of SOTRs. In a study of 31 heart transplant recipients, the seroconversion rate to TBE vaccine was markedly reduced compared with controls (35% vs 100%), but was not found to have any increased risk of adverse events compared with controls.[42] There is no TBE vaccine licensed in the United States, but for travelers with plans for significant exposure risks, inactivated TBE vaccination is available in Europe and Canada.[11]

Cholera

Overall there is low risk of cholera in most travelers; with only a single traveler diag-nosed with cholera out of 25,867 total ill travelers in the GeoSentinel database,[43] but the attack rate can be high in outbreak settings with poor sanitation. The greatest overall risk from cholera is rapid dehydration, which could be especially devastating to an SOTR, although there are no specific data available. There are inactivated oral cholera vaccines, but none available in the United States, and vaccine has not been studied in SOTRs. Travel to areas with cholera outbreaks should be discouraged, and for those SOTRs who plan on traveling anyway, obtaining vaccine from other sources should be investigated.

Routine Vaccinations

In addition to providing appropriate travel-related vaccines, the Infectious Diseases Society of America (IDSA) Travel Medicine guidelines give their highest recommenda-tion to the pretravel visit being used to update vaccinations that are routinely recom-mended according to US schedules and based on the traveler's age and underlying health status.[35]

Tetanus, diphtheria, and acellular pertussis

Tetanus exists in soil worldwide, and there is no specific increased risk in travel, aside from the potential increased risk of injury based on the traveler's activities and unfa-miliar surroundings. However, if an unvaccinated traveler sustains an injury overseas, tetanus toxoid is required, and it is preferable to avoid injections in many local health care settings. Diphtheria, on the other hand, is much more common in developing countries because of lack of vaccination in the local population. Outbreaks have occurred in Haiti and the Dominican Republic, but exist worldwide. It is a devastating illness even in the healthy host, with 5% to 10% mortality despite therapy.[11]

Seroprotection against tetanus after tetanus-diphtheria vaccination in SOTRs seems to be similar to that of healthy controls. However, seroprotection against diphtheria may wane more rapidly in this population.[29,44,45] All travelers vaccinated more than 10 years ago should routinely be vaccinated. For SOTRs traveling to areas where diphtheria is endemic, antibody titers should be checked and vaccine should be given if the titer is below the level of protection. If time allows, diphtheria antibody levels should be checked at least 4 weeks after vaccination. There are no specific data on pertussis response in SOTRs, but the current recommendation by the Advisory Committee on Immunization Practices (ACIP) is a one-time booster dose of tetanus, diphtheria, and acellular pertussis vaccine when tetanus boosting is indicated.[46]

Varicella zoster virus
The risk of exposure to varicella zoster virus (VZV) is higher in most other parts of the world than in the United States,[11] so travel is an important risk factor for primary varicella infections in those who are non-immune. In 1 study, 82% of cases of disseminated varicella in SOTRs were from primary infection and the mortality rate was 34%.[47] Both the varicella and herpes zoster vaccine are currently contraindicated in SOTRs, although there are small studies showing evidence of safety and relative efficacy of varicella vaccine use in pediatric SOTRs.[48]

Because SOTRs will have some degree of lifelong immunosuppression, there will be lifelong risk of VZV reactivation in those with history of varicella or varicella vaccine, and lifelong risk of primary varicella following exposure in those who are nonimmune. VZV prophylaxis with either valacyclovir or valganciclovir, as part of a preventive strategy for herpes viruses after solid-organ transplant, is known to be effective for short-term use during highest levels of immunosuppression, but there are insufficient data to recommend long-term VZV prophylaxis in SOTRs.[49] Although it has been studied in postexposure prophylaxis rather than preexposure prophylaxis, pooled immunoglobulin may offer some protection. Immunoglobulin is not approved for this indication, but may possibly provide some protection if it was given for reasons such as prevention of hepatitis A.

Measles, mumps, and rubella
Worldwide there are an estimated 20 million cases of measles each year,[11] and measles is still common in some parts of Europe, Asia, the Pacific, and Africa. In parts of the world where measles vaccination uptake is low, there is increased risk to susceptible travelers. Mumps is endemic in many areas of the world because mumps vaccine is used in only about 60% of the WHO member countries. The risk of travel exposure to mumps remains high in many developing and even industrialized countries, including the United Kingdom and Japan.[11] In SOTRs, measles has been implicated in acute graft rejection[50] and mumps has been shown to directly invade the graft and cause graft failure.[51]

In healthy patients more than 1 year of age, a single dose of measles, mumps, rubella (MMR) vaccine is approximately 80% effective against mumps and 95% effective against measles, and 2 doses are approximately 90% and 99% effective, respectively.[11] There are small studies of MMR vaccination in pediatric SOTRs, which have not shown evidence of graft rejection or disease from the vaccine-associated virus.[48] However, this has not been evaluated in adult SOTRs and would not currently be recommended. Ideally immunity should be assessed in the transplant candidate and vaccine given if non-immune.

Before travel to endemic areas, serologic evidence of immunity against measles, mumps, and rubella should be evaluated in all SOTRs. Immunoglobulin can be used temporarily to prevent or mitigate measles in a susceptible person, and may be considered in susceptible SOTRs traveling to endemic areas.[11] Immunoglobulin is not effective in preventing mumps infection after exposure and is not recommended.[11]

Hepatitis B

There are no specific data about the risk for hepatitis B infection among US travelers, but in worldwide international travelers presenting to GeoSentinel clinics, hepatitis B was the fourth most common vaccine-preventable illness, and the median trip duration of those presenting with hepatitis B was only a week and a half.[18] Hepatitis B is transmitted via body fluids, and the biggest risk to most travelers is through sexual encounters or unexpected need for local health care, where there may be risk of a contaminated blood supply and inadequately sterilized or reused equipment. Immunocompromised hosts are more likely to develop chronic infection after exposure.

In healthy adults not immune to hepatitis B undergoing standard 3-dose hepatitis B vaccination at 0, 1, and 6 months, a single vaccine gave seroprotective levels to only 7.5% of patients, the second brought seroprotection to 50%, and the third brought it to 92%.[52] The response rates in SOTRs or even solid-organ transplant candidates, however, are much poorer. Of those cirrhotic patients vaccinated before transplant, up to 35% of those who initially seroconverted before transplant have antibody levels below protective levels after liver transplantation.[53] Seroconversion in adults after transplant with standard 3-dose vaccine schedule is even worse, with rates less than 15%.[54–56] However, in a study of pediatric liver transplant recipients, 85% developed seroprotective hepatitis B surface antibody levels after immunization; 70% responded to the standard 3-dose series, and 50% of the primary nonresponders seroconverted after a double-dose booster.[57]

Various vaccine strategies have been used in SOTRs and other immunocompromised hosts, including alternative routes of administration, higher dosing, and experimental vaccine adjuvants, with varying degrees of success.[58,59] In hemodialysis and other immunocompromised patients, it is recommended to measure hepatitis B surface antibody titers at least 4 weeks after vaccination, with a titer greater than 10 mIU/mL considered protective; hemodialysis patients should be given a booster if the level is nonprotective.[60] Extrapolating from data and practice in hemodialysis patients, the American Society of Transplantation (AST) Infectious Diseases Community of Practice recommends that serial hepatitis B surface antibody titers should be assessed both before and every 6 to 12 months after transplantation to assess ongoing immunity.[19] Ideally, SOTRs who anticipate travel to areas with intermediate or high risk of hepatitis B transmission should start hepatitis B immunization at least 6 months before departure to give them the best chance of protection.

Influenza

In travelers presenting to GeoSentinel clinics, influenza was the third most common vaccine-preventable illness.[18] Influenza transmission is year round in the tropics, and the southern hemisphere has an opposite flu season to the northern hemisphere (April to September vs October to May).[11] Almost 3% of travelers to tropical and subtropical areas seroconvert, and 62% of them contracted influenza outside the season of their home country.[61] Cruises, which are frequently targeted by those with underlying medical issues including SOTRs as a safer form of travel, may confer increased risk of influenza throughout the year because there is often gathering of travelers from all over the world in a close contact environment.[11]

SOTRs are likely at increased risk of acquiring influenza and seem to be at increased risk of more severe infection. In 1 study, secondary bacterial pneumonia occurred in 17% of patients, and complications included myocarditis, myositis, and bronchiolitis obliterans. Of those that had biopsies, 62% showed some degree of acute allograft rejection.[62]

In terms of the efficacy of standard trivalent influenza vaccine in SOTRs, the results in the literature are mixed for both initial and persistent protection. One study of 165 renal transplant recipients showed similar rates of seroconversion following standard trivalent influenza vaccine compared with healthy controls, without any episodes of rejection.[63] In another study, more than 70% of lung transplant patients maintained seroprotective influenza titers to most influenza antigens from the previous season when tested just before their next annual vaccination. Seroprotection rates were similar compared with healthy controls.[64] There are also limited data on clinical outcomes in SOTRs for influenza vaccination. In 1 small study of heart transplant recipients, influenza-like illness was reported in about 30% of those who received influenza vaccine compared with about 60% of those receiving placebo.[65] In a retrospective analysis of pediatric liver transplant recipients vaccinated with 2009 pandemic H1N1 vaccine, the frequency of laboratory confirmed infection was 4% compared with 25% in unvaccinated patients.[66]

However, most studies show decreased seroprotection in SOTRs compared with healthy controls.[67] The decreased response in some studies was more pronounced in those receiving mycophenolate as part of their immunosuppressive regimen.[63,67] In terms of durability of seroprotection, a multicenter prospective study of 100 SOTRs showed only 30% of initial responders to the 2009 pandemic H1N1 vaccine maintained seroprotective titers at the start of the 2010 to 2011 flu season.[68]

Booster dosing of influenza vaccine has been examined as a method for increasing levels of protection, but has shown discrepancies in the literature,[63,68,69] and there is insufficient evidence at this time to recommend boosting except for those who were initially vaccinated within the first 3 months after solid-organ transplant.[70] There are also insufficient data to recommend high-dose, adjuvant, or intradermal vaccine to increase initial seroconversion or protect from waning immunity.[70]

Given the risk of influenza during travel, and the risk of more severe infection, SOTRs who have not been vaccinated within the past year should be vaccinated despite the possibly reduced efficacy, although vaccine may be more difficult to obtain after cessation of the influenza season domestically. The nasal live attenuated influenza vaccine is contraindicated in SOTRs.

Pneumococcus

Pneumococcal disease occurs worldwide, with reported rates higher in developing countries than in industrialized countries. Overall, pneumococcal disease is more common during winter and early spring, when respiratory viruses are circulating.[11] Compared with the general population, SOTRs have more than 12 times the incidence of invasive pneumococcal disease.[71]

In a study of 49 renal transplant recipients vaccinated using pneumococcal polysaccharide vaccine 23 (PPSV23), the 15-month total antibody concentration and the number of serotypes with protective antibodies decreased much more rapidly than in historic healthy controls.[72] Studies looking for strategies to increase the immunogenicity and durability of pneumococcal vaccination in SOTRs have not shown evidence of success. In a small study of heart and lung transplant recipients, 7-valent pneumococcal conjugate vaccine (PCV7) followed by PPSV23 did not provide any additional protection beyond the initial response to PCV7.[73] Similarly, in 130 liver transplant recipients, immunogenicity was not enhanced with PCV7 followed by a PPSV23 booster 8 weeks later, compared with vaccination with PPSV23 alone.[74]

However, based on a study of adults infected with HIV who showed decreased pneumococcal disease with PCV7,[75] in October 2012 the ACIP recommended that adults with compromised immune systems routinely receive the conjugate vaccine with 13-valent pneumococcal conjugate vaccine (PCV13). Adult SOTRs who are pneumococcal vaccine naive should receive a dose of PCV13 first, followed by a dose of PPSV23 at least 8 weeks later, followed by a second dose of PPSV23 5 years later. SOTRs previously vaccinated with PPSV23 should be given a PCV13 dose at least 1 year after the last PPSV23 dose. For those who require additional doses of PPSV23, the first such dose should be given no sooner than 8 weeks after PCV13 and at least 5 years after the most recent dose of PPSV23.[76]

Vaccination of Close Contacts of SOTRs

The SOTR's traveling companions should proceed with necessary vaccination, in part, with some vaccines, to protect the SOTR as well. Although live attenuated influenza vaccine (intranasal) should be avoided if the inactive version is available, other routine and travel-related live vaccines such as MMR, yellow fever, oral typhoid, varicella, and zoster vaccines are less likely to be transmitted and may be given to close contacts.[77] The 2009 AST solid-organ transplant vaccine guidelines actually recommend (although based on their lowest level of recommendation) that close contacts get MMR and varicella vaccination to help prevent exposure of the transplant recipient to higher levels of wild-type virus if the contact were to get natural infection.[19]

Traveler's Diarrhea and Other Food-Borne and Water-Borne Illnesses

Diarrhea is the most common illness of travelers, affecting around 50% of travelers to developing regions.[11] In travelers unwell enough to present to a GeoSentinel clinic, acute diarrhea was the second most common complaint; chronic diarrhea was the fourth most common presentation.[13,78] Enterotoxogenic *Escherichia coli* (ETEC) is the most common cause of diarrhea and usually resolves spontaneously in 3 to 5 days, but in SOTRs there is the potential for altered absorption of essential medications and dehydration, which can worsen renal function and increase the risk of drug toxicity and graft dysfunction. In terms of the other bacteria often the cause of traveler's diarrhea, a study from Turkey of SOTRs with diarrhea showed 12% had acute bacterial diarrhea with *Campylobacter*, *Shigella*, or *Salmonella*.[79] SOTRs, along with other immunocompromised hosts, have much higher rates of complications from salmonellosis, including bacteremia and metastatic foci, than normal hosts.[80] Higher levels of immunosuppression early after transplant or after episodes of rejection are associated with increased risk of salmonellosis and its complications. Relapses occur commonly despite prolonged antibiotic therapy, occasionally associated with graft loss and even death.[81] In the GeoSentinel database, bacterial diarrhea was most common in travelers returning from southeast Asia, and *Campylobacter* was the predominant cause.[13] *Campylobacter* infections in SOTRs may be more severe and harder to eradicate.[82]

To decrease the risk of developing traveler's diarrhea, SOTRs should be advised of the risks from unsafe food and water. They should avoid unbottled water in all of its hidden forms, fresh fruits and vegetables unless they are cooked or can be peeled, dairy foods, and undercooked meats and seafood. In general, it is likely safer to eat at pricier restaurants that are geared to tourists, because these establishments are looking for future returning customers and referrals. Street vendors should be avoided. Despite the traveler's best efforts, traveler's diarrhea often occurs because the preparation of food is usually out of their hands. The *Practice of Travel Medicine: Guidelines* by the IDSA recommend the provision of antibiotics, not for prevention, but to carry for self-treatment of traveler's diarrhea if it occurs.[35] This recommendation is based on evidence that self-treatment is about 80% effective,[78] and to avoid the potential complications of prophylactic antibiotic treatment (*C difficile*, arrhythmias, and so forth).

SOTRs who develop traveler's diarrhea should self-treat with a fluoroquinolone or azithromycin. However, all the recommended antibiotics for self-treatment of traveler's diarrhea have the added risk of QT prolongation and/or can alter drug levels for patients on tacrolimus. The risk of tendon rupture with quinolones is even greater in patients taking prednisone. There may be an advantage to levofloxacin over ciprofloxacin, because there are fewer significant drug interactions with mycophenolate, sirolimus, and the calcineurin inhibitors.[83] Azithromycin is generally used in travelers to south and southeast Asia, given the increased risk of fluoroquinolone-resistant *Campylobacter*. Similar to ciprofloxacin, azithromycin may prolong the QT interval and increase calcineurin inhibitor levels.[83] It is often recommended that calcineurin inhibitor levels be monitored more closely when used together with agents that may alter drug levels, however, that is rarely realistic in travelers.

In addition to antibiotic treatment of traveler's diarrhea, loperamide (or other antimotility agents) can be helpful for rapid symptom improvement. There are no reported interactions between loperamide and commonly used transplant-related medications. If diarrhea is bloody or accompanied by fever, however, antimotility agents should be used with caution because they may delay clearance of toxins from the gut. Oral rehydration is essential to decrease the risk of renal insufficiency and the potential for renally cleared drug toxicity. If diarrhea does not respond quickly to antibiotic self-treatment, especially if there is fever, blood in the stool, or inability to keep food down, the SOTR should seek medical attention.

There are good data to show that prophylactic antibiotics are effective at decreasing the risk of traveler's diarrhea, but again, the potential side effects of the medications usually outweigh the potential benefits. The IDSA travel guidelines give weak recommendations for prophylaxis in extenuating circumstances, such as in travelers in whom the risk for diarrhea is increased or the consequences of a diarrheal episode may be severe,[35] and it could be argued that some SOTRs may fit this scenario. If prophylactic antibiotics are prescribed, they should be recommended for no more than 2 to 3 weeks.[35] Fluoroquinolones are considered first choice agents given an abundance of evidence of their efficacy; they are given the highest recommendation in the guidelines.[35] Rifaximin, a nonabsorbable antibiotic approved by the US Food and Drug Administration for treatment of traveler's diarrhea caused by *E coli*, has demonstrated a 58% to 72% reduction in traveler's diarrhea in healthy travelers to limited areas where *E coli* is the major cause.[84–86] Use of subsalicylate bismuth (Pepto-Bismol) has been shown to reduce the rate of traveler's diarrhea by about 65%, but it requires 4 times daily use.[87] In addition, SOTRs with decreased renal function are at increased risk of developing salicylate toxicity from Pepto-Bismol.

Intestinal protozoa
Potentially contaminated food and water, encountered from drinking or sometimes recreational water activities, can be the source of many other infections, including intestinal protozoa.

Giardia intestinalis exists worldwide, but is most commonly diagnosed in travelers returning from South America, south Asia, and the Middle East. It accounts for more than one-quarter of the cases of infectious gastrointestinal disease in travelers returning to GeoSentinel clinics.[43] Although there are no reports of worse outcomes in SOTRs, in a Turkish series, 21% of SOTRs with diarrhea were diagnosed with giardiasis.[79]

Cryptosporidium parvum can be transmitted worldwide, although most travel-related cases come from Latin America and the Middle East. About 1% of travelers with infectious gastrointestinal disease presenting to GeoSentinel clinics were diagnosed with cryptosporidiosis.[43] Cryptosporidiosis is usually a self-limiting diarrheal illness in immunocompetent hosts, but can lead to chronic diarrhea with wasting and electrolyte imbalances, and even extraintestinal complications, in immunocompromised hosts. Although there are reports of cryptosporidiosis in SOTRs in the United States, most cases come from SOTRs in developing countries.[88] Studies of diarrhea in SOTRs in developing countries have found *Cryptosporidium* as the causative agent in up to 20% of patients.[79,89]

Cyclospora cayetanensis is reported in 1% of travelers with infectious gastrointestinal disease presenting to GeoSentinel clinics.[43] Cyclosporiasis is most common in tropical and subtropical regions.[11] There are a few case reports of cyclosporiasis causing diarrhea with wasting in renal transplant recipients.[90,91] The course does not seem to be different from that in immunocompetent hosts, but extrapolating from patients infected with HIV, the risk of acquisition may be higher in those with T-cell depression. The number of cases may be smaller than would otherwise be expected because the organism is susceptible to TMP/SMX.

Entamoeba histolytica occurs mainly in areas of Central and South America, Africa, and south Asia. *E histolytica* accounted for 12.5% of cases of diarrhea in returning travelers in the GeoSentinel database.[43] Although it has the potential to cause both intestinal and extraintestinal disease (primary liver abscesses) with increased risk in the immunocompromised host, only a few cases have been reported in SOTRs.[92]

Other Food Risks

SOTRs should be also counseled to avoid unpasteurized dairy products, which may be more commonly encountered during travel, and undercooked meats. The risk of listeriosis in SOTRs is more than 100 times greater than in healthy adults less than 65 years old,[93] with a mortality rate of about 25%.[94,95] Travelers taking TMP/SMX for routine prophylaxis are afforded some protection.[82,94,96] In addition, there have been case reports of *Mycobacteria bovis* infections[94,97,98] and brucellosis, including endocarditis[99] and neurobrucellosis, in renal transplant recipients.[100]

The SOTR should avoid undercooked meats to decrease the risk of acute toxoplasmosis, although most cases of primary toxoplasmosis in SOTRs are donor derived. In a series of febrile returned travelers, 1% were diagnosed with acute toxoplasmosis.[101] The acute infection in immunocompetent hosts generally causes a monolike illness, but can disseminate in immunocompromised hosts. In a case series of SOTRs, toxoplasmosis caused pneumonitis in 32%, myocarditis in 23%, brain involvement in 27%, and was disseminated at diagnosis in 23%, with an overall crude mortality of about 14%.[102] Avoiding undercooked meats also decreases the risk of the usual bacterial causes of traveler's diarrhea as well as the more unusual intestinal and extraintestinal helminthes in travelers.

Undercooked shellfish and seafood should also be avoided to decrease the risk of uncommon parasitic conditions such as anisakiasis and paragonimiasis, but also more common infections including hepatitis A, hepatitis E, and novorvirus.

Hepatitis E

Hepatitis E was the cause of 1% of cases of infectious gastrointestinal disease in the GeoSentinel surveillance system.[43] Epidemics of hepatitis E are principally caused by drinking fecally contaminated water, particularly in Africa and Asia. Sporadic disease in Japan, Europe, the Middle East, Asia, and South America is associated with eating inadequately cooked shellfish, venison, boar meat, and pig liver and sausage.[11] Hepatitis E usually causes acute self-limiting illness in normal hosts, but can cause fulminant hepatic failure in those with preexisting liver disease. Primary infection acquired by people who are immunosuppressed, such as after organ transplantation, may progress to chronic infection.[11] In a study of SOTRs presenting with unexplained increased liver enzymes, 6.5% tested positive for hepatitis E virus RNA. More than 50% of patients developed chronic hepatitis E infection.[103] SOTRs who are exposed to hepatitis E while traveling are presumably at increased risk of more severe acute disease, and at risk for the unusual development of chronic infection.

Norovirus

Norovirus seems to be increasing as a cause of traveler's diarrhea, with rates of up to 17% in returning travelers.[11] It is highly contagious from person to person, but raw or undercooked shellfish are also a frequent source of infection. Large norovirus outbreaks have been reported in hotels, airlines, and cruise ships.[11] This is important in SOTRs, because it has been shown that immunocompromised travelers presenting to travel clinics are more likely than nonimmunocompromised travelers to select cruise travel.[5] It is usually an acute self-limiting illness, but is more severe in immunocompromised hosts. Renal transplant patients are more likely to have electrolyte wasting and decreased renal function, and develop chronic infection than immunocompetent hosts.[104] Norovirus is associated with more weight loss, longer symptom duration, and higher rates of severe graft dysfunction than other causes of diarrhea in renal transplant recipients.[105] SOTRs should practice strict hand hygiene and avoid high-risk foods to decrease their risk of infection.

Malaria and Other Insect-Related Illnesses

Malaria

Malaria is the most common preventable infectious cause of death among returning travelers,[35] and is the leading identifiable cause of fever in travelers presenting to Geo-Sentinel clinics.[17] The greatest relative risk is in sub-Saharan Africa, followed by Oceania and south Asia.[106] The risk of malaria to travelers can change rapidly with the weather conditions, altitude, mosquito control efforts, and so forth. A useful source of the most up-to-date information available is the CDC malaria map (http://www.cdc.gov/malaria/map/index.html); areas can be searched for more specific malaria risk information and recommendations.

Immunocompromised travelers may be predisposed to more serious disease from malaria infection,[11] but there are no data on worse outcomes specifically in SOTRs. Although it is possible that SOTRs are at increased risk of malaria infection if exposed to a parasitized mosquito, most of the cases in the literature on malaria after transplant seem to be from donor-derived infections rather than de novo infections from mosquito exposure. Most cases in SOTRs have been described in renal transplant patients. *Plasmodium falciparum* has been the species in most cases, and is also associated with the most deaths.[92]

For certain regions of the world with increased risk of transmission, antimalarials are indicated in addition to other insect protection methods. There are several different choices of antimalarials, with the initial decision point coming from resistance patterns. There are only limited areas of the world where chloroquine is still effective, and there is emerging mefloquine resistance in southeast Asia. The next important factor in choosing antimalarials in the SOTR is drug interactions. Mefloquine may increase calcineurin inhibitor levels,[107,108] and may increase the risk of arrhythmias when given with TMP/SMX[107,109] or with tacrolimus.[107,108] When given with cyclosporine, mefloquine levels may increase causing increased risk of arrhythmias.[108] Chloroquine similarly may increase calcineurin inhibitor levels,[107,109] and increase the risk of arrhythmias with TMP/SMX[107,109] or tacrolimus.[107,108] Doxycycline may reduce mycophenolate levels[108] although it is not clear if this is clinically significant. Primaquine may increase calcineurin inhibitor levels.[107] Although atovaquone/proguanil is the most expensive option, there are fewer side effects and less risk of drug interactions in this travel population.

Other Insect-Transmitted Infections

Mosquitoes: dengue, chikungunya, West Nile virus

The geographic reach of dengue fever is growing, and it is commonly acquired in urban as well as rural settings. Dengue is the most common cause of fever in travelers returning from southeast Asia, but is also frequent in south Asia, Latin America, and the Caribbean.[17] The presentation in SOTRs seems to be similar to that in immunocompetent patients, although they may actually have less risk of dengue hemorrhagic shock syndrome because it is likely T-cell mediated,[110] a theory that is supported by small case series.[111] Chikungunya is another emerging infectious disease in tropical and subtropical areas, but there are no specific data on its course in SOTRs, and no specific prophylaxis aside from insect protective measures. Although recently the focus of West Nile virus has been in the United States, the virus has a widespread distribution in Africa, Asia, the Middle East, Europe, the Caribbean, and Latin America, and should be included in mosquito-borne risks to SOTR travelers. Although donor transmission has been reported, most cases are naturally acquired or through infected blood products. There is a high case fatality rate, and SOTRs are 40 times more likely to develop neuroinvasive disease.[92] There are currently no vaccinations or prophylactic medications available for any of these illnesses, so mosquito protection is crucial.

Sand flies: leishmaniasis

Leishmaniasis is an infection transmitted by sand flies with a high prevalence rate in southern Europe, India, Kenya, Sudan, and Brazil. Immunocompromised patients may develop de novo infection with a greater frequency than immunocompetent patients. More than 60 cases of visceral leishmaniasis in SOTRs have been described.[92] It is universally fatal in this population without treatment, and the death rate is approximately 20% to 30% even with treatment. Most cases have been described after renal transplant in patients who resided in or traveled to endemic areas without clear data on the route of transmission[110] although the fact that some infections occurred a decade after transplant makes de novo infection slightly more likely. Although there is treatment for leishmaniasis, there are no preventative medications or vaccines, so travelers to endemic regions should avoid outdoor activity from dusk to dawn, when the sand flies are most active, in addition to the other insect protective measures.

Tics: Rickettsia

Rickettsial infections were responsible for 2% of febrile illnesses in GeoSentinel patients presenting with fever.[17] The effect of immunosuppression on the development of complications caused by rickettsial infection is unknown, and Mediterranean spotted fever in a liver transplant recipient seemed to follow the usual clinical course.[112] Travelers taking doxycycline for malaria prophylaxis may have some protection against rickettsioses.

EXPOSURE TO SICK CONTACTS

The risk to most travelers of tuberculosis is small, however, the risk increases with long-term travel and visiting friends and relatives. Latent tuberculosis is 3 times more likely in those traveling for more than 6 months than those traveling for less than 1 month, and the highest rates of purified protein derivative conversion are in Africa.[15] Active tuberculosis was more than 60 times more common among immigrant travelers visiting friends and relatives than tourist travelers.[16] Although most cases of tuberculosis after solid-organ transplant are from reactivation, there are case reports of primary tuberculosis.[113,114] SOTRs are at higher risk of tuberculosis and have a higher mortality rate than healthy individuals.[115] For those SOTRs who may have prolonged exposure to tuberculosis through extended travel to endemic regions, especially those visiting friends and relatives, a pretravel test with an interferon gamma release assay should be considered, and if negative, repeated 8 to 10 weeks after returning from travel.[11] There may be benefit of the T-SPOT.TB test over the QuantiFERON-TB Gold In-Tube test in SOTRs, given the lower likelihood of indeterminate test results in immunocompromised hosts.[116]

Increased sexual promiscuity and casual relationships tend to occur during foreign travel, especially in long-term overseas travelers.[11] In addition to HIV, gonorrhea, chlamydia, syphilis, and hepatitis B, other infections such as acute CMV needs to be addressed in SOTRs. In 1 series, 2% of returning febrile travelers presented with acute CMV, a higher rate of infection than the rate for non–travel-related monolike illnesses.[101] Given the multitude of risks associated with CMV infection in SOTRs, in addition to HIV, hepatitis, syphilis, and so forth, it is crucial that the risks of sexually transmitted infections be discussed with SOTR travelers.

INHALATIONAL RISKS FROM THE ENVIRONMENT

SOTR travelers may be at risk for several endemic fungal infections depending on their destination and planned activities. *Coccidioides* species are endemic in semiarid to arid areas of North, Central, and South America. Rates of disseminated coccidioidomycosis beyond the lungs in SOTRs are as high as 75% in some series.[117] Coccidioidomycosis in SOTRs most often occurs due to reactivation of latent infection, with only rare case reports of naturally occurring infection.[118] Given the rarity of acute infection, even in patients relocating to areas of *Coccidioides* endemicity, there is unlikely a role for fluconazole prophylaxis in travelers.[119]

Histoplasma species are found worldwide. Although overall, histoplasmosis was seen in less than 0.5% of ill travelers in the GeoSentinel database, there are reports of exposure leading to infection in more than 50% of exposed travelers. These include, caving in Trinidad, Belize, Costa Rica, Nicaragua, and Peru,[120–125] church renovation in El Salvador,[126] and staying in a hotel with ongoing construction in Acapulco, Mexico.[125] Although reactivation can occur, histoplasmosis infections in SOTRs have been documented in several outbreak settings, suggesting acute infection from new exposure. Although the lungs are generally the route of exposure, in SOTRs dissemination is frequent, including the development of meningitis.[92,127]

Paracoccidioides brasiliensis exists in Latin America; most cases are found in Brazil. There are only rare case reports of paracoccidioidomycosis in SOTRs, but these cases were all more than 5 years after transplant, implying an increased likelihood of acute infection rather than reactivation. In these cases, the presentation and outcomes were similar to those in immunocompetent hosts. The low incidence of paracoccidioidomycosis in SOTRs in endemic areas may be partly explained by routine use of TMP/SMX prophylaxis, as it has activity against *Paracoccidioides brasiliensis* as well as *Pneumocystis jiroveci*.[92]

Penicillium marneffei is endemic in southeast Asia, and parts of east Asia, including Hong Kong and Taiwan. Several cases have been reported in travelers, mostly in immunocompromised hosts, and it is known to be a cause of severe disseminated opportunistic infections in hosts with T-cell deficiency.[128] There are few reports of *P marneffei* infection in SOTRs, and these cases may have been caused by reactivation rather than new exposure.[92] The specific exposure risk remains unclear, but the incidence in endemic areas increases during the rainy season.[129,130] Some have suggested advising immunocompromised travelers to avoid *P marneffei* endemic areas altogether,[131] but it may also be reasonable to advise those SOTRs who plan to travel to these areas to avoid travel during the rainy season.

To decrease the risks of these endemic fungi, the SOTR traveler should minimize exposure to outdoor dust and avoid hotels, restaurants, and other travel sites with active construction. They should avoid activities during travel that increase the risk of aerosolization of fungal spores such as caving, dirt biking, eco/adventure tourism. If traveling in dust-laden environments, SOTRs should choose transportation with enclosed air-conditioned cabs if possible.[11] In addition, they should be advised of the risk from livestock in local markets and farms. The AST guidelines outlining *Strategies for Safe Living Following Solid Organ Transplantation* give their weakest recommendation to wearing a mask if exposure to high-risk areas is unavoidable.[132]

RISKS FROM SKIN EXPOSURE AND WATER ACTIVITIES

SOTR travelers should also avoid walking barefoot and swimming in fresh water because of the risks of parasitic infections, bites, and cuts increasing the risk of bacterial infections.

Strongyloides stercoralis is a parasite found predominantly in the tropics and subtropics that can penetrate intact skin. In the GeoSentinel database, it was found in 6% of travelers presenting with infectious gastrointestinal disease.[43] For most immunocompetent hosts, the infection is completely asymptomatic. In immunocompromised patients, especially those on corticosteroids, hyperinfection can develop, with dissemination of larvae and gram-negative sepsis and meningitis, with resulting mortality rates as high as 85%.[92] Posttransplant strongyloidiasis may develop after primary infection or transmission via graft, although most transplant-related cases reported are from hyperinfection syndrome following accelerated autoinfection after immunosuppression from asymptomatic infection at the time of transplant.[92]

Schistosoma is a parasite that penetrates intact skin in fresh water in parts of South America, the Caribbean, and east and southeast Asia, but most travel-related infections come from sub-Saharan Africa.[11] *S mansoni* and *S japonicum* invade the liver, and *S haematobium* involves mainly the urinary tract and the kidney, and rarely they can disseminate to other organs including the brain and spinal cord. Of those travelers returning ill and presenting to the GeoSentinel Surveillance Network after travel to a region endemic for *Schistosoma*, 1.6% were diagnosed with active schistosomiasis.[133] However, the attack rate in individuals exposed to a body of water carrying *Schistosoma* is high. There are no data on naturally occurring cases in SOTRs, but for those who had donor-derived infection, or possible reactivation, the disease course seemed similar to that in immunocompetent hosts, and there does not seem to be increased risk of rejection.[92]

Although leptospirosis has a worldwide distribution, rates are highest in the tropics, and most travel-related cases have been seen in southeast Asia, the Caribbean Islands, and Latin America.[134] Leptospirosis was diagnosed in only 0.4% of febrile travelers in the GeoSentinel database,[17] but can have an attack rate of up to 40% in heavily exposed travelers.[135] Travelers participating in recreational water activities, particularly after heavy rainfall or flooding, are at highest risk. There are only a few cases of leptospirosis reported in SOTRs, but one-third of patients died, and all had severe disease characterized by acute renal failure, hepatic failure, and jaundice after exposure via water or rats.[136–138] SOTR travelers should be advised to avoid contact with potentially contaminated water. Although the benefit from chemoprophylaxis remains unclear given the mixed results in the literature,[139] the CDC recommends that adult travelers at increased risk for leptospirosis due to water exposure consider doxycycline prophylaxis (200 mg orally, weekly), started 1 to 2 days before and continuing throughout the period of exposure.[11]

NONINFECTIOUS RISKS

There are several noninfectious risks of travel, including injuries (the leading cause of preventable death in travelers), sunburn (with an increased risk of skin cancers in SOTRs), motion sickness (which may affect the ability to take medications), deep venous thrombosis (especially in intestinal transplant recipients and others known to have hypercoagulable states), and pollution (which may disproportionately affect lung and heart transplant recipients). Depending on the destination, altitude sickness may also be an issue. Travelers who rapidly ascend to altitude are at risk for altitude sickness, including those who fly directly into high-altitude airports. The illness can be a mild form of acute mountain sickness with nuance symptoms, but can also manifest itself in life-threatening high-altitude pulmonary edema or cerebral edema. In a small study of highly selected and carefully prepared liver transplant recipients, altitude was tolerated similarly to healthy climbers on Mount Kilimanjaro.[140] However, travel to altitude has not been studied more broadly in SOTRs and should likely be avoided especially in heart and lung transplant recipients. Acetazolamide decreases the risk and severity of altitude sickness and is offered as standard to travelers who will rapidly ascend to greater than 2500 m.[35] However, acetazolamide has not been studied in SOTRs and it may increase calcineurin inhibitor levels.[107]

SUMMARY

Many SOTRs are traveling internationally and may have greater risk of complications from typical travel-related illnesses and opportunistic infections not faced by healthy individuals. The risk for an individual SOTR depends on their net immunosuppression, graft status, medical comorbidities, and immunization history, along with the specific itinerary and activities of the trip. Transplant and travel providers have the best opportunity to help protect these high-risk travelers, through advice, medications, and safe and appropriate vaccinations, using the best currently available information about destination risks.

REFERENCES

1. United Nations World Tourism Organization (UNWTO). UNWTO tourism highlights. 2012 edition. UNWTO; 2012.
2. Uslan DZ, Patel R, Virk A. International travel and exposure risks in solid-organ transplant recipients. Transplantation 2008;86(3):407–12.

3. Roukens AH, Van Dissel JT, De Fijter JW, et al. Health preparations and travel-related morbidity of kidney transplant recipients traveling to developing countries. Clin Transplant 2007;21(4):567–70.
4. Boggild KA, Sano M, Humar A, et al. Travel patterns and risk behavior in solid organ transplant recipients. J Travel Med 2006;11(1):37–43.
5. Schwartz BS, Rosen J, Han P, et al. Immunocompromised international travelers from the United States, 2009-2011: preliminary analysis of demographic characteristics, travel destinations, and pre-travel health care from the global TravEpiNet consortium. Oral presentation, ID Week. San Diego (CA), October 19, 2012.
6. Ryan ET, Wilson ME, Kain KC. Illness after international travel. N Engl J Med 2002;347(7):505–16.
7. Wieten RW, Leenstra T, Goorhuis A, et al. Health risks of travelers with medical conditions: a retrospective analysis. J Travel Med 2012;19(2):104–10.
8. Baaten GG, Geskus RB, Kint JA, et al. Symptoms of infectious diseases in immunocompromised travelers: a prospective study with matched controls. J Travel Med 2011;18(5):318–26.
9. Kofidis T, Pethig K, Rüther G, et al. Traveling after heart transplantation. Clin Transplant 2002;16(4):280–4.
10. Fishman JA, the AST Infectious Diseases Community of Practice. Introduction: infection in solid organ transplant recipients. Am J Transplant 2009;9:S3–6.
11. Center for Disease Control and Prevention. CDC health information for international travel 2012. New York: Oxford University Press; 2012.
12. Mermin J, Ekwaru JP, Liechty CA, et al. Effect of co-trimoxazole prophylaxis, antiretroviral therapy, and insecticide-treated bednets on the frequency of malaria in HIV-1-infected adults in Uganda: a prospective cohort study. Lancet 2006; 367(9518):1256.
13. Freedman DO, Weld LH, Kozarsky PE, et al. Spectrum of disease and relation to place of exposure among ill returned travelers. N Engl J Med 2006;354(2): 119–30.
14. Leder K, Wilson ME, Freedman DO, et al. A comparative analysis of methodological approaches used for estimating risk in travel medicine. J Travel Med 2008;15(4):263–72.
15. Chen LH, Wilson ME, Davis X, et al. Illness in long-term travelers visiting GeoSentinel clinics. Emerg Infect Dis 2009;15(11):1773.
16. Ericsson CD, Hatz C, Leder K, et al. Illness in travelers visiting friends and relatives: a review of the GeoSentinel surveillance network. Clin Infect Dis 2006; 43(9):1185–93.
17. Wilson ME, Weld LH, Boggild A, et al. Fever in returned travelers: results from the GeoSentinel surveillance network. Clin Infect Dis 2007;44(12):1560–8.
18. Boggild AK, Castelli F, Gautret P, et al. Vaccine preventable diseases in returned international travelers: results from the GeoSentinel surveillance network. Vaccine 2010;28(46):7389–95.
19. Danzinger-Isakov L, Kumar D, the AST Infectious Diseases Community of Practice. Guidelines for vaccination of solid organ transplant candidates and recipients. Am J Transplant 2009;9:S258–62.
20. Kotton CN, Hibberd PL, the AST Infectious Diseases Community of Practice. Travel medicine and the solid organ transplant recipient. Am J Transplant 2009;9:S273–81.
21. Agarwal N, Ollington K, Kaneshiro M, et al. Are immunosuppressive medications associated with decreased responses to routine immunizations? A systematic review. Vaccine 2012;30(8):1413–24.

22. Ryan ET, Kain KC. Health advice and immunizations for travelers. N Engl J Med 2000;342(23):1716–25.
23. Vento S, Garofano T, Renzini C, et al. Fulminant hepatitis associated with hepatitis A virus superinfection in patients with chronic hepatitis C. N Engl J Med 1998;338(5):286–90.
24. Advisory Committee on Immunization Practices (ACIP), Centers for Disease Control and Prevention (CDC). Update: prevention of hepatitis A after exposure to hepatitis A virus and in international travelers. Updated recommendations the Advisory Committee on Immunization Practices (ACIP). MMWR Morb Mortal Wkly Rep 2007;56(41):1080–4.
25. Arslan M, Wiesner RH, Poterucha JJ, et al. Safety and efficacy of hepatitis A vaccination in liver transplantation recipients. Transplantation 2001;72(2):272–6.
26. Stark K, Günther M, Neuhaus R, et al. Immunogenicity and safety of hepatitis A vaccine in liver and renal transplant recipients. J Infect Dis 1999;180(6):2014–7.
27. Günther M, Stark K, Neuhaus R, et al. Rapid decline of antibodies after hepatitis A immunization in liver and renal transplant recipients. Transplantation 2001; 71(3):477–9.
28. Zlamy M, Elias J, Vogel U, et al. Immunogenicity of conjugate meningococcus C vaccine in pediatric solid organ transplant recipients. Vaccine 2011;29(37): 6163–6.
29. Huzly D, Neifer S, Reinke P, et al. Routine immunizations in adult renal transplant recipients. Transplantation 1997;63(6):839–45.
30. Huang DB, DuPont HL. Problem pathogens: extra-intestinal complications of *Salmonella enterica* serotype typhi infection. Lancet Infect Dis 2005;5(6):341–8.
31. Levine MM, Ferreccio C, Black RE, et al. Ty21a live oral typhoid vaccine and prevention of paratyphoid fever caused by *Salmonella enterica* serovar Paratyphi B. Clin Infect Dis 2007;45(Suppl 1):S24–8.
32. Kengsakul K, Sathirapongsasuti K, Punyagupta S. Fatal myeloencephalitis following yellow fever vaccination in a case with HIV infection. J Med Assoc Thai 2002;85(1):131–4.
33. Azevedo LS, Lasmar EP, Contieri FLC, et al. Yellow fever vaccination in organ transplanted patients: is it safe? A multicenter study. Transpl Infect Dis 2012; 14(3):237–41.
34. Veit O, Niedrig M, Chapuis-Taillard C, et al. Immunogenicity and safety of yellow fever vaccination for 102 HIV-infected patients. Clin Infect Dis 2009;48(5): 659–66.
35. Hill DR, Ericsson CD, Pearson RD, et al. The practice of travel medicine: guidelines by the Infectious Diseases Society of America. Clin Infect Dis 2006;43(12): 1499–539.
36. Srinivasan A, Burton EC, Kuehnert MJ, et al. Transmission of rabies virus from an organ donor to four transplant recipients. N Engl J Med 2005;352(11):1103–11.
37. Maier T, Schwarting A, Mauer D, et al. Management and outcomes after multiple corneal and solid organ transplantations from a donor infected with rabies virus. Clin Infect Dis 2010;50(8):1112–9.
38. Kopel E, Oren G, Sidi Y, et al. Inadequate antibody response to rabies vaccine in immunocompromised patient. Emerg Infect Dis 2012;18(9):1493.
39. Rodríguez-Romo R, Morales-Buenrostro LE, Lecuona L, et al. Immune response after rabies vaccine in a kidney transplant recipient. Transpl Infect Dis 2011; 13(5):492–5.
40. Cramer CH II, Shieck V, Thomas SE, et al. Immune response to rabies vaccination in pediatric transplant patients. Pediatr Transplant 2008;12(8):874–7.

41. Gibbons RV, Rupprecht CE. Postexposure rabies prophylaxis in immunosuppressed patients. JAMA 2001;285(12):1574–5.
42. Dengler TJ, Zimmermann R, Meyer J, et al. Vaccination against tick-borne encephalitis under therapeutic immunosuppression. Reduced efficacy in heart transplant recipients. Vaccine 1999;17(7–8):867–74.
43. Swaminathan A, Torresi J, Schlagenhauf P, et al. A global study of pathogens and host risk factors associated with infectious gastrointestinal disease in returned international travellers. J Infect 2009;59(1):19–27.
44. Enke BU, Bökenkamp A, Offner G, et al. Response to diphtheria and tetanus booster vaccination in pediatric renal transplant recipients. Transplantation 1997;64(2):237.
45. Pedrazzi C, Ghio L, Balloni A, et al. Duration of immunity to diphtheria and tetanus in young kidney transplant patients. Pediatr Transplant 1999;3(2):109–14.
46. Center for Disease Control and Prevention. Updated recommendations for use of tetanus toxoid, reduced diphtheria toxoid, and acellular pertussis (Tdap) vaccine in adults aged 65 years and older — Advisory Committee on Immunization Practices (ACIP), 2012. MMWR Morb Mortal Wkly Rep 2012;61(25):468–70.
47. Fehr T, Bossart W, Wahl C, et al. Disseminated varicella infection in adult renal allograft recipients: four cases and a review of the literature. Transplantation 2002;73(4):608–11.
48. Khan S, Erlichman J, Rand EB. Live virus immunization after orthotopic liver transplantation. Pediatr Transplant 2006;10(1):78–82.
49. Pergam SA, Limaye AP, the AST Infectious Diseases Community of Practice. Varicella zoster virus (VZV) in solid organ transplant recipients. Am J Transplant 2009;9:S108–15.
50. Sternfeld T, Spöri-Byrtus V, Riediger C, et al. Acute measles infection triggering an episode of liver transplant rejection. Int J Infect Dis 2010;14(6):e528–30.
51. Baas MC, Van Donselaar KA, Florquin S, et al. Mumps: not an innocent bystander in solid organ transplantation. Am J Transplant 2009;9(9):2186–9.
52. Joines RW, Blatter M, Abraham B, et al. A prospective, randomized, comparative US trial of a combination hepatitis A and B vaccine (Twinrix®) with corresponding monovalent vaccines (Havrix® and Engerix-B®) in adults. Vaccine 2001;19(32):4710–9.
53. Horlander JC Sr, Boyle N, Manam R, et al. Vaccination against hepatitis B in patients with chronic liver disease awaiting liver transplantation. Am J Med Sci 1999;318(5):304.
54. Chalasani N, Smallwood G, Halcomb J, et al. Is vaccination against hepatitis B infection indicated in patients waiting for or after orthotopic liver transplantation? Liver Transpl Surg 2003;4(2):128–32.
55. Feuerhake A, Muller R, Lauchart W, et al. HBV-vaccination in recipients of kidney allografts. Vaccine 1984;2(4):255–6.
56. Jacobson IM, Jaffers G, Dienstag JL, et al. Immunogenicity of hepatitis B vaccine in renal transplant recipients. Transplantation 1985;39(4):393.
57. Duca P, Del Pont JM, D'Agostino D. Successful immune response to a recombinant hepatitis B vaccine in children after liver transplantation. J Pediatr Gastroenterol Nutr 2001;32(2):168–70.
58. Bienzle U, Günther M, Neuhaus R, et al. Immunization with an adjuvant hepatitis B vaccine after liver transplantation for hepatitis B-related disease. Hepatology 2007;38(4):811–9.
59. Choy BY, Peiris J, Chan TM, et al. Immunogenicity of intradermal hepatitis B vaccination in renal transplant recipients. Am J Transplant 2002;2(10):965–9.

60. Center for Disease Control and Prevention. A comprehensive immunization strategy to eliminate transmission hepatitis B virus infection in the United States. MMWR 2006;55(RR16):1–25.
61. Mutsch M, Tavernini M, Marx A, et al. Influenza virus infection in travelers to tropical and subtropical countries. Clin Infect Dis 2005;40(9):1282–7.
62. Vilchez RA, McCurry K, Dauber J, et al. Influenza virus infection in adult solid organ transplant recipients. Am J Transplant 2002;2(3):287–91.
63. Scharpé J, Evenepoel P, Maes B, et al. Influenza vaccination is efficacious and safe in renal transplant recipients. Am J Transplant 2008;8(2):332–7.
64. Moran J, Rose W, Darga A, et al. Persistence of influenza vaccine-induced antibodies in lung transplant patients between seasons. Transpl Infect Dis 2011; 13(5):466–70.
65. Magnani G, Falchetti E, Pollini G, et al. Safety and efficacy of two types of influenza vaccination in heart transplant recipients: a prospective randomised controlled study. J Heart Lung Transplant 2005;24(5):588–92.
66. Goldschmidt I, Pfister ED, Becker M, et al. Acceptance and adverse events of the 2009 H1N1 vaccination in immunosuppressed pediatric liver transplant recipients. J Pediatr 2011;158(2):329–33.
67. Smith KG, Isbel NM, Catton MG, et al. Suppression of the humoral immune response by mycophenolate mofetil. Nephrol Dial Transplant 1998;13(1): 160–4.
68. Cordero E, Aydillo TA, Perez-Ordoñez A, et al. Deficient long-term response to pandemic vaccine results in an insufficient antibody response to seasonal influenza vaccination in solid organ transplant recipients. Transplantation 2012; 93(8):847–54.
69. Blumberg EA, Albano C, Pruett T, et al. The immunogenicity of influenza virus vaccine in solid organ transplant recipients. Clin Infect Dis 1996;22(2): 295–302.
70. Kumar D, Blumberg EA, Danziger-Isakov L, et al. Influenza vaccination in the organ transplant recipient: review and summary recommendations. Am J Transplant 2011;11(10):2020–30.
71. Kumar D, Humar A, Plevneshi A, et al. Invasive pneumococcal disease in solid organ transplant recipients: 10-year prospective population surveillance. Am J Transplant 2007;7(5):1209–14.
72. Lindemann M, Heinemann FM, Horn PA, et al. Long-term response to vaccination against pneumococcal antigens in kidney transplant recipients. Transplantation 2012;94(1):50–6.
73. Gattringer R, Winkler H, Roedler S, et al. Immunogenicity of a combined schedule of 7-valent pneumococcal conjugate vaccine followed by a 23-valent polysaccharide vaccine in adult recipients of heart or lung transplants. Transpl Infect Dis 2011;13(5):540–4.
74. Kumar D, Chen MH, Wong G, et al. A randomized, double-blind, placebo-controlled trial to evaluate the prime-boost strategy for pneumococcal vaccination in adult liver transplant recipients. Clin Infect Dis 2008;47(7):885–92.
75. French N, Gordon SB, Mwalukomo T, et al. A trial of a 7-valent pneumococcal conjugate vaccine in HIV-infected adults. N Engl J Med 2010;362(9):812–22.
76. Center for Disease Control and Prevention. Use of 13-valent pneumococcal conjugate vaccine and 23-valent pneumococcal polysaccharide vaccine for adults with immunocompromising conditions: recommendations of the Advisory Committee on Immunization Practices (ACIP). MMWR Morb Mortal Wkly Rep 2012; 61(40):816–9.

77. Center for Disease Control and Prevention. General recommendations on immunization: recommendations of the Advisory Committee on Immunization Practices (ACIP). MMWR Recomm Rep 2011;6(2):1–64.

78. Hill DR. Occurrence and self-treatment of diarrhea in a large cohort of Americans traveling to developing countries. Am J Trop Med Hyg 2000;62(5):585–9.

79. Arslan H, Inci EK, Azap OK, et al. Etiologic agents of diarrhea in solid organ recipients. Transpl Infect Dis 2007;9(4):270–5.

80. Ejlertsen T, Aunsholt NA. Salmonella bacteremia in renal transplant recipients. Scand J Infect Dis 1989;21(3):241–4.

81. Dhar J, Al-Khader A, Al-Sulaiman M, et al. Non-typhoid *Salmonella* in renal transplant recipients: a report of twenty cases and review of the literature. QJM 1991;78(3–4):235–50.

82. Kotton CN. Zoonoses in solid-organ and hematopoietic stem cell transplant recipients. Clin Infect Dis 2007;44(6):857–66.

83. Page RL II, Mueller SW, Levi ME, et al. Pharmacokinetic drug–drug interactions between calcineurin inhibitors and proliferation signal inhibitors with antimicrobial agents: implications for therapeutic drug monitoring. J Heart Lung Transplant 2011;30(2):124–35.

84. DuPont HL, Jiang ZD, Okhuysen PC, et al. A randomized, double-blind, placebo-controlled trial of rifaximin to prevent travelers' diarrhea. Ann Intern Med 2005;142(10):805.

85. Martinez-Sandoval F, Ericsson CD, Jiang Z, et al. Prevention of travelers' diarrhea with rifaximin in US travelers to Mexico. J Travel Med 2010;17(2):111–7.

86. Armstrong AW, Ulukan S, Weiner M, et al. A randomized, double-blind, placebo-controlled study evaluating the efficacy and safety of rifaximin for the prevention of travelers' diarrhea in US military personnel deployed to Incirlik air base, Incirlik, Turkey. J Travel Med 2010;17(6):392–4.

87. DuPont H, Ericsson C, Johnson P, et al. Prevention of travelers' diarrhea by the tablet formulation of bismuth subsalicylate. JAMA 1987;257(10):1347.

88. Bonatti H, Barroso Ii L, Sawyer R, et al. Cryptosporidium enteritis in solid organ transplant recipients: multicenter retrospective evaluation of 10 cases reveals an association with elevated tacrolimus concentrations. Transpl Infect Dis 2012;14(6):635–48.

89. Udgiri N, Minz M, Kashyap R, et al. Intestinal cryptosporidiasis in living related renal transplant recipients. Transplant Proc 2004;36(7):2128–9.

90. Kilbaş Z, Yenïcesu M, Araz E, et al. *Cyclospora cayetanensis* infection in a patient with renal transplant. Türk hijiyen ve deneysel biyoloji dergisi 2009;66(1):25–7.

91. Azami M, Sharifi M, Hejazi S, et al. Intestinal parasitic infections in renal transplant recipients. Ann Trop Med Publ Health 2011;4(1):29.

92. Martín-Dávila P, Fortún J, López-Vélez R, et al. Transmission of tropical and geographically restricted infections during solid-organ transplantation. Clin Microbiol Rev 2008;21(1):60–96.

93. Goulet V, Hebert M, Hedberg C, et al. Incidence of listeriosis and related mortality among groups at risk of acquiring listeriosis. Clin Infect Dis 2012;54(5):652–60.

94. Fernàndez-Sabé N, Cervera C, López-Medrano F, et al. Risk factors, clinical features, and outcomes of listeriosis in solid-organ transplant recipients: a matched case-control study. Clin Infect Dis 2009;49(8):1153–9.

95. Stamm AM, Dismukes WE, Simmons BP, et al. Listeriosis in renal transplant recipients: report of an outbreak and review of 102 cases. Rev Infect Dis 1982;4(3):665–82.

96. Wiesmayr S, Tabarelli W, Stelzmueller I, et al. Listeria meningitis in transplant recipients. Wien Klin Wochenschr 2005;117(5):229–33.
97. Chen SF, Gutierrez K. *Mycobacterium bovis* disease in a pediatric renal transplant patient. Pediatr Infect Dis J 2006;25(6):564–6.
98. Wyatt S, Morgan M, Nicholls A, et al. *Mycobacterium bovis* infection complicating renal transplantation. Nephrol Dial Transplant 1993;8(9):880–1.
99. Bishara J, Robenshtok E, Weinberger M, et al. Infective endocarditis in renal transplant recipients. Transpl Infect Dis 1999;1(2):138–43.
100. Yousif B, Nelson J. Neurobrucellosis–a rare complication of renal transplantation. Am J Nephrol 2001;21(1):66–8.
101. Bottieau E, Clerinx J, Van den Enden E, et al. Infectious mononucleosis-like syndromes in febrile travelers returning from the tropics. J Travel Med 2006;13(4): 191–7.
102. Fernàndez-Sabé N, Cervera C, Fariñas MC, et al. Risk factors, clinical features, and outcomes of toxoplasmosis in solid-organ transplant recipients: a matched case-control study. Clin Infect Dis 2012;54(3):355–61.
103. Kamar N, Selves J, Mansuy J, et al. Hepatitis E virus and chronic hepatitis in organ-transplant recipients. N Engl J Med 2008;358(8):811–7.
104. Mattner F, Sohr D, Heim A, et al. Risk groups for clinical complications of norovirus infections: an outbreak investigation. Clin Microbiol Infect 2006;12(1):69–74.
105. Roos-Weil D, Ambert-Balay K, Lanternier F, et al. Impact of norovirus/sapovirus-related diarrhea in renal transplant recipients hospitalized for diarrhea. Transplantation 2011;92(1):61–9.
106. Freedman DO. Malaria prevention in short-term travelers. N Engl J Med 2008; 359(6):603–12.
107. LexiComp Online. Lexi-drugs online. Hudson (OH): LexiComp; 2012. Available at: http://online.lexi.com/. Accessed December 28, 2012.
108. Epocrates Online Drugs. Epocrates online drugs. San Mateo (CA): Epocrates; 2012. Available at: http://www.epocrates.com/. Accessed December 28, 2012.
109. Micromedex Healthcare Series. Micromedex healthcare series. DRUGDEX system. Greenwood Village (CO): Thomson Healthcare; 2012. Available at: http://www.thomsonhc.com/. Accessed December 28, 2012.
110. Dana A, Antony A, Patel MJ. Vector-borne infections in solid organ transplant recipients. Int J Dermatol 2012;51(1):1–11.
111. Azevedo L, Carvalho D, Matuck T, et al. Dengue in renal transplant patients: a retrospective analysis. Transplantation 2007;84:792–4.
112. Barrio J, de Diego A, Ripoll C, et al. Mediterranean spotted fever in liver transplantation: a case report. Transplant Proc 2002;34(4):1255–6.
113. Skhiri H, Guedri Y, Souani Y, et al. Primary tuberculosis 1 year after conversion from azathioprine to mycophenolate in recipient kidney transplantation: a case report. Transplant Proc 2003;35(7):2678–9.
114. Bossert T, Bittner HB, Richter M, et al. Successful management of two heart transplant recipients with mycobacterial pulmonary infections. Ann Thorac Surg 2005;80(2):719–21.
115. Torre-Cisneros J, Doblas A, Aguado JM, et al. Tuberculosis after solid-organ transplant: incidence, risk factors, and clinical characteristics in the RESITRA (Spanish Network of Infection in Transplantation) cohort. Clin Infect Dis 2009; 48(12):1657–65.
116. Richeldi L, Losi M, D'Amico R, et al. Performance of tests for latent tuberculosis in different groups of immunocompromised patients. Chest J 2009;136(1): 198–204.

117. Holt CD, Winston DJ, Kubak B, et al. Coccidioidomycosis in liver transplant patients. Clin Infect Dis 1997;24(2):216–21.
118. Blair JE, Douglas DD. Coccidioidomycosis in liver transplant recipients relocating to an endemic area. Dig Dis Sci 2004;49(11):1981–5.
119. Blair JE. Coccidioidomycosis in patients who have undergone transplantation. Ann N Y Acad Sci 2007;1111(1):365–76.
120. Jülg B, Elias J, Zahn A, et al. Bat-associated histoplasmosis can be transmitted at entrances of bat caves and not only inside the caves. J Travel Med 2008; 15(2):133–6.
121. Buxton JA, Dawar M, Wheat LJ, et al. Outbreak of histoplasmosis in a school party that visited a cave in Belize: role of antigen testing in diagnosis. J Travel Med 2002;9(1):48–50.
122. Johnson J, Kabler J, Gourley M, et al. Cave-associated histoplasmosis: Costa Rica. MMWR Morb Mortal Wkly Rep 1988;37:312–3.
123. Weinberg M, Weeks J, Lance-Parker S, et al. Severe histoplasmosis in travelers to Nicaragua. Emerg Infect Dis 2003;9(10):1322.
124. Nasta P, Donisi A, Cattane A, et al. Acute histoplasmosis in spelunkers returning from Mato Grosso, Peru. J Travel Med 1997;4(4):176–8.
125. Morgan J, Cano MV, Feikin DR, et al. A large outbreak of histoplasmosis among American travelers associated with a hotel in Acapulco, Mexico, spring 2001. Am J Trop Med Hyg 2003;69(6):663–9.
126. Warren K, Weltman A, Hanks C, et al. Outbreak of histoplasmosis among travelers returning from El Salvador-Pennsylvania and Virginia, 2008. MMWR Morb Mortal Wkly Rep 2008;57(50):1349–53.
127. Cuellar-Rodriguez J, Avery R, Lard M, et al. Histoplasmosis in solid organ transplant recipients: 10 years of experience at a large transplant center in an endemic area. Clin Infect Dis 2009;49(5):710–6.
128. Carey J, Hofflich H, Amre R, et al. *Penicillium marneffei* infection in an immunocompromised traveler: a case report and literature review. J Travel Med 2005; 12(5):291–4.
129. Le T, Wolbers M, Chi NH, et al. Epidemiology, seasonality, and predictors of outcome of AIDS-associated *Penicillium marneffei* infection in Ho Chi Minh City, Viet Nam. Clin Infect Dis 2011;52(7):945–52.
130. Chariyalertsak S, Sirisanthana T, Supparatpinyo K, et al. Seasonal variation of disseminated *Penicillium marneffei* infections in northern Thailand: a clue to the reservoir? J Infect Dis 1996;173(6):1490–3.
131. Panackal AA, Hajjeh RA, Cetron MS, et al. Fungal infections among returning travelers. Clin Infect Dis 2002;35(9):1088–95.
132. Avery RK, Michaels MG, the AST Infectious Diseases Community of Practice. Strategies for safe living following solid organ transplantation. Am J Transplant 2009;9:S252–7.
133. Nicolls DJ, Weld LH, Schwartz E, et al. Characteristics of schistosomiasis in travelers reported to the GeoSentinel surveillance network 1997–2008. Am J Trop Med Hyg 2008;79(5):729–34.
134. Pavli A, Maltezou HC. Travel-acquired leptospirosis. J Travel Med 2008;15(6): 447–53.
135. Sejvar J, Bancroft E, Winthrop K, et al. Leptospirosis in "eco-challenge" athletes, Malaysian Borneo, 2000. Emerg Infect Dis 2003;9(6):702.
136. Khosravi M, Bastani B. Acute renal failure due to leptospirosis in a renal transplant recipient: a brief review of the literature. Transplant Proc 2007;39(4): 1263–6.

137. Gerasymchuk L, Swami A, Carpenter CF, et al. Case of fulminant leptospirosis in a renal transplant patient. Transpl Infect Dis 2009;11(5):454–7.
138. Manfro RC, Boger MV, Kopstein J, et al. Acute renal failure due to leptospirosis in a renal transplant patient. Nephron 1993;64(2):317.
139. Brett-Major DM, Lipnick RJ. Antibiotic prophylaxis for leptospirosis. Cochrane Database Syst Rev 2009;(3):CD007342.
140. Pirenne J, Van Gelder F, Kharkevitch T, et al. Tolerance of liver transplant patients to strenuous physical activity in high-altitude. Am J Transplant 2004; 4(4):554–60.

Perspectives on Liver and Kidney Transplantation in the Human Immunodeficiency Virus-Infected Patient

Peter Chin-Hong, MD[a], George Beatty, MD, MPH[b],
Peter Stock, MD, PhD[c],*

KEYWORDS

- Human immunodeficiency virus • Transplantation • Hepatitis B • Hepatitis C • Liver
- Kidney

KEY POINTS

- HIV disease following liver and kidney transplantation remains well controlled despite the immunosuppressive requirements.
- Early outcomes following kidney transplantation in HIV infected recipients are comparable to HIV negative recipients in recipients with well controlled HIV.
- Although outcomes following liver transplantation in HIV/HBV coinfected recipients are outstanding, the 3 year outcomes in HIV/HCV coinfected patients are problematic related to issues with recurrent HCV.
- Rejection rates following both kidney and liver transplantation are surprisingly high, and suggest a dysregulated immune system in the HIV infected recipients.

INTRODUCTION

Infection with human immunodeficiency virus (HIV) is no longer considered a contraindication for liver and kidney transplantation in patients with advanced organ failure. There were historical and legitimate fears that the immunosuppression needed after transplantation would exacerbate an already compromised immune system and result in considerable mortality and morbidity in patients. There were also concerns that using scarce organs in this population would not be a good use of resources.[1,2]

Several factors led to a positive change in thinking by the transplantation community. First, the remarkable advances in the treatment of HIV-infected patients over

[a] Department of Medicine, University of California at San Francisco, 13 Parnassus Avenue, S410, San Francisco, CA 94143-0654, USA; [b] UCSF Positive Health Care Program, Building 80, Ward 84, San Francisco, CA 94143-0874, USA; [c] Department of Surgery, University of California, 505 Parnassus Avenue, M884, San Francisco, CA 94143-0780, USA
* Corresponding author.
E-mail address: peter.stock@ucsfmedctr.org

Infect Dis Clin N Am 27 (2013) 459–471
http://dx.doi.org/10.1016/j.idc.2013.02.010
0891-5520/13/$ – see front matter © 2013 Elsevier Inc. All rights reserved.

the past 3 decades have resulted in improved survival.[3] Second, there has been a tremendous improvement in the understanding and implementation of the prophylaxis of opportunistic infections that afflict both populations of patients with HIV as well as patients undergoing transplantation. There has been an increasing proportion of HIV-infected patients with advanced kidney and liver disease, and hence an increased demand for organs.[3-5] Liver transplantation in the HIV-infected population has been driven mainly by complications of coinfection with hepatitis B virus (HBV) and hepatitis C virus (HCV), which both share similar modes of transmission to HIV. Liver disease is now a major cause of mortality in HIV-infected individuals. There has also been an increase in demand for kidney transplantation from HIV-associated nephropathy, immunoglobulin A nephropathy, and glomerulonephritis as a result of HIV coinfection with HBV and HCV.

The initial published reports of outcomes of transplantation in HIV-infected patients came from single-patient experiences or case series by single institutions.[6,7] Multiple centers providing retrospective and then prospective studies provided more robust and generalizable data.[8-11] This increasing knowledge base has led to refinements in the way HIV-infected patients are selected for transplantation, particular antiretroviral agents are recommended, immunosuppressive regimens are chosen, and complications in these patients after transplant are anticipated. This article first reviews the latest outcomes in liver and kidney transplantation worldwide, focusing on the experiences in the era of highly active antiretroviral therapy (HAART). Then, in keeping with the theme of this issue of emerging infectious disease issues in solid organ transplantation, some of the key issues and controversies that have recently arisen in the field are reviewed.

OUTCOMES IN LIVER TRANSPLANTATION
Overall Survival

Summarizing several of the early experiences of transplantation of HIV-infected persons since the widespread use of HAART in 1996, a report by the US Scientific Registry of Transplant Recipients (SRTR) described 1-year survival rates in liver transplant recipients from 60% to 100%.[12-15] In the largest experience reported in this document,[14] investigators combined data in HIV-infected patients undergoing transplantation from several centers in Pittsburgh, Miami, San Francisco, Minneapolis, and London. They then compared outcomes in this group to age-matched and race-matched cohorts of HIV-uninfected transplant patients from the United Network for Organ Sharing. There was no appreciable difference in cumulative survival at 1, 2, and 3 years in the HIV-infected patients (87%, 73%, and 73%) compared with the matched HIV-uninfected patients (87%, 82%, and 78%) (Table 1). Among the HIV-infected patients, lower survival was associated with HCV infection, not being able to tolerate HIV medications after transplant, and CD4+ T-cell counts less than 200 after transplant. Although HCV infection was associated with higher mortality in HIV-infected patients, this was not statistically different from survival in the HIV-uninfected HCV-positive controls.

Hepatitis B

Outcomes in HIV-HBV coinfected patients are excellent after transplantation. The largest report compared the experience of a prospective cohort of 22 HIV-HBV coinfected patients transplanted between 2001 and 2007 with 20 HBV monoinfected patients.[8] Patient/graft survival at 4 years was 85% in the HIV-HBV group compared with 100% in the HBV monoinfected group after transplantation ($P = .09$). After

Table 1
Rates of patient and graft survival at 1 year and 3 years among HIV-infected compared with HIV-uninfected individuals in published multicenter cohort studies

Location	Organ	N (HIV + Patients)	Patient Survival (%)				Graft Survival (%)				Reference
			At 1 y		At 3 y		At 1 y		At 3 y		
			HIV+	HIV−	HIV+	HIV−	HIV+	HIV−	HIV+	HIV−	
United States	Liver	24	87	87	73	78					14
United States	Liver (HBV)	22	85	100	85	100	85	100	85	100	8
Spain	Liver (HCV)	84	88	90	62	76	86	85	60	69	9
United States	Liver (HCV)	89	76	92	60	79	72	88	53	74	11
United States	Kidney	150	95		88		90		74		10

Missing values in table not provided in respective studies.

transplantation, all patients received hepatitis B immune globulin (HBIG) (continued indefinitely with a decrease in dose frequency after 12 months) as well as anti-HBV nucleoside or nucleotide analogues. All patients remained hepatitis B surface antigen and HBV DNA negative after transplantation (median follow-up of 3.5 years). The data in recipients coinfected with hepatitis B and HIV show that if there is suitable control of the copathogen, HIV infection does not negatively affect allograft and patient survival. This finding is in contrast to the results after liver transplantation in recipients coinfected with HCV and HIV, in whom the copathogen is more challenging to control.

Hepatitis C

Outcomes in HIV-HCV coinfected patients are more variable and depend on the selection criteria used. In a study of 84 HCV-HIV patients who underwent transplantation in Spain, 5-year survival rates were 54% compared with 71% in HCV monoinfected transplant patient controls.[9] Another US prospective, multicenter study compared patient and graft survival for 89 patients coinfected with HCV and HIV with 2 control groups (235 HCV monoinfected liver transplant patients, and all transplant recipients in the United States who were 65 years or older).[11] Patient survival rates at 1 and 3 years were 76% and 60% in the HCV-HIV group compared with 92% and 79% in the HCV monoinfected liver transplant group. Graft survival at 3 years was 53% and 74% in both groups, respectively. Independent predictors of graft loss among HCV-HIV transplant recipients included older age, combined kidney-liver transplant, an anti-HCV-positive donor, and a body mass index (BMI, calculated as weight in kilograms divided by the square of height in meters) less than 21 kg/m². If patients with HCV-HIV did not have a combined kidney-liver transplant or an anti-HCV-positive donor, and had a BMI of 21 kg/m² or higher, patient and graft survival were similar to HCV monoinfected patients.

OUTCOMES IN KIDNEY TRANSPLANTATION

Several studies have shown excellent survival in HIV-infected kidney transplant recipients.[10,15–18] In the largest of the published studies (N = 150), investigators reported patient survival at 1 and 3 years of 95% and 88% and allograft survival of 90% and 74%.[10] The survival of HIV-infected kidney transplant recipients was between that of all kidney transplant recipients and those older than 65 years, as reported by SRTR.

HIV-SPECIFIC OUTCOMES AFTER TRANSPLANTATION

Studies have generally shown no evidence of HIV-disease progression to AIDS or HIV-opportunistic infections after transplant. However, depending on the type of immunosuppressive agents used, CD4+ T-cell counts may be affected. In 1 prospective cohort study of kidney transplant recipients, HIV-infected patients who received induction with thymoglobulin had a higher median decline in CD4+ T cells at 1 year after transplant, compared with those who did not receive this agent (−239 vs −135 cells/mm³).[10] At 3 years, there was no difference in the change of CD4+ T cells from baseline between the 2 groups.

There have been few HIV-associated opportunistic infections after transplantation. In the US multicenter study of 125 HIV-infected liver and 150 kidney transplant patients, there have been only 4 cases of Kaposi sarcoma, 2 cases of *Pneumocystis jiroveci* pneumonia, 1 case of cryptosporidiosis, and 6 cases of esophageal candidiasis. A history of opportunistic infections was not independently associated with mortality.[19] In a Spanish study of 84 liver transplant recipients coinfected with HCV and

HIV, severe infection was an independent risk factor for mortality among these patients (hazard ratio 2.6, $P<.01$).[9] However, there was no difference in the occurrence of infection as a cause of death when comparing the coinfected transplant patients with those who were HIV uninfected (8% vs 6%).

EMERGING ISSUES
Eligibility Criteria

Based on the accumulating data from observational studies, the eligibility criteria for potential HIV-infected transplant candidates is evolving (**Box 1**). In many senses, it is becoming liberalized, particularly with respect to permitting a history of opportunistic infections in potential transplant candidates.[2] However, opportunistic infections for which there are no reliable therapeutic options after transplantation remain a contraindication to transplantation. These infections include progressive multifocal leukoencephalopathy, chronic cryptosporidiosis, primary central nervous system lymphoma, and drug-resistant fungal infections (such as *Scedosporium prolificans*).

However, long-term outcomes in patients coinfected with HCV and HIV who have received liver transplants are leading to a refinement of selection criteria in this population. Potential HCV-HIV transplant candidates who have a BMI of at least 21 kg/m^2 and do not need a concomitant kidney transplant may have a better probability of patient and graft survival than sicker patients.[11] Older donors and donors who are HCV-infected are associated with eventual graft loss in this study, and should be used with caution in this population. The use of older donors yields poorer results in HCV mono-infected recipients as well.

The absolute CD4+ T-cell count continues to be an important component of potential candidates for transplantation. For kidney transplantation, most centers require that HIV-infected patients have a CD4+ T-cell count greater than 200 cells/mL, any time in the 16 weeks before transplantation. For HIV-infected patients with

---

Box 1
Eligibility criteria for HIV-infected transplant candidates

Meet center-specific criteria for specific organ transplant

HIV-related criteria

    Kidney: CD4+ T-cell count greater than 200 cells/μL

    Liver: CD4+ T-cell count greater than 100 cells/μL (CD4+ T-cell count >200 cells/μL if history of opportunistic infection or malignancy)

    HIV RNA suppressed for kidney transplant recipients

    HIV RNA suppressed for liver transplant recipients, or expected to be suppressed if unable to tolerate cART

    Stable antiretroviral regimen

    No active opportunistic infection or neoplasm

    No history of chronic cryptosporidiosis, primary central nervous system lymphoma or progressive multifocal leukoencephalopathy

Other

    Liver (HCV): BMI greater than 21 kg/m^2, no need for combined kidney transplant, no HCV+ donor

advanced liver disease, we permit a lower absolute CD4+ T-cell cutoff of greater than 100 cells/mL (except if there is a history of opportunistic infection or malignancy, in which case, the cutoff is 200 cells/mL). This strategy allows for presumed splenic sequestration of T lymphocytes, based on the observation of patients with portal hypertension and splenomegaly, particularly those with high MELD (Model for End-Stage Liver Disease) scores. For children, the percentage of CD4+ T cells is more important. For children 1 to 2 years of age, the CD4+ percentage should be greater than 30. For children between 2 and 10 years, the CD4+ percentage should be greater than 20.

The HIV-1 RNA also continues to be important in the evaluation of potential transplant candidates who are HIV-infected. Most centers require that patients have an undetectable HIV RNA, based on the most recent level checked at least 16 weeks before the transplant date. Some liver transplant candidates are unable to tolerate HAART because of drug-associated hepatotoxicity. In these cases, the requirement for an undetectable HIV RNA may be waived if an experienced HIV clinician can confidently predict that viral suppression could occur after transplantation with the available options.

Immunosuppression Considerations

Multiple immunosuppressive regimens have been used in the treatment of HIV-infected patients after transplant. However, it is not clear whether 1 regimen is superior to another. For induction, most centers avoid lymphocyte-depleting regimens (ie, thymoglobulin) for induction agents, given the profound effect on CD4+ T cells that these lymphocyte-depleting agents can have. As a result of the high occurrence of rejection episodes in the HIV-infected kidney transplant population,[10] many centers have used the interleukin 2 receptor inhibitors for induction therapy.[2] Most centers have been able to avoid the use of lymphocyte-depleting induction agents in HIV-infected liver transplant patients, given that steroids and adjustments in maintenance therapy have been generally been successful in managing rejection episodes that arise.

Most centers use a maintenance therapy regimen of steroids, a calcineurin inhibitor (tacrolimus or cyclosporin A), and the antiproliferative agent mycophenolate mofetil (MMF). We use steroids at standard doses in the HIV-infected transplant recipient. Cyclosporine has been a common agent used because of both antiretroviral and immunomodulatory properties.[20,21] In addition, because of the lower risk of glucose intolerance compared with tacrolimus, cyclosporine was favored by many centers. However, there is recent evidence of an association of cyclosporine with graft rejection, although there was no impact on graft survival.[10] We target similar calcineurin trough levels to those in the HIV-uninfected transplant population. Like cyclosporine, MMF has antiretroviral properties and synergizes with didanosine, abacavir, and tenofovir.[22,23]

The target of rapamycin inhibitor sirolimus is an alternative to the calcineurin inhibitors and is of interest for several reasons. It is an effective antiproliferative agent for Kaposi sarcoma.[24] Given these anticancer properties, it may also be useful in cases of patients who develop malignancies after transplant.[25] It also downregulates the expression of C-C chemokine receptor type 5 (CCR5) on CD4+ T cells and synergizes with the antiretroviral agents enfuvirtide and maraviroc, which inhibit viral entry or CCR5 chemokine coreceptor-facilitated attachment.[26] Also, because many HIV-infected patients have some degree of renal impairment that is HIV associated or from other causes, sirolimus may be a useful agent when compared with the calcineurin inhibitors.

Antiretroviral Considerations

As in other HIV-infected patients, we generally use 3 active drugs from among the classes of antiretroviral medications. These drugs include the nucleoside analogue reverse transcriptase inhibitors (NRTIs), the nonnucleoside analogue reverse transcriptase inhibitors (NNRTIs), HIV-protease inhibitors (PIs), entry inhibitors, and integrase inhibitors. The goal is to devise a regimen that can be delivered in the posttransplant setting that provides continuous suppression of HIV, ensures adequate therapeutic levels of the immunosuppressive medications, and minimizes overlapping drug toxicities (**Table 2**).

The ability to concomitantly administer both a potent antiretroviral regimen with a combination of immunosuppressive and opportunistic infection prophylactic drugs remains a challenge. This situation is because of multiple bidirectional drug interactions between antiretroviral and immunosuppressive regimens.[27] The immunosuppressive agents (cyclosporine, tacrolimus, and sirolimus) require adjustment depending on which antiretroviral drug is chosen (see **Box 1**). PIs commonly inhibit the cytochrome P450 3A4 (CYP450) system, and patients require a decreased dose of immunosuppression (eg, 1 mg tacrolimus orally weekly).[28] Patients on NNRTI-based regimens require an increase in the dose of calcineurin inhibitors or sirolimus, because of the induction of P450 3A4. The induction of P450 3A4 by NNRTIs is not as strong as the inhibition by PIs. Therefore, when both a PI and an NNRTI are used, the doses of immunosuppression are adjusted as if a PI alone was used (ie, reduction of the dose of immunosuppression).

There has been some systematic study of these drug interactions. One study[29] reported the experience of 35 HIV-infected patients after transplant who were on various drug regimens (NNRTIs, PIs, or both). The investigators showed that patients on PIs needed lower doses of cyclosporine, tacrolimus, or sirolimus using longer dosing intervals compared with those not on PIs. Adjustment was an ongoing process for those on PIs: the area under the curve for cyclosporine continued to change over a 2-year period, with continual need for dose adjustment. Conversely, patients on cyclosporine and efavirenz required higher doses of cyclosporine.

Chemokine Receptors and Transplantation

There has been great interest in evaluating the role of CCR5 chemokine receptor antagonists in transplantation. CCR5 is a coreceptor that HIV uses to enter the target cell. HIV-infected individuals who are homozygous for the CCR5 δ 32 mutation (1% of Whites) have a nonfunctional receptor and are highly resistant to HIV infection.[30,31] CCR5 also plays an important role in alloreactivity. There is some evidence that these individuals also have reduced rates of rejection and improved survival after transplantation. In 1 study of 1227 kidney transplant recipients, those who were homozygous for CCR5 δ 32 (2% of this population) had improved survival compared with those who were either heterozygous for CCR5 δ 32 or homozygous for wild-type CCR5.[32] In another study of 158 liver transplant recipients,[33] patients who were homozygous for CCR5 δ 32 had no rejection episodes, compared with 13% of those homozygous for CCR5 δ 32, and 31% in the CCR5 wild-type patients. Modifying the CCR5 receptor pharmacologically with a CCR5 receptor antagonist may also be beneficial. Investigators added a 33-day course of the CCR5 receptor antagonist maraviroc to graft-versus-host disease (GVHD) prophylaxis in 35 patients undergoing hematopoietic stem cell transplantation.[34] An unusually low proportion of patients in this study developed grade III or IV GVHD by day 180 (6%). The mechanisms underlying these observations are unclear. In the GVHD study, investigators showed that maraviroc was

Table 2
Antiretroviral considerations in the transplant setting for specific drugs

Antiretroviral Class/Agent	General Considerations	Adjustment in Immunosuppression
NRTIs	Avoid NRTIs with mitochondrial toxicity (eg, didanosine, stavudine, and zidovudine) if MMF is used concomitantly	None
Abacavir	Theoretically avoid if donor is HLA B5701+ because of risk of hypersensitivity reaction. Not commonly used in clinical practice	
Abacavir	Associated with decreased response to recurrent hepatitis C treatment (ribavirin phosphorylation impaired)	
Abacavir	May have synergistic effect against HIV if MMF concomitantly used[23]	
Tenofovir	Associated with proximal tubular dysfunction and Fanconi syndrome in the nontransplant setting. Limited data regarding risk of renal toxicity after kidney transplantation	
Tenofovir	May exacerbate osteopenia and osteoporosis associated with advanced liver and kidney disease before transplant and steroid use after transplant	
Zidovudine	May worsen bone marrow suppression if MMF is used at the same time	
NNRTIs		Require increases in cyclosporine, tacrolimus, or sirolimus
Nevirapine	Avoid in patients undergoing liver transplantation because of fears of drug-associated hepatotoxicity	
Integrase inhibitors		None
Raltegravir	Associated with low occurrence of rejection	Favored. Relative absence of drug interactions after transplant
PIs	May exacerbate hyperlipidemia that occurs after transplantation, as well as calcineurin inhibitor associated hyperglycemia	Require lower dose and increase in dosing interval of cyclosporine, tacrolimus, or sirolimus
Atazanavir	Avoid. Proton pump inhibitors frequently required indefinitely after transplant and this is contraindicated with atazanavir	

associated with impaired lymphocyte chemotaxis without impact on lymphocyte function. As CCR5 receptor antagonists continue to be developed for HIV treatment, there is promise for its future use in transplantation, even in individuals who are not HIV infected.

Prophylaxis for Opportunistic Infections

Prophylaxis for cytomegalovirus (CMV), *Pneumocystis jiroveci* pneumonia (PCP), and fungal infections is routinely given to all patients for several months after transplantation. In addition, we recommend additional opportunistic infection prophylaxis for the HIV-infected transplant patient (**Table 3**). Screening and treatment of latent tuberculosis infection follows routine guidelines in HIV-infected patients. Immunizations for HIV-infected patients are the same as recommended for transplant patients who are not HIV infected.

Management of Hepatitis B Coinfection

Outcomes in the HBV-HIV transplant patients undergoing liver transplantation have been excellent, as reviewed earlier. We recommend following the same guidelines for treatment of HBV after transplant as in the published studies. This procedure involves using HBIG and antiretrovirals that also have activity against HBV. HBIG is continued indefinitely using a standard tapering protocol. Antiretrovirals that are

Table 3
Opportunistic infection prophylaxis for HIV-infected transplant recipients

Opportunistic Infection	Preferred Agent	Primary Prophylaxis[a]	Secondary Prophylaxis[b]
Pneumocystis jiroveci pneumonia	Trimethoprim/ sulfamethoxaxole	Lifelong	Lifelong
CMV	Valganciclovir	No HIV-specific indication. Follow standard center-specific prophylactic regimens for transplant recipients (eg, 6 mo valganciclovir for CMV-negative recipients of CMV-positive donors)	CD4+ T cell <75–100 cells/mL Discontinue when CD4+ T cells >200 cells/mL for 3–6 mo
Cryptococcosis	Fluconazole	No HIV-specific indication	CD4+ T cell <200 cells/mL Discontinue when CD4+ T cells >200 cells/mL for 3–6 mo
Mycobacterium avium complex	Azithromycin	CD4+ T cells <50 cells/mL Discontinue when CD4+ T cells >100 cells/mL for 3–6 mo	CD4+ T cell <50 cells/mL Discontinue when CD4+ T cells >100 cells/mL for 3–6 mo
Toxoplasmosis	Trimethoprim/ sulfamethoxaxole	Toxoplasmosis IgG-positive donor or recipient CD4+ T cells <100 cells/mL	CD4+ T cell <200 cells/mL Discontinue when CD4+ T cells >100 cells/mL for 3–6 mo

[a] No history of infection.
[b] Previous history of infection. Apart from following CD4+ T-cell criteria, we recommend secondary prophylaxis for at least 1 month after transplantation, and for 1 month after treatment of rejection.

commonly used include tenofovir plus either lamivudine or emtricitabine and that have HBV as well as HIV activity. In cases in which entecavir may be needed for additional HBV activity after transplant, it is important to ensure that HIV is concomitantly suppressed. This strategy is because entecavir may select for HIV resistance, despite not having specific anti-HIV activity.[35] This management strategy for patients with HBV-HIV had led to control of HBV recurrence after transplant, and corresponding good outcomes in terms of patient and graft survival.

Management of Hepatitis C Coinfection

In contrast to the excellent outcomes seen in the HBV-HIV transplant patients, patients with HCV-HIV have had high rates of HCV recurrence after transplantation, with lower patient and graft survival in general. In response to the poorer outcomes, some centers have revised their selection criteria, as discussed earlier. In general, the recommendations for management of HCV reactivation after transplant are similar regardless of HIV status. We usually initiate HCV treatment when there is histologic evidence of progression or severe recurrence. There are challenges in using interferon and ribavirin after transplant in a population at risk for thrombocytopenia and lymphopenia, and many patients require growth products and antidepressants. There is limited experience so far with the new class of direct-acting HCV antivirals such as telaprevir and boceprevir in this population. Although promising in general, the use of these new agents will be complicated by substantial drug interactions[36] and there are limited data at this point to guide clinical practice in the HIV-HCV coinfected transplant patient. Spontaneous clearance of HCV in several of the coinfected patients has been observed, although there has not been a good explanatory model.

Rejection

HIV-infected patients mount a vigorous alloimmune response after transplant. This finding is supported by the observation that rejection rates in HIV-infected patients are 2 to 3 times higher than in HIV-uninfected patients after transplant. In a multisite observational study of 150 HIV-infected kidney transplant patients, 1-year and 3-year rejection rates were 31% and 41%, compared with a control rate of 12% in the general kidney transplant population.[10] This finding did not seem to affect graft function in the period observed, because there was no statistical difference in graft function between the HIV-infected and uninfected populations. In a study of 89 HCV-HIV liver transplant recipients, 3-year rejection rates were 39%, higher than the 24% of HIV-negative HCV patients observed.[11] More than 50% of the rejection episodes occurred in the first 21 days after liver transplantation. The reasons for the higher rate of rejection seen in HIV-infected patients are likely multifactorial. Drug interactions between antiretroviral agents (particularly PIs) and calcineurin inhibitors may have led to lower total drug exposure of immunosuppression. Even although there was a careful attempt to adjust dosing of calcineurin inhibitors based on troughs, the substantially longer intervals between doses could have led to subtherapeutic levels of drug. In the HIV kidney transplant study referenced earlier,[10] use of cyclosporine was independently associated with rejection. In the HIV liver transplant study discussed earlier,[11] lower tacrolimus trough levels were associated with rejection. Alternatively, it could be that the immune activation and general immune dysregulation found in HIV could have led to a heightened and nonspecific enhancement of alloimmunity. Use of integrase inhibitors, as well as avoidance of PIs, may minimize drug-drug interactions. More long-term follow-up is needed to determine whether these episodes of rejection translate into graft loss.

SUMMARY

HIV infection is not an absolute contraindication to kidney and liver transplantation in patients with advanced organ disease. Compared with the general transplant population, several observational studies have revealed equivalent patient and graft survival outcomes in kidney and selected liver transplants in the HIV-infected population. To ensure the best outcomes, patients need to be selected carefully with well-controlled HIV, and posttransplant complications need to be aggressively managed. As new information becomes available, selection criteria continue to be refined. Emerging issues in the HIV-infected transplant field include determining the best drug combinations of antiretrovirals and immunosuppressive medications to administer, optimally treating hepatitis C recurrence after transplantation, and after long-term outcomes in patients. As these cohorts mature, they will also give valuable information about malignancies (particularly those that are virally mediated like HPV-associated neoplasia) in this growing population.[37] Nevertheless, demand for organs continue to outstrip supply. Demand for organs will only increase as the HIV-infected population ages, given comorbidities in this population such as hypertension, diabetes mellitus, and chronic hepatitis. New ways of increasing organ availability such as transplantation of HIV-positive donors and recipients will continue to be hot discussion topics.[38]

ACKNOWLEDGMENTS

We thank Rodney Rogers for his formidable organizational skills.

REFERENCES

1. Spital A. Should all human immunodeficiency virus-infected patients with end-stage renal disease be excluded from transplantation? The views of U.S. transplant centers. Transplantation 1998;65(9):1187–91.
2. Stock PG, Roland ME. Evolving clinical strategies for transplantation in the HIV-positive recipient. Transplantation 2007;84(5):563–71.
3. Palella FJ Jr, Delaney KM, Moorman AC, et al. Declining morbidity and mortality among patients with advanced human immunodeficiency virus infection. HIV Outpatient Study Investigators [see comments]. N Engl J Med 1998;338(13): 853–60.
4. Feinberg MB. Changing the natural history of HIV disease. Lancet 1996; 348(9022):239–46.
5. Kaplan JE, Hanson D, Dworkin MS, et al. Epidemiology of human immunodeficiency virus-associated opportunistic infections in the United States in the era of highly active antiretroviral therapy. Clin Infect Dis 2000;30(Suppl 1):S5–14.
6. Erice A, Rhame FS, Heussner RC, et al. Human immunodeficiency virus infection in patients with solid-organ transplants: report of five cases and review. Rev Infect Dis 1991;13(4):537–47.
7. Trullas JC, Cofan F, Tuset M, et al. Renal transplantation in HIV-infected patients: 2010 update. Kidney Int 2011;79:825–42.
8. Coffin CS, Stock PG, Dove LM, et al. Virologic and clinical outcomes of hepatitis B virus infection in HIV-HBV coinfected transplant recipients. Am J Transplant 2010; 10(5):1268–75.
9. Miro JM, Montejo M, Castells L, et al. Outcome of HCV/HIV-coinfected liver transplant recipients: a prospective and multicenter cohort study. Am J Transplant 2012;12:1866–76.

10. Stock PG, Barin B, Murphy B, et al. Outcomes of kidney transplantation in HIV-infected recipients. N Engl J Med 2010;363(21):2004–14.
11. Terrault NA, Roland ME, Schiano T, et al. Outcomes of liver transplant recipients with hepatitis C and human immunodeficiency virus coinfection. Liver Transpl 2012;18(6):716–26.
12. Neff GW, Bonham A, Tzakis AG, et al. Orthotopic liver transplantation in patients with human immunodeficiency virus and end-stage liver disease. Liver Transpl 2003;9(3):239–47.
13. Prachalias AA, Pozniak A, Taylor C, et al. Liver transplantation in adults coinfected with HIV. Transplantation 2001;72(10):1684–8.
14. Ragni MV, Belle SH, Im K, et al. Survival of human immunodeficiency virus-infected liver transplant recipients. J Infect Dis 2003;188(10):1412–20.
15. Stock PG, Roland ME, Carlson L, et al. Kidney and liver transplantation in human immunodeficiency virus-infected patients: a pilot safety and efficacy study. Transplantation 2003;76(2):370–5.
16. Abbott KC, Swanson SJ, Agodoa LY, et al. Human immunodeficiency virus infection and kidney transplantation in the era of highly active antiretroviral therapy and modern immunosuppression. J Am Soc Nephrol 2004;15(6):1633–9.
17. Kumar MS, Sierka DR, Damask AM, et al. Safety and success of kidney transplantation and concomitant immunosuppression in HIV-positive patients. Kidney Int 2005;67(4):1622–9.
18. Qiu J, Terasaki PI, Waki K, et al. HIV-positive renal recipients can achieve survival rates similar to those of HIV-negative patients. Transplantation 2006;81(12): 1658–61.
19. Beatty G, Barin B, Fox L, et al. HIV-related predictors and outcomes in 275 liver and/or kidney transplant recipients. Presented at 6th IAS conference on HIV pathogenesis, treatment, and prevention. Rome (Italy), July 17–20, 2011.
20. Schwarz A, Offermann G, Keller F, et al. The effect of cyclosporine on the progression of human immunodeficiency virus type 1 infection transmitted by transplantation–data on four cases and review of the literature. Transplantation 1993; 55(1):95–103.
21. Streblow DN, Kitabwalla M, Malkovsky M, et al. Cyclophilin a modulates processing of human immunodeficiency virus type 1 p55Gag: mechanism for antiviral effects of cyclosporin A. Virology 1998;245(2):197–202.
22. Heredia A, Margolis D, Oldach D, et al. Abacavir in combination with the inosine monophosphate dehydrogenase (IMPDH)-inhibitor mycophenolic acid is active against multidrug-resistant HIV-1. J Acquir Immune Defic Syndr 1999;22(4):406–7.
23. Margolis D, Heredia A, Gaywee J, et al. Abacavir and mycophenolic acid, an inhibitor of inosine monophosphate dehydrogenase, have profound and synergistic anti-HIV activity. J Acquir Immune Defic Syndr 1999;21(5):362–70.
24. Stallone G, Schena A, Infante B, et al. Sirolimus for Kaposi's sarcoma in renal-transplant recipients. N Engl J Med 2005;352(13):1317–23.
25. Heredia A, Amoroso A, Davis C, et al. Rapamycin causes down-regulation of CCR5 and accumulation of anti-HIV beta-chemokines: an approach to suppress R5 strains of HIV-1. Proc Natl Acad Sci U S A 2003;100(18):10411–6.
26. Gilliam BL, Heredia A, Devico A, et al. Rapamycin reduces CCR5 mRNA levels in macaques: potential applications in HIV-1 prevention and treatment. AIDS 2007; 21(15):2108–10.
27. Izzedine H, Launay-Vacher V, Baumelou A, et al. Antiretroviral and immunosuppressive drug-drug interactions: an update. Kidney Int 2004;66(2):532–41.

28. Frassetto L, Baluom M, Jacobsen W, et al. Cyclosporine pharmacokinetics and dosing modifications in human immunodeficiency virus-infected liver and kidney transplant recipients. Transplantation 2005;80(1):13–7.
29. Frassetto LA, Browne M, Cheng A, et al. Immunosuppressant pharmacokinetics and dosing modifications in HIV-1 infected liver and kidney transplant recipients. Am J Transplant 2007;7(12):2816–20.
30. Doranz BJ, Rucker J, Yi Y, et al. A dual-tropic primary HIV-1 isolate that uses fusin and the beta-chemokine receptors CKR-5, CKR-3, and CKR-2b as fusion cofactors. Cell 1996;85(7):1149–58.
31. Dean M, Carrington M, Winkler C, et al. Genetic restriction of HIV-1 infection and progression to AIDS by a deletion allele of the CKR5 structural gene. Hemophilia Growth and Development Study, Multicenter AIDS Cohort Study, Multicenter Hemophilia Cohort Study, San Francisco City Cohort, ALIVE Study. Science 1996; 273(5283):1856–62.
32. Fischereder M, Luckow B, Hocher B, et al. CC chemokine receptor 5 and renal-transplant survival. Lancet 2001;357(9270):1758–61.
33. Heidenhain C, Puhl G, Moench C, et al. Chemokine receptor 5Delta32 mutation reduces the risk of acute rejection in liver transplantation. Ann Transplant 2009; 14(3):36–44.
34. Reshef R, Luger SM, Hexner EO, et al. Blockade of lymphocyte chemotaxis in visceral graft-versus-host disease. N Engl J Med 2012;367(2):135–45.
35. McMahon MA, Jilek BL, Brennan TP, et al. The HBV drug entecavir effects on HIV-1 replication and resistance. N Engl J Med 2007;356(25):2614–21.
36. Luetkemeyer AF, Havlir DV, Currier JS. Complications of HIV disease and antiretroviral therapy. Top Antivir Med 2012;20(2):48–60.
37. Nissen NN, Barin B, Stock PG. Malignancy in the HIV-infected patients undergoing liver and kidney transplantation. Curr Opin Oncol 2012;24(5):517–21.
38. Muller E, Kahn D, Mendelson M. Renal transplantation between HIV-positive donors and recipients. N Engl J Med 2010;362(24):2336–7.

Pharmacologic Issues of Antiretroviral Agents and Immunosuppressive Regimens in HIV-infected Solid Organ Transplant Recipients

Jennifer Primeggia, MD*, Joseph G. Timpone Jr, MD, Princy N. Kumar, MD

KEYWORDS

- HIV • Immunosuppression • Organ transplantation • Drug interactions

KEY POINTS

- Most nucleoside reverse transcriptase inhibitors are excreted via the renal system and drug interactions with immunosuppression based on hepatic metabolism are not observed; concomitant use may, however, be limited by additive toxicities (myelosuppression, nephrotoxicity, lactic acidosis).
- Drug interactions between nonnucleoside reverse transcriptase inhibitors (NNRTIs) and immunosuppressants are difficult to predict and data on second-generation NNRTIs are lacking.
- Etravirine has unpredictable drug interactions; clinicians may choose to avoid this medication in the posttransplant period.
- Protease inhibitors inhibit cytochrome P-450, leading to elevated levels of calcineurin inhibitors; dose adjustments are required when used concomitantly.
- Raltegravir has been successfully coadministered with calcineurin inhibitors and no toxicities have been observed.
- Drug-drug interactions should be carefully considered in HIV-positive patients when choosing an ARV regimen and drug levels should be closely monitored in the posttransplant period; close collaboration between the HIV primary care provider and the transplant team is encouraged.

No disclosures.

Author Contributions: Drafting article (J. Primeggia); Critical revision of the article, approval of article (J. Timpone); Concept/design, critical revision, approval of the article (P. Kumar).

Georgetown University Medical Center, Division of Infectious Diseases, Department of Medicine, 3800 Reservoir Road Northwest, 5PHC, Washington, DC 20007-2113, USA

* Corresponding author.

E-mail address: jxprime@gmail.com

Infect Dis Clin N Am 27 (2013) 473–486

http://dx.doi.org/10.1016/j.idc.2013.02.011

id.theclinics.com

INTRODUCTION

Patients with HIV are at risk of developing end-stage organ disease, partly from the disease itself and partly from the toxicity of antiretrovirals (ARVs). The Data Collection on Adverse Events of Anti-HIV Drugs study, composed of data from 893 person-years of follow-up in 23,441 HIV-positive patients found that 14.5% of deaths were from liver-related causes, making liver disease the most frequent cause of non-AIDS–related death.[1] An analysis conducted in 2000 among 822 HIV-positive patients also identified a high risk of death from liver disease in this population; the proportion of deaths attributable to end-stage liver disease in HIV-infected persons were 1.2% in those with HIV alone, 22% in those with hepatitis B virus coinfection, and 31% in those with hepatitis C virus (HCV) coinfection.[2] The effects of ARVs on the progression of hepatic fibrosis in HIV monoinfected and HIV-HCV coinfected individuals are still not well understood. One study that followed monoinfected and HIV/HCV coinfected patients investigated the relationship between highly active antiretroviral therapy exposure and hepatic fibrosis (using the aspartate aminotransferase-to-platelet ratio index as a surrogate marker of significant hepatic fibrosis) found that ARV use was associated with increased hepatic fibrosis only in patients with HIV/HCV coinfection, highlighting the importance of treatment of HCV in those with HIV coinfection.[3]

Prolonged ARV use may lead to the development of renal and cardiovascular complications as well. Broadly speaking, there are 4 main metabolic complications associated with ARV use: dyslipidemia, insulin resistance and diabetes mellitus, lipodystrophy, and vitamin D deficiency.[4] Lipid abnormalities have been reported in up to 74% of HIV-infected patients treated with protease inhibitors, and diabetes in up to 14% of patients 1 year after the initiation of ARVs.[4] Cardiovascular disease, metabolic disorders and their sequelae, as well as bone health are already comorbid conditions that an aging population faces. An aging population further faces progression of underlying renal and hepatic disease confounded by HIV itself and by ARV use. Renal disease related to HIV may be caused directly by HIV, leading to conditions such as HIV-associated nephropathy, HIV-associated thrombotic microangiopathy, and HIV-associated, immune-mediated glomerulonephritis.[5] Renal disease may also be directly and indirectly associated with ARV use. Nephropathy may result indirectly from impaired glucose tolerance in the setting of ARV use, as with diabetic nephropathy. ARVs may also cause direct nephrotoxicity. Classic associations include indinavir with crystalluria and nephrolithiasis and tenofovir with Fanconi syndrome.[5] With so many variables affecting renal function, the true prevalence of chronic kidney disease in HIV infection is unknown, although various studies report rates of proteinuria of approximately 30%.[6] ARVs, HIV, and HIV coinfection with HBV or HCV may all increase the risk of development of end-stage renal and liver disease.

Once considered an absolute contraindication to transplantation, HIV-positive patients with undetectable viral loads are now transplanted successfully.[7,8] The 1-year and 3-year graft survival rates for patients with HIV who undergo kidney transplantation are reported at 95% and 88%, respectively.[8] Among liver transplant recipients, the United Network for Organ Sharing database reported a 2-year survival probability of 70% compared with 81% among patients without HIV.[8] Higher success rates, however, have been compromised by increased rates of rejection and by toxicities from combined immunosuppressive and ARV regimens.[7,8] Drug-drug interactions between immunosuppressives and ARVs alter plasma levels, which can lead to toxic plasma drug levels, HIV virologic breakthrough, and organ rejection. Awareness of drug-drug interactions is important, as close monitoring may avoid some adverse outcomes.

When considering drug-drug interactions, some general principles may be applied. The mainstay of immunosuppression in solid organ transplantation includes depleting protein immunosuppressive agents (against T cells and/or B cells), calcineurin inhibitors (cyclosporine [CsA] and tacrolimus), target-of-rapamycin inhibitors (sirolimus), and inhibitors of nucleotide synthesis (mycophenolate mofetil [MMF]).[9] **Table 1** describes the metabolism of agents commonly used in posttransplant immunosuppressive regimens, as well as side effects and toxicities, particularly in the setting of increased drug exposure. **Table 2** provides a summary of drug interactions between ARVs and immunosuppressants. In general, protease inhibitors (PIs) inhibit cytochrome P-450, leading to markedly elevated levels of calcineurin inhibitors. Nonnucleoside reverse transcriptase inhibitors (NNRTIs), on the other hand, induce P-450, leading to more rapid elimination of calcineurin inhibitors. Most nucleoside reverse transcriptase inhibitors (NRTIs) are excreted by the renal system and interactions based on hepatic metabolism are not readily encountered. Broadly speaking, however, the extent of these drug interactions is not well characterized. Although interactions may be predicted based on pharmacokinetics, much has been learned from in vivo observations after combining ARVs and immunosuppressive regimens posttransplantation. With this review, we characterize these interactions as they have thus far been described in the literature.

NRTIS

As most NRTIs are excreted via the renal system, interactions with immunosuppressive agents based on hepatic metabolism are not observed. NRTI use may be limited, however, by side-effect profiles, particularly when combined with immunosuppressants. For example, azathioprine and MMF are associated with leucopenia and neutropenia.[9] When they are combined with zidovudine, there is an additive myelotoxicity.[11] Although tenofovir is safe in patients without comorbid conditions (with a serious adverse event rate as low as 0.5%), there is an increased risk of renal toxicity in patients with comorbid conditions, such as diabetes and hypertension.[12] These comorbidities are extremely common and are often the cause of renal transplantation. Additionally, the calcineurin inhibitors have also been associated with the development of these metabolic complications.[13] Cyclosporine, tacrolimus, and sirolimus are all associated with nephrotoxicity.[12,14,15] There is an additional risk of nephrotoxicity in patients who receive tenofovir with concomitant nephrotoxic agents.[16] Therefore, in patients with calcineurin nephrotoxicity posttransplantation, concurrent tenofovir use may further contribute to nephrotoxicity.

There may, however, be advantages to combining certain NRTIs with immunosuppressive agents. An interesting interaction between NRTIs, MMF, and the HIV virus itself has been described in vitro. MMF is a prodrug that releases mycophenolic acid, which inhibits inosine monophosphate dehydrogenase, an enzyme in purine synthesis.[9] This results in depletion of intracellular deoxyguanosine triphosphate. Synergy was observed between abacavir and MMF in the inhibition of HIV-1 viral replication in both mononuclear cells and macrophages via depletion of cellular guanosine pools, which resulted in increased intracellular concentrations of abacavir.[17] This antiviral effect was also observed with didanosine, and to a lesser extent with lamivudine and zalcitabine.[17] Increased intracellular concentrations of abacavir and didanosine, however, may also increase the risk of toxicity. Posttransplant lactic acidosis was described in a liver transplant recipient who received didanosine and MMF; the investigators speculated that concomitant administration of NRTIs and MMF may have

Table 1
Characteristics of commonly used immunosuppressive drugs in solid organ transplantation

Drug	Mechanism of Action	Metabolism/ Transporter	Side Effects and Toxicities Associate with Increased Drug Exposure
Cyclosporine	Binds to cyclophilin, preventing dephosphorolation of NF-AT and its translocation from the cell cytoplasm to the nucleus, thereby preventing activation of promoters of T-cell activation.[10]	CYP3A P-gp transporter	Acute or chronic nephrotoxicity, hyperkalemia, hypomagnesemia, hyperuricemia, hypertension, hyperlipidemia, hepatotoxicity, thrombocytopenia, thrombotic microangiopathy, hirsutism, gum hyperplasia, tremor[10]
Tacrolimus (FK506)	Binds to intracellular protein FKBP-12 forming a complex of tacrolimus-FKBP-12, calcium, calmodulin, and calcineurin and inhibiting the phosphatase activity of calcineurin. This prevents the dephosphorylation and translocation of NF-AT, thereby preventing activation of promoters of T-cell activation.	CYP3A	Acute or chronic nephrotoxicity, Posterior Reversible Encephalopathy Syndrome, delirium, coma, headache, tremors, paresthesias, myocardial hypertrophy
Sirolimus (Rapamycin)	Binds to FKBP12; this complex binds to and inhibits activation of the mammalian target of rapamycin, a regulatory kinase. This inhibition suppresses cytokine-driven T-cell proliferation	CYP3A P-gp transporter	Acute or chronic nephrotoxicity, hemolytic-uremic syndrome, thrombotic thrombocytopenic purpura, thrombotic microangiopathy, hepatotoxicity, peripheral edema, hypertriglyceridemia, hypertension, interstitial lung disease
Mycophenolate mofetil	Converted to mycophenolic acid, the active form of the drug, it reversibly inhibits inosine monophosphate dehydrogenase, the enzyme that controls the rate of de novo synthesis of guanine monophosphate, which is critical to B-lymphocyte and T-lymphocyte proliferation	Glucuronyl transferase	Neutropenia, pure red cell aplasia, gastrointestinal intolerance (nausea, vomiting, diarrhea)
Prednisone	Binds with high affinity to cytoplasmic receptors, ultimately inhibiting production of IL-1 (a co-stimulus for helper T-cell activation and IL-6 (inducer of B-cell activation)	CYP3A4	Elevation of blood pressure, salt and water retention, increased potassium excretion Exacerbation of systemic fungal infections Adrenocortical insufficiency may result from rapid withdrawal

Abbreviations: IL, interleukin; NF-AT, nuclear factor of activated T-lymphocytes; P-gp, P-glycoprotein.
Data about drugs derived from the manufacturer's inserts for health care professionals unless otherwise indicated.

Table 2
Metabolism of antiretrovirals and effect on selected immunosuppressants

Antiretroviral	Metabolism	Effect on Immunosuppressant Levels
Nucleoside reverse transcriptase inhibitors		
Abacavir Didanosine Emtricitabine Lamivudine Stavudine Tenofovir Zidovudine	No significant metabolism via the P450 system. Renal excretion.	No change in levels of cyclosporine, tacrolimus, sirolimus, or MMF
Nonnucleoside reverse transcriptase inhibitors	**Metabolized via CYP3A4**	
Efavirenz	Substrate and inducer of CYP3A4, CYP2B6	↓ Cyclosporine[22] ↓ Tacrolimus[23] ↓ Sirolimus No change in MMF
Nevirapine	Substrate and inducer of CYP3A	No change in cyclosporine[20,21] ↓ Tacrolimus ↓ Sirolimus No change in MMF
Etravirine	Substrate for CYP3A, CYP2C9, CYP2C19 Inducer of CYP3A Inhibitor of CYP2C9, CYP2C19, P-glycoprotein	Effect on cyclosporine, tacrolimus, sirolimus, and MMF unpredictable[25,26]
Rilpivirine	Substrate for CYP3A	No change in levels of cyclosporine, tacrolimus, sirolimus or MMF anticipated[27]
Protease inhibitors	**Metabolized via CYP3A4**	
Atazanavir	Substrate and inhibitor of CYP3A4 Inhibitor of UGT1A1	↑ Cyclosporine ↑ Tacrolimus[38] ↑ Sirolimus No change in MMF
Darunavir	Inhibitor of CYP3A4	↑ Cyclosporine ↑ Tacrolimus[34] ↑ Sirolimus No change in MMF
Fosamprenavir	Inhibitor of CYP3A4	↑ Cyclosporine ↑ Tacrolimus[33] ↑ Sirolimus[33] No change in MMF
Indinavir	Inhibitor of CYP3A4	↑ Cyclosporine[30] ↑ Tacrolimus ↑ Sirolimus No change in MMF

(continued on next page)

Table 2
(continued)

Antiretroviral	Metabolism	Effect on Immunosuppressant Levels
Lopinavir/ritonavir	Substrate and inhibitor of CYP3A4 Inducer of glucuronidation	↑ Cyclosporine[30] ↑ Tacrolimus[31] ↑ Sirolimus No change in MMF
Nelfinavir	Substrate and inhibitor of CYP3A4 Substrate and inhibitor of P-gp[33]	↑ Cyclosporine, but effect may be difficult to predict[35] ↑ Tacrolimus, but effect may be difficult to predict ↑ Sirolimus, but effect difficult to predict[36] No change in MMF
Ritonavir	Inhibitor of CYP3A4, CYP1A2, CYP2C9, CYP2C19, CYP2B6 and other enzymes including glucuronosyltransferase Inhibitor of CYP3A4 Inhibitor of CYP2D6	↑ Cyclosporine[28] ↑ Tacrolimus ↑ Sirolimus No change in MMF
Saquinavir	Inhibitor of CYP3A4 Substrate for P-gp	↑ Cyclosporine ↑ Tacrolimus ↑ Sirolimus No change in MMF
Tipranavir	Substrate and inhibitor of CYP3A4 Substrate and inducer of P-gp Weak inhibitor of P-gp	↑ Cyclosporine ↑ Tacrolimus ↑ Sirolimus No change in MMF
Integrase inhibitors		
Elvitegravir/cobicistat Raltegravir	Glucuronidation	No change in levels of cyclosporine, tacrolimus, sirolimus, or MMF anticipated
CCR5 antagonists		
Maraviroc	Substrate for CYP3A Substrate for P-gp	No change in levels of cyclosporine, tacrolimus, sirolimus, or MMF anticipated
Fusion inhibitor		
Enfuvirtide	Undergoes catabolism to its constituent amino acids	No change in levels of cyclosporine, tacrolimus, sirolimus, or MMF anticipated

Abbreviations: MMF, mycophenolate mofetil; P-gp, permeability glycoprotein; UGT1A1, UDP glucuronosyltransferase 1 family, polypeptide A1; ↑, increased drug level; ↓, decreased drug level.
 Data about drugs derived from the manufacturer's inserts for health care professionals unless otherwise indicated.

played a role.[18] In vitro data have also demonstrated that the concomitant use of thymidine analogs (such as zidovudine or stavudine) with MMF resulted in antagonism.[17] Although this has been observed in vitro, there has been no evidence of increased virologic failure in renal transplant recipients receiving MMF and zidovudine in the largest trial noted to date.[7]

NNRTIS

The current NNRTIs include delavirdine, efavirenz, nevirapine, etravirine, and rilpivirine. All NNRTIs are metabolized by the liver and are substrates of CYP3A4. Efavirenz and nevirapine are also inducers of this enzyme, which theoretically leads to more rapid elimination of calcineurin inhibitors. Therefore, pharmacokinetic principles predict that patients receiving efavirenz or nevirapine should require much higher doses of calcineurin inhibitors to achieve goal trough levels.[19] However, an in vivo pharmacokinetic study by Frassetto and colleagues[20] demonstrated that patients on either nevirapine or efavirenz required doses of CsA similar to those of non-HIV transplant patients, suggesting a minimal impact of NNRTIs on CsA pharmacokinetics. In a separate pharmacokinetic study, Stock and colleagues[21] also found no change in CsA level in patients who received nevirapine as part of their regimen. Compared with nevirapine, the use of efavirenz required a small but clinically significant increase in CsA dosing.[22] Additionally, when efavirenz was added to a tacrolimus regimen, 4 recipients of a liver transplant required only a small change in the daily dose of tacrolimus.[23] This effect may have been observed because efavirenz is a liver-specific inducer of CYP3A and does not alter intestinal CYP3A; therefore, tacrolimus bioavailability is not altered.[24]

Etravirine, a relatively new NNRTI, which is a substrate and an inducer of several CYP enzymes, has unpredictable drug interactions[25,26] and should be used cautiously in the posttransplant period. Rilpivirine is another second-generation NNRTI and was approved by the Food and Drug Administration (FDA) in May 2011. It is primarily metabolized by CYP3A. It is not an inducer of the P450 system and theoretically should not exert an effect on immunosuppressant drug levels.[27] To our knowledge, there are no published reports of the use of either of these agents in the posttransplant period.

PROTEASE INHIBITORS

Multiple studies have demonstrated drug-drug interactions between PIs and immunosuppressants in vivo. The largest pharmacokinetic study, conducted in 35 HIV-positive subjects who underwent liver or kidney transplantation, found that subjects on any PI-containing regimen required a fourfold to fivefold lower CsA dose and a 50% increase in dosing interval compared with those on CsA with an NNRTI.[22] For PI regimens that included ritonavir, the dosing requirement was further decreased with an even greater dosing interval.[22] Although interactions between PIs and immunosuppressants are known, the degree of interaction and the magnitude of such interactions are more difficult to predict.

Of all the PIs, ritonavir is known to be the most potent of P450 inhibitors. Drug-drug interactions are observed, even when doses as low as 100 mg daily are used as part of an ARV-boosting regimen.[28] Ritonavir blocks P-glycoprotein (P-gp) and cytochrome P450, both of which are critically involved in the metabolism of CsA and tacrolimus.[28] In comparing dose adjustments of immunosuppressants after resuming boosted and unboosted PIs, Guaraldi and colleagues[28] found more rapid increases in immunosuppressant trough concentrations 48 hours after initiating ritonavir-boosted PI therapy. Additionally, a median 7.5-fold decrease in immunosuppressant dosage was required for patients receiving a boosted regimen compared with a 2.9-fold decrease for an unboosted regimen.[28] Although an unboosted regimen appears to exert less of an effect on immunosuppressive drug levels, boosting is now an essential part of first-line PI-based treatment regimens.[29]

With significant dose adjustments, patients have been managed successfully with ritonavir-boosted regimens after transplantation. Lopinavir/ritonavir is a potent inhibitor of P450 and significant interactions have been characterized when used in combination with both tacrolimus and CsA. CsA in conjunction with either lopinavir/ritonavir or indinavir/ritonavir necessitated a dose decrease of 80% to 95% in CsA[30]; however, close monitoring of CsA therapy via drug trough levels resulted in safe and rejection-free immunosuppression over a mean of 15 months in one pharmacokinetic profile investigation.[30] Outside of a controlled pharmacokinetic study, the pharmacokinetics of concomitant PIs and immunosuppressants are less predictable. Two liver transplant recipients who received lopinavir/ritonavir required significant dose modification; they received a final dose of 0.5 mg weekly and 1.0 mg weekly.[31] Another liver transplant recipient was noted to have a tacrolimus concentration of 71.7 ng/mL (trough reference range 5–20 ng/mL) after 48 hours of therapy with lopinavir/ritonavir and no tacrolimus dose adjustment; further doses of tacrolimus were held for 35 days.[32] In yet another liver transplant recipient, despite a 50% dose-reduction of tacrolimus, after 5 doses of lopinavir/ritonavir, a trough tacrolimus level of 49 ng/mL was noted and the patient did not require further dosing of tacrolimus for 38 days.[31] Unfortunately, these patients experienced neurotoxic side effects (insomnia, tremors, headaches, altered mental status) consistent with the known adverse effects of tacrolimus; symptoms resolved as tacrolimus levels decreased.[31,32] These cases highlight the difficulties in predicting an individual response to combination therapy and the adverse outcomes that may result. A preemptive decrease in tacrolimus dosing by at least 50% the day before starting ARVs is an option for patients; decreasing or holding tacrolimus for several days after initiating ARVs has also been suggested.[31,32]

Profound interactions between immunosuppressants and fosamprenavir/ritonavir and darunavir/ritonavir have been observed as well. The coadministration of tacrolimus with fosamprenavir/ritonavir resulted in a 10-fold increase in tacrolimus half-life and an increased time to steady state of 2 days; goal tacrolimus serum concentrations were achieved with a dosing regimen of 0.5 mg every 4 days.[33] A similar interaction was noted with sirolimus coadministered with ritonavir-boosted fosamprenavir. An increased time to steady state of 10 days was noted and the patient was maintained at goal serum concentrations with 1 mg of sirolimus weekly.[33] In one kidney transplant recipient, when darunavir/ritonavir was used in combination with tacrolimus, a trough as high as 106.7 ng/mL was observed and the patient developed acute kidney injury; adequate trough levels were achieved with a significant dose reduction in tacrolimus to 0.5 mg per week, 3.5% of the usual dose.[34] Caution in administration is advised with both of these regimens.

Less predictable than other protease inhibitors is nelfinavir. Frassetto and colleagues[35] examined the degree of interaction between nelfinavir and CsA; both drugs are substrates and inhibitors of the cytochrome P450 system and the P-gp system, making the degree of interaction difficult to anticipate. Although intravenous CsA had little effect on oral nelfinavir pharmacokinetics, oral CsA given concomitantly with nelfinavir was noted to alter the in vivo levels of nelfinavir; similar trends were also observed with indinavir.[35] This study demonstrated a high degree of variability in pharmacokinetics among the study participants; this makes predictions difficult and provides compelling evidence for close therapeutic monitoring of patients receiving CsA and nelfinavir.[35] Similar interactions were observed with concomitant nelfinavir and sirolimus as well. A liver transplant recipient who received both nelfinavir and sirolimus demonstrated increased trough concentration and prolongation of the half-life of sirolimus even when one-fifth of the recommended dose of nelfinavir was administered.[36]

In vitro studies have demonstrated that atazanavir is an inhibitor and inducer of P-gp and a potent inhibitor of CYP3A.[37] In a recent case report, Tsaperas and colleagues[38] described the interaction between tacrolimus and unboosted atazanavir in an HIV-positive renal transplant recipient. The patient ultimately required 1.5 mg twice daily of tacrolimus, a much lower dose compared with similar patients who did not receive atazanavir.[38] Other studies, however, have found that lower doses of tacrolimus were needed when patients received other PIs.[33,34] It is speculated that the reason for this difference is twofold. First, atazanavir may not be as potent an inhibitor of CYP3A4 as other protease inhibitors. Second, atazanavir may decrease tacrolimus bioavailability, resulting in higher dosing requirements.[38] Although a steady dosing regimen for atazanavir may be advantageous for patient adherence, atazanavir may not be preferable for posttransplant recipients who receive proton pump inhibitors. Patients who take proton pump inhibitors must separate atazanavir temporally, as atazanavir solubility decreases as gastric pH increases; this adds another level of complexity to their medication regimen.[39] Therefore, the routine use of atazanavir in the posttransplant setting should be avoided.

Prednisone is metabolized via the cytochrome P450 system, and concomitant use with CYP3A inhibitors, such as ritonavir and indinavir, have the potential to result in increased plasma concentrations of corticosteroids.[40] The association of steroids with the development of adrenal suppression and Cushing syndrome is already well described in nontransplant HIV-positive patients who receive ritonavir.[41–43] Solid organ transplant recipients remain on steroids for a prolonged time after their surgery and increased steroid exposure is a concern. In a pharmacokinetic analysis of a single 20-mg dose of prednisone combined with lopinavir/ritonavir, Busse and colleagues[44] observed elevated plasma concentrations of prednisolone (the measured metabolite) compared with HIV-positive patients not receiving ARVs. ARVs may alter the pharmacokinetics of steroids and this is an important consideration in transplant recipients.[41–44]

INTEGRASE INHIBITORS

Raltegravir avoids many of the major drug-drug interactions seen with the PIs, as it is metabolized primarily by glucuronidation rather than by the P450 system. No drug-drug interactions have thus far been observed when raltegravir was used in combination with tacrolimus or CsA, MMF, and steroids.[45] The largest retrospective review of outcomes of 13 HIV-positive patients who underwent either liver or kidney transplantation demonstrated excellent tolerability, prompt attainment of goal trough levels with standard doses of tacrolimus and CsA, no episodes of acute rejection, good graft function, and good control of HIV over a 9-month follow-up period, making raltegravir an attractive agent for use in transplant recipients.[45]

More recently, success with raltegravir has also been demonstrated in patients undergoing simultaneous pancreas-kidney transplantation. After successful transplantation and initiation of tacrolimus, an ARV regimen of raltegravir and 2 NRTIs was instituted; target plasma levels were achieved at a doses similar to doses used in HIV-negative recipients.[46] HIV-1 was adequately controlled under the raltegravir-based regimen over a 9-month follow-up period.[46] Similar success has been reported with the coadministration of raltegravir and sirolimus in an HIV-infected liver transplant recipient who developed renal impairment after transplantation: after the development of calcineurin-related nephrotoxicity, his immunosuppressive regimen was changed to sirolimus, whereas his ARV regimen was changed from stavudine, lamivudine, and abacavir to raltegravir, lamivudine, and abacavir.[47] Twelve weeks after transplantation, the patient's renal function improved, as did his CD4 count; the HIV viral load remained below 50 copies.[47]

The successful coadministration of raltegravir and CsA has also been described. At 4 weeks, after changing from enfuvirtide to raltegravir, a patient demonstrated maintenance of suppression of the HIV viral load, improvement in CD4 count, and maintenance of goal trough levels with a minimal dose adjustment.[26] Raltegravir levels were obtained at this time and plasma concentrations were comparable with patients who were not exposed to immunosuppressives. Furthermore, no toxicities related to either ARV or immunosuppressive therapies were noted in the patient.[26] Overall, a raltegravir-based regimen seems to be an attractive option, especially when seeking to avoid the deleterious side effects of protease inhibitors, particularly when combined with calcineurin inhibitors. Raltegravir is known to have a low genetic barrier to resistance and long-term follow-up data are lacking, however.

Elvitegravir is a new integrase inhibitor that has been coformulated with cobicistat and tenofovir/emtricitabine as a single tablet once daily, known as Stribilid. Both elvitegravir and cobicistat are metabolized by CYP3A4. Additionally, cobicistat is a potent selective inhibitor of CYP3A, which results in increased systemic exposure of elvitegravir. Although the use of this medication has not been described in solid organ transplantation, it is likely that it will exert an effect similar to ritonavir, owing to CYP3A inhibition.[48]

CCR5 ANTAGONISTS

Maraviroc, a CCR5 antagonist approved by the FDA for treatment of HIV in 2007, is a substrate of CYP3A and P-gp. As a result, drug interactions with calcineurin inhibitors are not anticipated.[49] Maraviroc provides 2 unique advantages in the setting of transplantation. First, the CCR5 receptor itself appears to play a role in the pathogenesis of graft-versus-host disease (GVHD) and solid-organ rejection.[50,51] CCR5 is important for lymphocyte recruitment and maraviroc blockade has been found to inhibit lymphocyte trafficking.[51] When maraviroc was added to a conventional GVHD prophylaxis regimen after allogeneic hematopoietic stem-cell transplantation, a lower incidence of visceral GVHD was observed.[51] A second advantage to the use of maraviroc may be the potential synergy with sirolimus (Rapamycin) in the treatment of HIV. Administration of sirolimus to primates has been observed to decrease CCR5 messenger RNA expression in peripheral blood mononuclear cells and cervicovaginal tissues, supporting the notion that sirolimus in conjunction with CCR5 antagonists, such as maraviroc, may be a strategy for treatment of HIV infection, although further studies are needed.[52]

SUMMARY

The concern for drug-drug interactions in HIV-positive solid organ transplant recipients lies in the increased risks of toxicities of the medications leading to adverse events. Although synergy against HIV replication has been described with certain combinations of therapy in vitro, additive toxicities have also been observed. Despite difficulties achieving therapeutic windows of immunosuppressants, overall favorable posttransplant outcomes have been reported. As more ARV regimens are cautiously initiated in the posttransplant period, we will continue to further our knowledge of drug-drug interactions in the transplant population and to improve long-term survival rates.

Given the very complicated pharmacologic interactions between ARV therapies and immunosuppressive regimens, close collaboration must exist between the transplant team and the HIV primary care provider. This becomes especially important when there is a need to change an ARV regimen in the posttransplantation period. For example, a change from a PI-based regimen to an NNRTI-based regimen could result in a dramatic decrease in calcineurin levels, precipitating allograft rejection. Based on the current literature, it appears that with close monitoring, ARVs can be safely administered with immunosuppressive therapies without the risk of significant drug-associated toxicity or HIV disease progression.[7,8] Transplant surgeons and HIV primary care providers must be knowledgeable of these important drug interactions when caring for this patient population.

ACKNOWLEDGMENTS

The authors thank Dr Lan Duong, Pharm D, Georgetown University Hospital.

REFERENCES

1. Weber R, Sabin CA, Friss-Moller N, et al. Liver-related deaths in persons infected with human immunodeficiency virus: the D:A:D study. Arch Intern Med 2006;166: 1632–41.
2. Salmon-Ceron D, Lewden C, Morlat P, et al. Liver disease as a major cause of death among HIV infected patients: role of hepatitis C and B viruses and alcohol. J Hepatol 2005;42:799–805.
3. Moodie EE, Pant Pai N, Klein MB. Is antiretroviral therapy causing long-term liver damage? A comparative analysis of HIV-mono-infected and HIV/Hepatitis C co-infected cohorts. PLoS One 2009;4:e4517. http://dx.doi.org/10.1371/journal. pone.0004517.
4. Hester EK. HIV medications: an update and review of metabolic complications. Nutr Clin Pract 2012;27:51–64.
5. Roline G, Schmid H, Fischereder M, et al. HIV-associated renal disease and highly active antiretroviral therapy-induced nephropathy. Clin Infect Dis 2006; 42:1488–95.
6. Gupta SK, Eustace JA, Winston JA, et al. Guidelines for the management of chronic kidney disease in HIV-infected patients: recommendations of the HIV Medicine Association of the Infectious Disease Society of America. Clin Infect Dis 2005;40:1559–85.
7. Stock PG, Barin B, Murphy B, et al. Outcomes of kidney transplantation in HIV-infected recipients. N Engl J Med 2010;363:2004–14.
8. Mindikoglu AL, Regev A, Magder LS. Impact of human immunodeficiency virus on survival after liver transplantation: analysis of United Network for Organ Sharing database. Transplantation 2008;85:359–68.
9. Halloran PF. Immunosuppressive drugs for kidney transplantation. N Engl J Med 2004;351:2715–29.
10. Tedesco D, Haragsim L. Cyclosporine: a review. J Transplant 2012;2012:230386. http://dx.doi.org/10.1155/2012/230386, 7.
11. Roland ME, Stock PG. Liver transplantation in HIV-infected recipients. Semin Liver Dis 2006;26:273–84.
12. Nelson MR, Katlama C, Montaner JS, et al. The safety of tenofovir disoproxil fumarate for the treatment of HIV infections in adults: the first 4 years. AIDS 2007;21: 1273–81.
13. Guitard J, Rostaing L, Kamar N. New-onset diabetes and nephropathy after renal transplantation. Contrib Nephrol 2011;170:247–55.

14. Marti HP, Frey FJ. Nephrotoxicity of rapamycin: an emerging problem in clinical medicine. Nephrol Dial Transplant 2005;20:13–5.
15. Chapman JR. Chronic calcineurin inhibitor nephrotoxicity—lest we forget. Am J Transplant 2011;11:693–7.
16. Castellano C, Williams W, Kepler TB, et al. Clinical predictors of tenofovir-associated nephrotoxicity in HIV-1-infected patients. Paper presented at: XVII International AIDS Conference [abstract WEAB0104]. Mexico City (Mexico), August 3–8, 2008.
17. Margolis D, Heredia A, Gaywee J, et al. Abacavir and mycophenolic acid, an inhibitor of inosine monophosphate dehydrogenase, have profound and synergistic anti-HIV activity. J Acquir Immune Defic Syndr 1999;21:362–70.
18. Antoniades C, Macdonald C, Knisely A, et al. Mitochondrial toxicity associated with HAART following liver transplantation in an HIV-infected recipient. Liver Transpl 2004;10:699–702.
19. Marfo K, Greenstein S. Antiretroviral and immunosuppressive drug-drug interactions in human immunodeficiency virus-infected liver and kidney transplant recipients. Transplant Proc 2009;41:3796–9.
20. Frassetto L, Baluom M, Jacobeson W, et al. Cyclosporine pharmacokinetics and dosing modifications in human immunodeficiency virus-infected liver and kidney transplant recipients. Transplantation 2005;80:13–7.
21. Stock PG, Roland ME, Carlson L, et al. Kidney and liver transplantation in human immunodeficiency virus-infected patients: a pilot safety and efficacy study. Transplantation 2003;76:370–5.
22. Frassetto LA, Browne M, Cheng A, et al. Immunosuppressant pharmacokinetics and dosing modifications in HIV-1 infected liver and kidney transplant recipients. Am J Transplant 2007;7:2816–20.
23. Teicher E, Vincent I, Bonhomme-Faivre L, et al. Effect of highly active antiretroviral therapy on tacrolimus pharmacokinetics in hepatitis C virus and HIV co-infected liver transplant recipients in the ANRS CH-08 study. Clin Pharmacokinet 2007;46:941–52.
24. Mouly S, Lown KS, Kornhauser D, et al. Hepatic but not intestinal CYP3A4 displays dose-dependent induction by efavirenz in humans. Clin Pharmacol Ther 2002;72:1–9.
25. Kakuda TN, Scholler-Gyure M, Hoetelmans RM. Pharmacokinetic interactions between etravirine and non-antiretroviral drugs. Clin Pharmacokinet 2011;50:25–39.
26. Di Biagio A, Rosso R, Siccardi M, et al. Lack of interaction between raltegravir and cyclosporine in an HIV-infected liver transplant recipient. J Antimicrob Chemother 2009;64:874–5.
27. Edurant (rilpivirine) tablets [package insert]. Raritan, NJ: Tibotec Pharmaceuticals; 2011.
28. Guaraldi G, Cocchi S, Motta A, et al. Differential dose adjustments of immunosuppressants after resuming boosted versus unboosted HIV-protease inhibitors postliver transplant. Am J Transplant 2009;9:2429–34.
29. Panel on Antiretroviral Guidelines for Adults and Adolescents. Guidelines for the use of antiretroviral agents in HIV-1-infected adults and adolescents. Department of Health and Human Services; 2011. p. 1–166. Available at: http://www.aidsinfo.nih.gov/ContentFiles/AdultandAdolescentGL.pdf. Accessed August 1, 2011.
30. Vogel M, Voigt E, Michaelis HC, et al. Management of drug-to-drug interactions between cyclosporine A and the protease-inhibitor lopinavir/ritonavir in liver-transplanted HIV-infected patients. Liver Transpl 2004;20:939–44.

31. Jain AB, Venkataramanan R, Eghtesad B, et al. Effect of coadministered lopinavir and ritonavir (Kaletra) on tacrolimus blood concentration in liver transplantation patients. Liver Transpl 2003;9:954–60.

32. Schonder KS, Schullo MA, Okusanya O. Tacrolimus and lopinavir/ritonavir interaction in liver transplantation. Ann Pharmacother 2003;37:1793–6.

33. Barau C, Blouin P, Creput C, et al. Effect of coadministered HIV-protease inhibitors on tacrolimus and sirolimus blood concentrations in a kidney transplant recipient. Fundam Clin Pharmacol 2009;23:423–5.

34. Meretz D, Battegay M, Marzolini C, et al. Drug-drug interaction in a kidney transplant recipient receiving HIV salvage therapy and tacrolimus. Am J Kidney Dis 2009;54:e1–4.

35. Frassetto L, Thai T, Aggarwal AM, et al. Pharmacokinetic interactions between cyclosporine and protease inhibitors in HIV+ subjects. Drug Metab Pharmacokinet 2003;18:114–20.

36. Jain AK, Venkataramanan R, Fridell JA, et al. Nelfinavir, a protease inhibitor, increases sirolimus levels in a liver transplantation patient: a case report. Liver Transpl 2002;8:838–40.

37. Perloff ES, Duan SX, Skolnik PR, et al. Atazanavir: effects on P-glycoprotein transport and CYP3A metabolism in vitro. Drug Metab Dispos 2005;33:764–70.

38. Tsaperas DS, Webber AB, Aull MJ, et al. Managing the atazanavir-tacrolimus drug interaction in a renal transplant recipient. Am J Health Syst Pharm 2011; 15:138–42.

39. Reyataz (atazanavir sulfate) capsules [package insert]. Princeton, NJ: Bristol-Myers Squibb; 2011.

40. Prednisone [package insert]. Columbus, OH: Roxane Laboratories, Inc; 2009.

41. Dort K, Padia S, Wispelwey B, et al. Adrenal suppression due to an interaction between ritonavir and injected triamcinolone: a case report. AIDS Res Ther 2009;6:10.

42. Herold MA, Gunthard HF. Cushing syndrome after steroid-infiltration in two HIV-patients with antiretroviral therapy. Praxis 2010;99:863–5.

43. Molloy A, Matheson NJ, Meyer PA, et al. Cushing's syndrome and adrenal axis suppression in a patient treated with ritonavir and corticosteroid eye drops. AIDS 2011;25:1337–9.

44. Busse KH, Formentini E, Alfar R, et al. Influence of antiretroviral drugs on the pharmacokinetics of prednisolone in HIV-infected individuals. J Acquir Immune Defic Syndr 2008;15:561–6.

45. Tricot L, Teicher E, Peytavin G, et al. Safety and efficacy of raltegravir in HIV-infected transplant patients cotreated with immunosuppressive drugs. Am J Transplant 2009;9:1946–52.

46. Miro JM, Ricart MJ, Trullas JC, et al. Simultaneous pancreas-kidney transplantation in HIV-infected patients: a case report and literature review. Transplant Proc 2010;42:3887–91.

47. Moreno A, Barcena R, Quereda C, et al. Safe use of raltegravir and sirolimus in an HIV-infected patient with renal impairment after orthotopic liver transplantation. AIDS 2008;22:547–8.

48. Stribilid (elvitegravir, cobicistat, emtricitabine, tenofovir disoproxil fumarate) tablets [package insert]. Foster City, CA: Gilead Sciences, Inc; 2012.

49. Selzentry (maraviroc) tablets [package insert]. Freiburg, Germany: Pfizer Manufacturing Deutschland GmbH; 2010.

50. Heidenhain C, Pulh G, Moench C, et al. Chemokine receptor 5Δ32 mutation reduces the risk of acute rejection in liver transplantation. Ann Transplant 2009; 14:36–44.

51. Reshef R, Luger SM, Hexner EO, et al. Blockade of lymphocyte chemotaxis in visceral graft-versus-host disease. N Engl J Med 2012;367:135–45.
52. Gilliam BL, Heredia A, Devico A, et al. Rapamycin reduces CCR5 mRNA levels in macaques: potential applications in HIV-1 prevention and treatment. AIDS 2007; 21:2108–10.

Index

Note: Page numbers of article titles are in **boldface** type.

A

Acinetobacter baumannii
    impact on patients considered for lung transplantation, 347–348
Adenovirus
    in IMVTx recipients, 367
Alimentary protozoa
    in SOTRs, 413–414
Amebic infections
    donor-derived
        diagnostic and management strategies for, 265–266
Amoeba(s)
    free-living
        in SOTRs, 412–413
Antiretroviral agents
    in HIV–infected SOTRs, **473–486**. *See also* Solid organ transplant recipients (SOTRs),
        HIV–infected, antiretroviral agents and immunosuppressive regimens in
Aspergillus spp.
    A. terreus
        impact on patients considered for lung transplantation, 352
    infections related to
        donor-derived
            diagnostic and management strategies for, 265
        in IMVTx recipients, 370–371

B

Babesiosis
    in SOTRs, 414
Bacterial infections
    in CTA recipients
        prevention of, 389
    donor-derived
        diagnostic and management strategies for, 259–261
            bloodstream infection in organ donors, 259–260
            TB, 260–261
BK virus
    virology of, 272
BK virus nephropathy (BKVN)
    in renal transplant recipient, **271–283**
        clinical manifestations of, 274–276
        diagnosis of, 276
        incidence of, 272–273

Infect Dis Clin N Am 27 (2013) 487–500
http://dx.doi.org/10.1016/S0891-5520(13)00035-4
0891-5520/13/$ – see front matter © 2013 Elsevier Inc. All rights reserved.

Moving?

Make sure your subscription moves with you!

To notify us of your new address, find your **Clinics Account Number** (located on your mailing label above your name), and contact customer service at:

Email: journalscustomerservice-usa@elsevier.com

800-654-2452 (subscribers in the U.S. & Canada)
314-447-8871 (subscribers outside of the U.S. & Canada)

Fax number: 314-447-8029

Elsevier Health Sciences Division
Subscription Customer Service
3251 Riverport Lane
Maryland Heights, MO 63043

*To ensure uninterrupted delivery of your subscription, please notify us at least 4 weeks in advance of move.

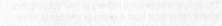

Printed and bound by CPI Group (UK) Ltd, Croydon, CR0 4YY

03/10/2024

01040441-0007